This book is to be returned on or before
the last date stamped below

HAMMERSMITH CARDIOLOGY WORKSHOP SERIES
VOLUME 3

Hammersmith Cardiology Workshop Series

Series Editor: Attilio Maseri

Volume 1: *A. Maseri and J. F. Goodwin, editors. 352 pp. 1984*
Volume 2: *A. Maseri, editor. 272 pp. 1985*
Volume 3: *A. Maseri, B. E. Sobel, S. Chierchia, editors. 320 pp. 1987*

Hammersmith Cardiology Workshop Series

Volume 3

Editors

Attilio Maseri, M.D., F.R.C.P., F.A.C.C.
Royal Postgraduate Medical School
Hammersmith Hospital
London, England

Burton E. Sobel, M.D., F.A.C.C.
Washington University School of Medicine
St. Louis, Missouri

Sergio Chierchia, M.D.
Royal Postgraduate Medical School
Hammersmith Hospital
London, England

Raven Press  New York

Raven Press, 1185 Avenue of the Americas, New York, New York 10036

Made in the United States of America

International Standard Book Number 0–88167–283–1
International Standard Series Number 0891–9755

The material contained in this volume was submitted as previously unpublished material, except in the instances in which credit has been given to the source from which some of the illustrative material was derived.

Great care has been taken to maintain the accuracy of the information contained in the volume. However, Raven Press cannot be held responsible for errors or for any consequences arising from the use of the information contained herein.

Materials appearing in this book prepared by individuals as part of their official duties as U.S. Government employees are not covered by the above-mentioned copyright.

9 8 7 6 5 4 3 2 1

D
616
HAM

Preface to the Series

New data and new concepts appear in the medical literature at an ever-increasing rate. Physicians face the difficult task of the overall synthesis of this growing volume of information and not infrequently are presented with conflicting but apparently authoritative views on various topics.

This European and American Cardiology Series has accepted the challenge of following the exciting developments in cardiology and its related disciplines by bringing together, in a public forum, leading authorities from both sides of the ocean who present and discuss the most relevant advances and controversial aspects of cardiovascular research and clinical practice.

The salient feature of the course is the considerable time reserved for discussion after each presentation and at the end of each session. The lively exchange of opinions among speakers, discussants, and audience provides a unique opportunity for perceiving the areas of consensus and for developing a balanced view of controversial issues.

This series gives an account of the presentations of invited speakers, a précis of the discussion, and an editorial view of both. The reports of the presentations of the speakers constitute a synthesis of new data or personal views of complex issues. The debate among invited speakers, discussants, and audience is summarized, highlighting unresolved issues and those where new agreement has been reached. The editorial comment is separately presented in an attempt to steer the reader through these difficult areas.

It is intended that "European and American Cardiology at the Hammersmith" will be an annual event and the proceedings will be published yearly.

Preface to Volume 3

This volume of the Hammersmith Cardiology Workshop Series presents the proceedings of the third European and American Cardiology Course at the Hammersmith and is devoted to advances and controversies in ischemic heart disease.

The first part of the course covered the mechanisms of ischemic cardiac pain, the significance of painless ischemia, and the various mechanisms of dynamic stenosis and coronary occlusion in infarction. The central part of the course ranged from techniques used in detecting myocardial ischemia, to coronary thrombolysis, to antiplatelet and anticoagulant therapy, to an update of organization and policies in coronary care units. The final part of the course covered the determinants of prognosis in ischemic heart disease and the results of medical treatment of coronary surgery and angioplasty.

This volume, like the previous two, has no pretensions of providing comprehensive reviews. Rather, it offers a series of introductory lectures particularly chosen to stimulate discussion. The précis of the discussions and the editorial comments that follow each section give an account of consensus or disagreement in controversial areas among world authorities.

Acknowledgments

The organizers of the 1985 European and American Cardiology Course at the Hammersmith wish to express their gratitude to Schwarz Pharmaceuticals UK and Pharma Schwarz GmbH for their generous support, which made the organization of the course and publication of the proceedings possible. We also wish to thank Shiley Limited for its sponsorship of the surgical session.

Contents

Routine Techniques for the Detection of Transient Ischemia

Regional Myocardial Metabolic Abnormalities

Update: Organization and Policies in CCU

Special Lecture

Antiplatelet and Anticoagulant Therapy

Medical Treatment of Ischemic Heart Disease

Determinants of Prognosis in Ischemic Heart Disease

Contributors

Luis Araujo, M.D.
Cardiovascular Research Unit
Royal Postgraduate Medical School
Hammersmith Hospital
London W12 OHS, England

Raphael Balcon, M.D., M.R.C.P.
London Chest Hospital
London E2 9JX, England

G. Baroldi, M.D.
Institute Biomedical Science
Institute Clinical Physiology CNR
20162 Milan, Italy

**Michel E. Bertrand, M.D.,
F.A.C.C.**
Hopital Cardiologique
Lille University
59037 Lille, France

G. V. R. Born, F.R.C.P., F.R.S.
Department of Pharmacology
King's College
London WC2R 2LS, England

Paolo Camici, M.D.
CNR Institute of Clinical Physiology and
  Istituto di Patologia Speciale Medica I
University of Pisa
56100 Pisa, Italy

D. A. Chamberlain, M.D., F.R.C.P.
Department of Cardiology
Royal Sussex County Hospital
Brighton BN2 5BE, England

Sergio Chierchia, M.D.
Cardiovascular Research Unit
Royal Postgraduate Medical School
Hammersmith Hospital
London W12 OHS, England

Djamel Chitour, M.D.
Unité de Recherches de Neurophysiologie
  Pharmacologique de l'INSERM (U.161)
75014 Paris, France

**P. Collins, M.A., M.B., B.Chir.,
M.R.C.P.(U.K.)**
Departments of Cardiology, Radiology,
  and Pharmacology
University of Wales College of Medicine
Cardiff CF4 4XN, Wales

C. Richard Conti, M.D., F.A.C.C.
Division of Cardiovascular Medicine
University of Florida
College of Medicine
Gainesville, Florida 32610

Filippo Crea, M.D.
Cardiovascular Research Unit
Royal Postgraduate Medical School
Hammersmith Hospital
London W12 OHS, England

**Graham J. Davies, M.D.,
M.R.C.P.**
Cardiovascular Unit
Royal Postgraduate Medical School
Hammersmith Hospital
London W12 OHS, England

J. A. Davies, M.D., F.R.C.P.
University Department of Medicine
The General Infirmary
Leeds LS1 3EX, England

**Michael J. Davies, M.D., M.R.C.S.,
M.C.Path.**
Cardiovascular Pathology Unit
St. George's Hospital Medical School
London SW17 ORE, England

Colin T. Dollery, M.B., F.R.C.P.
Department of Clinical Pharmacology
Royal Postgraduate Medical School
Hammersmith Hospital
London W12 OHS, England

D. H. Edwards
Departments of Cardiology, Radiology,
  and Pharmacology
University of Wales College of Medicine
Cardiff CF4 4XN, Wales

J. L. Fourrier, M.D.
Hopital Cardiologique
Lille University
59037 Lille, France

K. M. Fox, M.D., M.R.C.P.
National Heart Hospital
London W1M 8BA, England

James J. Glazier, M.B., B.Ch.,
M.R.C.P.I., M.R.C.P.
Cardiovascular Research Unit
Royal Postgraduate Medical School
Hammersmith Hospital
London W12 OHS, England

U. Goldbourt, M.D.
Heart Institute
Chaim Sheba Medical Center
52621 Tel Hashomer, Israel

John L. Gordon, Ph.D.
Department of Vascular Biology
MRC Clinical Research Center
Harrow HA1 3UJ, England

T. M. Griffith, M.A., M.B., B.Ch.,
M.R.C.P., F.R.C.P.
Departments of Cardiology, Radiology,
  and Pharmacology
University of Wales College of Medicine
Cardiff CF4 4XN, Wales

William Grossman, M.D., F.A.C.C.
Cardiovascular Division
Harvard-Thorndike Laboratory
Beth Israel Hospital
Boston, Massachusetts 02215

Andrew H. Henderson, M.D.,
F.R.C.P.
Department of Cardiology
University of Wales College of Medicine
Cardiff CF4, 4XN, Wales

Paul G. Hugenholtz, M.D.,
F.A.C.C.
Thoraxcenter
Erasmus University
Academic Hospital
3000 Rotterdam DR, The Netherlands

T. Jones, D.Sc.
MRC Cyclotron Unit
Hammersmith Hospital
London W12 OHS, England

Desmond G. Julian, M.D., F.R.C.P.
Department of Cardiology
The University of Newcastle upon Tyne
Freeman Hospital
Newcastle upon Tyne NE7 7DN, England

Juan Carlos Kaski, M.D.
Cardiovascular Research Unit
Royal Postgraduate Medical School
Hammersmith Hospital
London W12 OHS, England

David T. Kelly, M.D.
Hallstrom Institute of Cardiology
University of Sydney
Camperdown NSW 2050, Australia

Spencer B. King III, M.D.
Cardiovascular Laboratory
Emory University
Atlanta, Georgia 30322

Gerry A. Klassen, M.D.
Departments of Medicine and Physiology
  and Biophysics
Dalhousie University and Victoria General
  Hospital
Halifax, Nova Scotia B3H 2Y9, Canada

Wolfgang Kübler, M.D.
Abteilung Innere Medizin III (Kardiologie)
Medizinische Universitätsklinik
6900 Heidelberg 1, Federal Republic of
Germany

Jean M. Lablanche, M.D.
Hopital Cardiologique
Lille University
59037 Lille, France

K. Laird-Meeter, M.D.
Thoraxcenter
Erasmus University
Academic Hospital
3000 Rotterdam DR, The Netherlands

Adriaan A. Lammertsma, M.D.
MRC Cyclotron Unit
Hammersmith Hospital
London W12 OHS, England

Daniel Le Bars, M.D.
Unité de Recherches de Neurophysiologie
Pharmacologique de l'INSERM (U.161)
75014 Paris, France

M. J. Lewis, M.B., B.Ch., Ph.D.
Departments of Cardiology, Radiology,
and Pharmacology
University of Wales College of Medicine
Cardiff CF4 4XN, Wales

Paul R. Lichtlen, M.D., F.A.C.C.
Division of Cardiology
Hannover Medical School
LD-3000 Hannover, Federal Republic of
Germany

Floyd D. Loop, M.D.
Department of Thoracic and
Cardiovascular Surgery
The Cleveland Clinic Foundation
Cleveland, Ohio 44106

Alberto Malliani, M.D.
Istituto Ricerche Cardiovascolari, CNR
Patologia Medica, Ospedale "L.Sacco"
Università Milano
20157 Milan, Italy

Attilio Maseri, M.D., F.R.C.P.,
F.A.C.C.
Division of Cardiovascular Diseases
Royal Postgraduate Medical School
Hammersmith Hospital
London W12 OHS, England

Lawson McDonald, M.D.,
F.R.C.P., F.A.C.C.
National Heart Hospital
London W1M 8BA, England

Henry N. Neufeld, M.D.
Heart Institute
Chaim Sheba Medical Center
52621 Tel Hashomer, Israel

Celia M. Oakley, M.D., F.R.C.P.,
F.A.C.C.
Division of Cardiovascular Diseases
Royal Postgraduate Medical School
Hammersmith Hospital
London W12 OHS, England

Dieter Opherk, M.D.
Abteilung Innere Medizin III (Kardiologie)
Medizinische Universitätsklinik
69 Heidelberg, Federal Republic of
Germany

Nina Rehnqvist, M.D.
Department of Medicine
Danderyd Hospital
S-182 88 Danderyd, Sweden

William C. Roberts, M.D.
Pathology Branch
National Heart, Lung, and Blood
Institute
National Institutes of Health
Bethesda, Maryland 20205

J. R. T. C. Roelandt, M.D.
Thoraxcenter
Erasmus University
Academic Hospital
3000 Rotterdam DR, The Netherlands

Patrick W. Serruys, M.D.
Thoraxcenter
Erasmus University
Academic Hospital
3000 Rotterdam DR, The Netherlands

**Desmond J. Sheridan, M.D.,
  M.R.C.P.**
Department of Cardiology
St. Mary's Hospital
London W2 1NY, England

Burton E. Sobel, M.D.
Cardiovascular Division
Washington University School of Medicine
St. Louis, Missouri 63110

Terry Spinks, Ph.D.
MRC Cyclotron Unit
Hammersmith Hospital
London W12 OHS, England

H. William Strauss, M.D.
Nuclear Medicine Division
Massachusetts General Hospital
Boston, Massachusetts 02114

Kenneth M. Taylor, M.D., F.R.C.S.
Department of Cardiac Surgery
Royal Postgraduate Medical School
Hammersmith Hospital
London W12 OHS, England

Harald Tillmanns, M.D.
Abteilung Innere Medizin III (Kardiologie)
Medizinische Universitätsklinik
*6900 Heidelberg 1, Federal Republic of
  Germany*

G. Traisnel, M.D.
Hopital Cardiologique
Lille University
59037 Lille, France

Luis Villanueva, M.D.
*Unité de Recherches de Neurophysiologie
  Pharmacologique de l'INSERM (U.161)*
75014 Paris, France

Babette B. Weksler, M.D.
Department of Medicine
SCOR Center in Thrombosis
*The New York Hospital-Cornell Medical
  Center*
New York, New York 10021

A. Y. K. Wong, M.D.
*Departments of Medicine and Physiology
  and Biophysics*
*Dalhousie University and Victoria General
  Hospital*
Halifax, Nova Scotia B3H 2Y9, Canada

HAMMERSMITH CARDIOLOGY WORKSHOP SERIES
VOLUME 3

Hammersmith Cardiology Workshop Series, Vol. 3,
edited by A. Maseri, B. E. Sobel, and S. Chierchia.
Raven Press, New York © 1987.

Afferent Nervous Impulses During Acute Myocardial Ischemia

Alberto Malliani

*Istituto Ricerche Cardiovascolari, CNR; Patologia Medica, Ospedale "L. Sacco";
Università Milano, 20157 Milan, Italy*

The afferent fibers running in the cardiac sympathetic nerves are generally considered the only essential pathway for the transmission of cardiac pain. This concept has arisen from observing that a high thoracic sympathectomy was able to induce surgical relief of anginal pain in humans (12) or the abolition of animal reactions, suggestive of pain, accompanying coronary occlusion (10).

Almost two decades have elapsed since electrophysiological investigations into the properties of afferent sympathetic cardiac fibers have started to afford direct evidence on the nature of the stimuli capable of exciting them (1,6). Cardiac sympathetic afferent fibers have a tonic impulse activity and subserve cardiovascular reflexes that are mainly excitatory in nature (1,6). I shall restrict my analysis to the properties of ventricular sympathetic afferent fibers (either small myelinated or unmyelinated), that is, the afferent fibers that are most likely to convey cardiac nociception.

VENTRICULAR SYMPATHETIC AFFERENT FIBERS

It now seems established that these ventricular receptors always possess some mechanosensitivity that attributes to their fibers some degree of spontaneous impulse activity (if the hemodynamic conditions are in the normal range) and a responsiveness to normal hemodynamic events (1,6). In addition, these afferent fibers are also markedly excited by bradykinin or other chemical substances (4–8), thus displaying properties of "polymodal" receptors, a term indicating that the receptive zone is considered to be sensitive to both mechanical or chemical stimuli.

Coronary occlusion (2,6) or the administration of bradykinin (1,4,5), a natural algesic substance suspected to take part in the genesis of cardiac pain, markedly excited the ventricular sympathetic afferent fibers; however, a recruitment of silent afferent fibers could never be appreciated (5,7). In more explicit terms, these experimental findings negated the existence of a population of ventricular sympathetic afferent fibers normally devoid of a spontaneous impulse activity, being

1

unresponsive to physiologic hemodynamic stimuli, but, conversely, excitable during coronary occlusion or during other stimulations of possible algogenic significance. That is, the ventricular receptors with a merely nociceptive function were unlikely to exist, at least on the basis of our experimental results (5–8).

To understand the relevance of a similar conclusion, it is essential to recall that the peripheral mechanisms for nociception, either somatic or visceral, have been analyzed throughout the years in relation to two main hypotheses proposing, respectively, "intensity" or "specificity" (7,8).

The "intensity" mechanism, the most obvious and probably the first to be formulated, assumes that pain results from an excessive stimulation of receptive structures. Alternatively, pain may be conceived of as a "specific" sensation that is the product of the excitation of a well-defined nociceptive apparatus, the functional characteristics of which make it responsive only to a limited class of events, the "noxious" stimuli.

As to the soma, there are experimental observations indicating that both certain primary afferent units and certain higher order cells to which they project are excited solely or most effectively by stimuli strong enough to threaten the integrity of the tissue. Yet, these findings, suggesting some degree of "specificity," do not deny the importance of the modulation played by other neural mechanisms upon nociceptive information (11).

On the visceral side, the "intensity" mechanism appears by far the most likely candidate. However, such a general view, which denies the existence of specific sensors for visceral pain, is unable to explain in simple terms some recent and quite unexpected findings. Indeed, it seemed a consolidated notion that the intracoronary injection of bradykinin had to elicit signs of pain; however, this observation is likely to pertain only to animals that are recovering from recent surgery. In fact, behavioral reactions were never displayed by conscious unanesthetized animals after full recovery from surgery (8,9). Hence, a massive excitation of cardiac sympathetic afferent fibers induced by bradykinin, intense enough to produce a striking excitatory cardiovascular reflex (9), was inadequate to trigger overt signs of pain. Thus, we proposed a modified version of the "intensity" theory (8). Cardiac pain would result from the extreme excitation of a spatially restricted population of afferent sympathetic fibers.

According to this hypothesis, the intracoronary injection of bradykinin would produce a too widespread excitation of cardiac sympathetic afferent fibers and, therefore, would not elicit pain. In general, any activation of sympathetic afferent fibers widely distributed, such as during an increase in systemic arterial pressure, would be modulated by central inhibitory mechanisms, preventing the breakthrough of pain. The facilitatory influence apparently played by recent surgery, suggesting a spatially localized mechanism of convergence at the spinal level, from the soma and from the heart, is consistent with this view. It is our very recent experimental observation that signs of pain can be elicited in the conscious dog, also after full recovery from surgery, by mechanically distending a very small area of the coronary adventitia.

IS THERE AN "ALARM SYSTEM"?

In clinics, the heart has been regarded, for years, as possessing an alarm system (3) of which myocardial ischemia has been considered the exquisite trigger. This view is now untenable. Tissue damage too often does not represent an adequate stimulus for eliciting pain, as in the case of myocarditis, valve ulcerations, or silent myocardial ischemia. Although all these events are likely to alter the impulse activity of sympathetic afferent fibers, we must accept the mysterious gap that still separates the peripheral receptive process and the onset of pain, which is a conscious experience.

The afferent sympathetic fibers probably recognize, as their primary function, that of mediating reflexes; this is a likely hypothesis for their biological development, surely more likely than signaling cardiac pain in animals. Thus, this afferent system would work as an alarm system only in some conditions. It is clear that we would like to understand what opens the door to the conscious perception of pain. We have to know more analytical details about the peripheral abnormalities, which we suspect to be mainly mechanical in nature, that trigger the event. We have to know more about central modulating factors, which should, incidentally, by definition, be far from stable. In this sense, the capability of the central nervous system, of changing the gains of all of its circuits is likely to contribute to the increasingly recognized instability of the so-called stable angina.

In conclusion, during myocardial ischemia, afferent sympathetic fibers innervating the ventricles increase their firing. This increased afferent barrage produces excitatory cardiovascular reflexes, whether or not they might prevail (6). However, only some episodes of transient myocardial ischemia are accompanied by pain. Hence, the alarm system has a porosity which would make it, technically, very poor. From an even more general point of view, the difference is quite clear between tissue injury to the soma and to the heart: A man who could severely wound his arm without feeling pain would be considered "unusual." A man undergoing serious cardiac damage without feeling pain is absolutely "usual." An alarm system that does not work consistently and predictably is not an alarm system. The fact that in clinics cardiac pain acts, at times, as an ally is only a sign that options are sometimes useful.

REFERENCES

1. Bishop, V. S., Malliani, A., and Thorèn, P. (1983): Cardiac mechanoreceptors. In: *Handbook of Physiology. Section 2. The Cardiovascular System, Vol. III. Peripheral Circulation and Organ Blood Flow*, pp. 497–555, edited by J. T. Sheperd, F. M. Abboud, and S. R. Geiger. American Physiological Society, Washington, D.C.
2. Brown, A. M. (1967): Excitation of afferent cardiac sympathetic nerve fibers during myocardial ischemia. *J. Physiol.*, 190:35–53.
3. Cohn, P. F. (1980): Silent myocardial ischemia in patients with a defective anginal warning system. *Am. J. Cardiol.*, 45:697–702.

4. Coleridge, J. C. G., and Coleridge, H. M. (1979): Chemoreflex regulation of the heart. In: *Handbook of Physiology. Section 2. The Cardiovascular System, Vol. 1. The Heart,* pp. 653–676, edited by R. M. Berne, N. Sperelakis, and S. R. Geiger. American Physiological Society, Washington, D.C.
5. Lombardi, F., Della Bella, P., Casati, R., and Malliani, A. (1981): Effects of intracoronary administration of bradykinin on the impulse activity of afferent sympathetic unmyelinated fibers with left ventricular endings in the cat. *Circ. Res.,* 48:69–75.
6. Malliani, A. (1982): Cardiovascular sympathetic afferent fibers. *Rev. Physiol. Biochem. Pharmacol.,* 94:11–74.
7. Malliani, A., and Lombardi, F. (1982): Consideration of the fundamental mechanisms eliciting cardiac pain. *Am. Heart J.,* 103:575–578.
8. Malliani, A., Pagani, M., and Lombardi, F. (1984): Visceral versus somatic mechanisms. In: *Textbook of Pain,* pp. 100–109, edited by P. D. Wall and R. Melzack. Churchill Livingstone, Edinburgh.
9. Pagani, M., Pizzinelli, P., Furlan, R., Guzzetti, S., Rimoldi, O., Sandrone, G., and Malliani, A. (1985): Analysis of the pressor sympathetic reflex produced by intracoronary injections of bradykinin in conscious dogs. *Circ. Res.,* 56:175–183.
10. Sutton, D. C., and Lueth, H. C. (1930): Experimental production of pain on excitation of the heart and great vessels. *Arch. Intern. Med.,* 45:827–867.
11. Wall, P. D., and Melzack, R., (editors) (1984): *Textbook of Pain.* Churchill Livingstone, Edinburgh.
12. White, J. C. (1957): Cardiac Pain. Anatomic pathways and physiologic mechanisms. *Circulation,* 16:644–655.

Hammersmith Cardiology Workshop Series, Vol. 3,
edited by A. Maseri, B. E. Sobel, and S. Chierchia.
Raven Press, New York © 1987.

Mechanisms of Cardiac Pain

Graham J. Davies

*Department of Cardiology, Royal Postgraduate Medical School, Hammersmith Hospital,
London W12 OHS, England*

Painless myocardial infarction is a well-recognized phenomenon, the incidence of which has been reported to be approximately 20% in the Framingham study (1). Painless, transient myocardial ischemia has been recognized and reported with increasing frequency in recent years (2–6), its incidence estimated to be approximately 70% of ischemic episodes in both patients with unstable angina (6) and those with chronic stable angina (7,8). However, there is considerable variation among patients and in the same patient from day to day. The mechanism of cardiac pain remains unknown and is presumably complex. Although evidence exists to suggest modulation of the transmission of painful stimuli both at spinal cord and cerebral levels, the exact nature of the stimulus, receptors, afferent fibers, and modulatory mechanisms is obscure (9,10).

STIMULUS, RECEPTORS, AND AFFERENCE PATHWAYS

Two main theories exist regarding the nature of the *stimulus* eliciting pain. The mechanical theory, proposed by Colbeck (11), implicates mechanical stretch, while the chemical hypothesis (12) implicates the release of chemical substances as the painful stimuli. Opinions are also divided regarding the nature of sensory *receptors*. Nonspecific stimulation of sensory receptors (9,13) forms the basis of the "intensity" hypothesis, but the "specificity" hypothesis is based on the existence of receptors, termed nociceptors (14), which are specifically sensitive to noxious stimuli. Whatever the exact nature of the stimulus and receptor, transmission of the potentially painful stimuli occurs in the sympathetic cardiac nerves, synapsing with fibers of the spinothalamic tracts, which also receive afferent somatic input. It appears likely that the central transmission of potentially painful stimuli are facilitated or inhibited within the spinal cord by other afferent impulses, as described by Melzack and Wall (15) in the "gate control" theory of pain. At this level they may also be modified by descending inhibitory stimuli.

PERCEPTION OF PAIN

It is apparent that patients with painless myocardial infarction and ischemia may have low sensitivity to pain. This was suggested in clinical studies reported by Babey (16) and Roseman (17), and supported by quantitative studies of pain threshold (18,19). The results of recent studies have confirmed these findings. Glazier et al. (20) found the pain threshold in response to cold, electrical skin stimulation, and forearm ischemia to be significantly higher in patients whose ischemic episodes were predominantly painless than in those with predominantly painful episodes. However, there was considerable overlap between the two groups; hence, this mechanism of silent ischemia cannot explain all cases.

Apart from a higher pain threshold, more complex factors may influence the perception of pain. Patients with painless ischemia may differ in personality (19). A reduced tendency to complain has been reported with lower scores for nervousness and excitability on a personality questionnaire (19).

THE PAINFUL STIMULUS

Duration

A certain duration of ischemia is necessary for pain to appear. A study by Chierchia et al. (21) of patients with variant or unstable angina showed that episodes of myocardial ischemia of less than three min were invariably silent. However, episodes of longer duration could be either painless or painful. A recent study of spontaneous and ergometrine-induced ischemia shows that painless episodes are generally shorter than painful episodes, but there is a large overlap between the groups (22). Similar results in patients with chronic stable angina pectoris were found by Deanfield et al. (7) using ambulatory electrocardiographic monitoring.

Severity

There is no clear relationship between the severity and extent of myocardial ischemia and angina pectoris. Evidence of severe ischemia in the absence of pain has been reported. In these patients, during painless episodes, the severity of ischemia has been documented by thallium-201 scintigraphy (23), rubidium-82 uptake (24), and an increase in end-diastolic pressure and myocardial oxygen extraction (6). Chierchia et al. (21) showed that ischemic episodes were painless when the associated increase in left ventricular end-diastolic pressure was less than 7 mm Hg, but episodes with larger increases in pressure could be either painful or painless. Monitoring left ventricular volume and function during spontaneous and ergometrine-induced ischemia has shown no difference in the magnitude of stroke volume change between painful and painless ischemic episodes (22). It would, therefore, appear that a certain duration and severity of myocardial ischemia are necessary but not sufficient conditions for the occurrence of angina pectoris.

The Nature of the Stimulus

Whether the stimulus is chemical or mechanical remains unknown. However, with regard to the former, large intracoronary doses of bradykinin (25) or ventridine (26) do not cause pain reactions in the dog. The massive left ventricular dilatation, observed during spontaneous and ergometrine-induced ischemia (22), should be sufficient to activate mechanoreceptors and yet may not be associated with pain. Furthermore, there does not appear to be a relationship between the rate of change of left ventricular volume and pain (22).

CONCLUSION

The mechanism of cardiac pain is complex. A certain duration and severity of ischemia are necessary but not sufficient to account for pain. Neither chemical nor mechanical stimulation of cardiac receptors may be sufficient to induce pain. Summation of subliminal stimuli may be involved, and it is probable that different impulses are modulated both within the spinal chord and at higher levels.

REFERENCES

1. Kannel, W. B., and Abbott, R. D. (1984): Incidence and prognosis of unrecognized myocardial infarction. *N. Engl. J. Med.,* 311:1144–1147.
2. Guazzi, M., Fiorentini, C., Polese, A., and Margini, F. (1970): Continuous electrocardiographic recording in Prinzmetal's variant angina pectoris. A report of four cases. *Br. Heart J.,* 32:611–616.
3. Cohn, P. F. (1977): Severe, asymptomatic coronary artery disease: a diagnostic, prognostic and therapeutic puzzle. *Am. J. Med.,* 62:565–568.
4. Schang, S. J., and Pepine, C. J. (1977): Transient asymptomatic ST segment depression during daily activity. *Am. J. Cardiol.,* 39:396–402.
5. Maseri, A., Severi, S., De Nes, M., L'Abbate, A., Chierchia, S., Marcilli, M., Ballestra, A. M., Parodi, O., Biagini, A., and Distante, A. (1978): "Variant" angina: one aspect of a continuous spectrum of vasospastic myocardial ischemia. *Am. J. Cardiol.,* 42:1019–1033.
6. Chierchia, S., Brunelli, C., Simonetti, I., Lazzari, M., and Maseri, A. (1980): Sequence of events in angina at rest: primary reduction in coronary flow. *Circulation,* 61:759–768.
7. Deanfield, J. E., Maseri, A., Selwyn, A. P. (1983): Myocardial ischemia during daily life in patients with stable angina: its relation to symptoms and heart rate changes. *Lancet,* 2:753–8.
8. Chierchia, S., Gallino, A., and Smith, G. (1984): The role of heart rate in the pathophysiology of chronic stable angina. *Lancet,* 2:1353–1358.
9. Gooddy, W. (1957): On the nature of pain. *Brain,* 80:118–131.
10. Malliani, A., Pagani, M., and Lombardi, F. (1984): Visceral versus somatic mechanisms. In: *Textbook of Pain,* pp. 100–109, edited by P. D. Wall and R. Melzack. Churchill Livingstone, Edinburgh.
11. Colbeck, E. H. (1903): Angina pectoris: a criticism and a hypothesis. *Lancet,* 1:793–795.

12. Lewis, T. (1932): Pain in muscular ischemia—its relation to anginal pain. *Arch. Intern. Med.*, 49:713–727.
13. Noordenbos, W. (1959): Pain. Elsevier, Amsterdam.
14. Perl, E. R. (1971): Is pain a specific sensation? *J. Psychiatr. Res.*, 8:273–87.
15. Melzark, R., and Wall P. D. (1965): Pain mechanisms: a new theory. *Science*, 150:971–9.
16. Babey, A. M. (1939): Painless acute infarction of the heart. *N. Engl. J. Med.*, 220:410–412.
17. Roseman, M. D. (1954): Painless myocardial infarction: a review of the literature and analysis of 220 cases. *Ann. Intern. Med.*, 41:1–8.
18. Procacci, P., Zoppi, M., Padeletti, L., and Maresca, M. (1976): Myocardial infarction without pain. A study of the sensory function of the upper limbs. *Pain*, 2:309–313.
19. Droste, C., and Roskamm, H. (1983): Experimental pain measurements in patients with asymptomatic myocardial ischemia. *J. Am. Coll. Cardiol.*, 1:940–945.
20. Galazier, J. J., Chierchia, S., Brown, M. J., Maseri, A. (1986): Importance of generalized defective perception of painful stimuli as a cause of silent myocardial ischaemia in chronic stable angina pectoris. *Am. J. Cardiol.*, 58:667–72.
21. Chierchia, S., Lazzari, M., Freedman, S. B., Brunelli, C., and Maseri, A. (1983): Impairment of myocardial perfusion and function during painless myocardial ischemia. *J. Am. Coll. Cardiol.*, 1:924–930.
22. Davies, G. J., Chierchia, S., and Bencivelli, V. (1987): Sequence and magnitude of ventricular volume changes in painful and painless myocardial ischemia assessed by a precordial probe. *Circulation (in press)*.
23. Maseri, A., Parodi, O., Severi, S., and Pesola, A. (1976): Transient transmural reduction of myocardial blood flow, demonstrated by thallium-201 scintigraphy, as a cause of variant angina. *Circulation*, 54:280–288.
24. Deanfield, J. E., Shea, M., and Kensett, M. (1984): Silent myocardial ischemia due to mental stress. *Lancet*, 2:1001–1005.
25. Guzman, F., Braun, C., and Lim, R. K. S. (1962): Visceral pain and the pseudoaffective response to intra-arterial infection of bradykinin and other elgesic agents. *Arch. Int. Pharmacodyn. Ther.*, 136:353–384.
26. Barron, K. W., and Bishop, V. S. (1982): Reflex cardiovascular changes with veratridine in the conscious dog. *Am. J. Physiol.*, 242:H810–H817.

Hammersmith Cardiology Workshop Series, Vol. 3,
edited by A. Maseri, B. E. Sobel, and S. Chierchia.
Raven Press, New York © 1987.

Central Modulation of Pain: Physiological Approach in Animals

Daniel Le Bars, Luis Villanueva, and Djamel Chitour

Unité de Recherches de Neurophysiologie Pharmacologique de l'INSERM (U. 161),
75014 Paris, France

The transmission of nociceptive messages is powerfully modulated as early as the first relays of the central nervous system, i.e., at the levels of the spinal dorsal horn or trigeminal nucleus. The "gate control" theory (80) was an attempt to summarize schematically the data relevant to these controls, and, although its details have been subject to debate (85,113), it is now well established that, from a general point of view, the transmission of nociceptive messages is under the influence of both segmental mechanisms and systems involving supraspinal structures. Most relevant to the clinical and therapeutical approaches to pain is the physiological observation that somatic or visceral stimuli can trigger these controls, which indicates that highly complex interactions occur before a noxious message reaches the brain. Schematically, at least three main types of systems seem to be involved in these controls, depending on the part of the neuraxis implicated: Inhibitory processes could involve either segmental, propriospinal, or supraspinal mechanisms.

Such inhibitory effects have been particularly studied on convergent neurons, i.e., those cells that respond to both innocuous and noxious stimuli applied to a well-delimited area of the body (excitatory receptive field). Without excluding a role of noxious specific neurons (25) in the transmission of nociceptive information, we believe that convergent neurons are of prime importance, the most convincing argument for their role in nociception being their clear ability to be influenced by converging excitatory and inhibitory mechanisms in a fashion that can be related to clinical observations. For example, viscerosomatic convergence (12,33,35, 37,38,43,46,49,83,92,102,104) could explain clinical referred pain (100), and most of the manipulations that result in hypoalgesia or analgesia in humans also result in a reduction of nociceptive responses of convergent neurons in animals. These manipulations include systemic or intrathecal morphine administration (17,55,58,69,71,72,120) and, as detailed below, dorsal column stimulation, transcutaneous electrical stimulation, stimulation of periaqueductal or periventricular structures, and heterotopic noxious stimulation.

9

INHIBITORY PROCESSES TRIGGERED BY
SEGMENTAL MECHANISMS

It is now well established that the electrical activation of large diameter peripheral myelinated fibers is able to inhibit the firing of dorsal horn neurons induced by noxious stimulation (15,23,44,50,81,93,111). Such inhibitory effects are essentially metameric in nature, but analogous inhibitory effects can also be induced by the stimulation of the dorsal columns (36,50,53,75), which activate the same kind of fibers and, via antidromic processes, would probably trigger the same mechanisms. Finally, the activities of a large proportion of convergent neurons can be inhibited by the application of innocuous mechanical stimuli to an area surrounding the excitatory receptive field (inhibitory receptive field) (7,53,111,112).

The nature of the inhibitions observed in electrophysiological experiments has been a controversial subject. It is generally accepted today that they involve both presynaptic and postsynaptic mechanisms. Finally, neurons located within the substantia gelatinosa—SG, lamina II of Rexed (95,96)—are most probably involved in at least some of these effects (9,22,114).

These electrophysiological data could represent the neuronal basis of hypoalgesia obtained in humans by high-frequency low-intensity electrical stimulation of peripheral nerves and dorsal roots (19,76,82,86,101,115) or dorsal columns (84,87,103). It is important to note, however, that the time constants of these clinical and physiological phenomena are quite different; pain can be alleviated for hours in patients whereas neuronal inhibitions last, at best, for several seconds.

INHIBITORY PROCESSES TRIGGERED BY
PROPRIOSPINAL MECHANISMS

There exist some propriospinal inhibitory mechanisms triggered by noxious inputs (16,34,40). For example, in unanesthetized spinal rats, some activities (e.g., responses to a sustained pinch) of convergent neurons can be depressed to some extent by distant conditioning noxious stimuli (16). By comparison, with diffuse noxious inhibitory controls (see below) observed in intact animals, these inhibitions appear to concern only some convergent neurons (roughly 50%), to be weaker, and to adapt to base-line levels within 30 sec. In addition, these inhibitory effects, although concerning several metameres, are more marked for conditioning noxious stimuli applied to structures proximal to the excitatory receptive field than for stimuli applied more distally. For example, noxious stimuli applied to the tail or the contralateral hindpaw are much more effective than identical stimuli applied on the forepaws for reducing responses of a neuron whose excitatory receptive field is located on the ipsilateral hindpaw. The circuitry and pharmacology of such a propriospinal inhibitory system is, as yet, unknown.

"STIMULATION-PRODUCING ANALGESIA"

It is well established (3,4,8,10,31,73,78,79) that strong analgesia can be elicited by the electrical stimulation of brainstem structures such as the periaqueductal gray (PAG) and certain raphe nuclei. These analgesic effects are most probably, at least in part, the result of the activation of descending inhibitory pathways that block the spinal transmission of nociceptive messages, especially those transported by convergent neurons: PAG stimulation induced strong inhibitory effects upon dorsal horn convergent neurons (20,21,30,47,51,74,88). Such an action appears to be indirect since PAG shows few spinal projections. On the basis of both anatomical and electrophysiological evidence, it is generally accepted that the spinal inhibitory effects induced by PAG stimulation result from the activation of the nucleus raphe magnus (NRM).

Furthermore, the electrical stimulation of the NRM induces both stronger analgesic effects than those originating from the PAG (89,91) and important depressions of the activity of convergent neurons (2,5,6,30,32,39,48,54,70,77,97,98,119).

The NRM projects massively and directly toward the spinal cord, with a certain proportion of this projection belonging to serotonergic neurons. These fibers travel through the dorsolateral funiculus (DLF), the section of which counteracts the inhibitory effects induced on dorsal horn neurons by NRM stimulation (2,32,119). Such inhibitory effects are also reduced in animals pretreated with a blocker of serotonin synthesis, para-chlorophenylalanine (pCPA) (98). In addition, microelec-trophoretic application of 5-hydroxytryptamine (5-HT) induced a depression of dorsal horn neuronal responses to noxious inputs (6,45,52,56,57,94), and these effects are particularly clear when 5-HT is applied within the superficial layers of the dorsal horn, where dense 5-HT fiber terminals have been found.

These data tend to suggest that the stimulation of NRM might exert its inhibitory effects by releasing 5-HT within the dorsal horn; this has actually been demonstrated (99). Such an action can be mimicked by means of intrathecal injection of 5-HT which, indeed, induced noticeable hypoalgesic effects (116,121).

In addition, endogenous opioids could be involved in these phenomena since the systemic administration of the opiate antagonist, naloxone, has been shown to partly block the inhibitory processes triggered by the stimulation of NRM (90, 97,122). A spinal site of naloxone action is supported by the high density of enkephalinergic terminals and opiate receptors in the upper regions of the dorsal horn, one of the principal terminal sites of projection from the NRM. Finally, in behavioral studies, intrathecal naloxone was reported to block the analgesia induced by NRM stimulation (123).

DIFFUSE NOXIOUS INHIBITORY CONTROLS (DNIC)

The activity of certain dorsal horn neurons can be strongly inhibited by noxious inputs. Since such effects do not appear to be somatotopically organized but do

concern the entire body, they have been called diffuse noxious inhibitory controls (DNIC) (64,65). Indeed, convergent neurons (i.e., those receiving both low- and high-threshold afferents), whether recorded in the dorsal horn or in its homologous structure for the face (the trigeminal nucleus caudalis), are under the influence of DNIC (27,64). These controls have been observed in the anesthetized intact rat: The activities of almost all convergent neurons, including those projecting toward the thalamus (26), can be blocked by various noxious stimuli when these are applied to parts of the body distant from the excitatory receptive fields. These inhibitory effects concern all types of neuronal activity, whether spontaneous or induced by noxious or innocuous stimuli. Finally, this property appears to be specific to convergent neurons since the other neuronal types commonly encountered within the dorsal horn or the trigeminal nucleus caudalis (noxious-specific neurons, nonnoxious neurons, cold responsive neurons, or proprioceptive neurons) are not affected by DNIC (27,65).

For example, when studying lumbar convergent neurons with peripheral receptive fields located on the ipsilateral hindpaw extremities, this type of inhibition can be triggered from widespread areas of the body: the tail, the contralateral hindpaw, the forepaws, the ears, the nose, or the viscera. Although nonnoxious stimuli are totally ineffective, very strong inhibitions are observed during the application of various noxious stimuli from mechanical, thermal, chemical, or electrical origin. In addition, long-lasting aftereffects commonly follow the period of conditioning stimulation. Both the strength and long duration of these inhibitions are illustrated in Fig. 1, in which the response of a convergent neuron to repetitive electrical stimulation of its receptive field is conditioned by various distant noxious stimuli.

The strength of the effect is actually related to the strength of the conditioning stimulus. For example, the threshold for triggering DNIC by a thermal stimulus is found between 40°C and 44°C and, beyond, a very significant correlation is observed between the conditioning temperature (44–52°C) and the degree of inhibition (61,109). This observation strongly suggests that the recruitment of peripheral nociceptors is essential to trigger DNIC.

Since DNIC disappears in anesthetized animals with a cervical section of the spinal cord ("spinal animals") (65), one can conclude that the underlying mechanisms are not confined to the spinal cord and involve pathways ascending from and descending to it. The ascending pathways involved in the triggering of DNIC are mainly crossed and are confined to the ventrolateral quadrant (110); the descending pathways are mainly, if not entirely, confined to the DLF (108).

Further evidence gives credence to the hypothesis that diffuse noxious inhibitory controls are mediated via the bulbospinal serotonergic system: They are strongly reduced following NRM electrolytic lesion (28), 5-HT depletion by a pretreatment with pCPA (29), or blockade of 5-HT receptors (24). Conversely, the systemic administration of 5-hydroxytryptophan, the precursor of 5-HT synthesis, was found to potentiate DNIC.

Neurochemical experiments clearly demonstrate that bulbospinal 5-HT systems can be activated by NRM stimulation (14,99). The same systems are probably

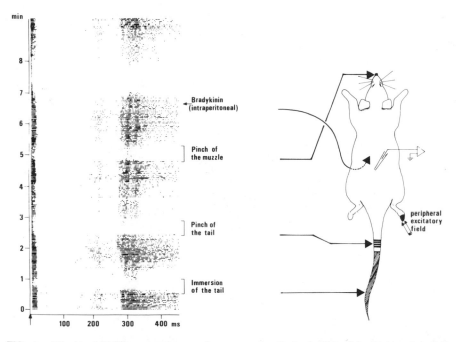

FIG. 1. Effects of DNIC on responses of convergent units to Aα-fiber (short latency) and C-fiber (long latency) inputs are illustrated as a dot-display analysis of responses induced by regular suprathreshold electrical stimulation applied to a rat's peripheral excitatory receptive field. Each spike is represented by a dot and the successive responses are accumulated with time running upward. Note that application of thermal (immersion of the tail in a 52°C water bath), mechanical (pinch of tail and muzzle), and chemical (i.p. administration of 8 μg bradykinin) noxious stimuli resulted in strong inhibitions of responses to both types of fiber inputs. (From ref. 29.)

activated by noxious peripheral inputs. Indeed, the bilateral stimulation of the sciatic nerve in the cat, with current intensities high enough to recruit Aδ and/or C fibers, induced a 5-HT release within the subarachnoid space, and this effect disappeared during thoracic cold block (105). In addition, noxious stimuli applied to the tail of rats resulted in a large 5-HT synthesis increase within the dorsal horn, with minimal effects within the ventral horn (117). These experimental data are in keeping with the clinical observation of higher concentrations of 5-hydroxyindoleacetic acid in the lumbar cerebrospinal fluid of patients suffering from chronic or acute pain than for patients exhibiting no pain (41).

The parallelism between the two modalities of activation (from central and peripheral origin) of bulbospinal systems is further substantiated by another of their properties, their naloxone susceptibility. Diffuse noxious inhibitory controls are depressed by naloxone (0.3 mg/kg i.v.), and by comparing these results (63) with those of Rivot et al. (97) concerning NRM stimulation studied in the same species (rat), one is struck by the fact that the antagonistic effects in each case, of equivalent doses of naloxone, are very similar. Since naloxone is a relatively specific opiate antagonist, at least in low doses, these data suggest the participation of endogenous opioid(s), most probably enkephalins, in DNIC.

We have stressed the fact that DNIC affect all activities of convergent neurons; for instance, neuronal responses to both the activation of A and C peripheral fibers are influenced by DNIC. These properties suggest that a final postsynaptic mechanism is responsible for the inhibitions. This is also suggested by the fact that DNIC strongly depress convergent neuron excitation induced by the direct microelectrophoretic application of glutamate (106,107). Since such amino acid is known to directly excite the neuronal membrane, it is most probable that a hyperpolarization of the neuronal membrane is the ultimate mechanism sustaining DNIC. Once again, the parallelism between DNIC and the inhibitions triggered by NRM stimulation can be emphasized since the latter has been observed to produce an inhibitory postsynaptic potential (IPSP) during the recording of convergent spinothalamic neurons (42). However, complementary presynaptic mechanisms cannot be excluded.

IS PAIN TRIGGERED BY A GRADIENT OF ACTIVITY IN A NEURONAL POPULATION?

The electrophysiological data related to DNIC demonstrate that a noxious stimulus applied to a body area triggers not only a chain of excitatory events but, also, via a supraspinal loop, diffuse inhibitory processes concerning all spinal and trigeminal convergent neurons not directly excited by the initial stimulus. The fact that a noxious stimulus seems able to trigger certain brainstem structures and thus inhibit convergent neurons, whereas such a stimulus is obviously perceived as painful, suggests that DNIC might be involved in nociception.

Knowing that convergent neurons are not only activated by noxious inputs but also, in a nonnegligible fashion, by light mechanical stimuli (60), thus giving rise to a "basic somesthetic activity," we proposed (65) a model in which pain could be triggered by a contrast signal between excitatory information emanating from both the segmental pool of convergent and nociceptive-specific neurons and the DNIC-mediated silencing of the remaining convergent neuronal population (Fig. 2). As an intense noxious stimulus is applied to an area of the body, the convergent and nociceptive-specific neurons in the corresponding segmental zone will be activated (Fig. 2B) and then give rise to excitatory messages transmitted to higher centers (Fig. 2C). This signal will, in turn, induce DNIC (Fig. 2D), which will inhibit those convergent spinal and trigeminal neurons not directly influenced by the initial stimulus (Fig. 2E). By these means, a high level of contrast will be attained between the activities of the excited segmental neurons and the depressed activity of the rest of the pool of convergent cells.

This "contrasting phenomenon" could also apply to the mediation of anginal pain and the pain that accompanies myocardial infarction. The excitatory events have been studied extensively on thoracic spinothalamic and spinoreticular neurons

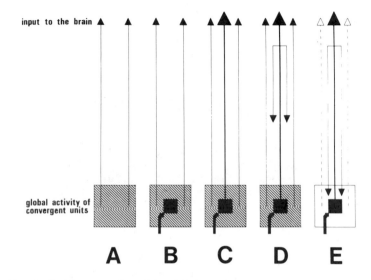

input to the brain

global activity of
convergent units

A   B   C   D   E

FIG. 2. Hypothetical interpretation of the global activity of spinal and trigeminal neurons involved in nociception at spinal and trigeminal levels. Taken as a whole, this activity would be of a reasonably high order in freely moving animals because of the properties of convergent neurons, sending a "basic somesthetic activity" toward the brain **(A).** A noxious stimulus activates both noxious-only and convergent neurons **(B),** which send an excitatory input to the brain **(C).** These inputs trigger the DNIC system **(D),** consequently reducing the activity of the remaining nonsegmental convergent units not directly affected by the initial stimulus **(E).** Hence, a contrast signal is set up. (From ref. 67.)

by Foreman and colleagues (11–13,37). Figure 3 illustrates the possible inhibitory facet of cardiac pain: The intracardiac administration of bradykinin (2 μg/kg), which stimulates sympathetic afferent nerve endings (1), induced a strong inhibition of a convergent neuron recorded within the nucleus caudalis of the trigeminal system.

We have proposed that the brain is able to recognize this contrast message and so, consequently, DNIC can be interpreted as a filter allowing the extraction of a nociceptive message from the overall activity of convergent neurons. The theoretical framework of such a hypothesis, including its possible relationship with morphine analgesia, has been developed elsewhere (62,66–68). We believe that a functional role of DNIC is supported by the clinical and experimental observations of the masking of a pain by the experience of pain at another locus (18,59,118).

If convergent neurons indeed play an important role in the transmission of nociceptive messages, one could postulate that, in terms of pain sensation, the concomitant application of two distinct noxious stimuli would result in the attenuation of the pain resulting from the weaker stimulus. It is as if the central nervous system temporarily eliminates, in the same manner as the "basic somesthetic activity," the transmission of the less urgent weaker stimulus. In such a system, the final sensation would be dependent not only on a balancing effect between

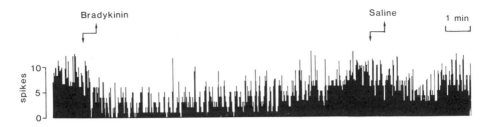

FIG. 3. Possible "inhibitory facet" induced by cardiac pain. The intracardiac administration of bradykinin (2 μg/kg, *arrow*) via a catheter implanted in the right jugular vein induced strong inhibitions of C-fiber responses of a convergent neuron recorded in the nucleus caudalis of the trigeminal system. Note that the inhibitory effects lasted several minutes after the end of bradykinin administration. The injection of the same volume of saline induced minimal changes in the neuronal responses.

two peripheral noxious inputs to the brain, but also on the relative contribution of these inputs to the silencing of the background activity of convergent neurons. On the basis of this hypothesis, the complexity of certain forms of clinical pain and the variety and range of syndromes observed could be the result of a double process of coding of the nociceptive information, an excitatory and an inhibitory facet, the latter produced by DNIC.

ACKNOWLEDGMENT

The authors are very grateful to Mrs. M. Hoch for the dactylogram.

REFERENCES

1. Baker, D. G., Coleridge, H. M., Coleridge, J. C. G., and Nerdrum, T. (1980): Search for a cardiac nociceptor: stimulation by bradykinin of sympathetic afferent nerve endings in the heart of the cat. *J. Physiol. (Lond.)*, 306:519–536.
2. Basbaum, A. I., Clanton, C. H., and Fields, H. L. (1976): Opiate and stimulus produced analgesia: functional anatomy of medullospinal pathway. *Proc. Natl. Acad. Sci., (U.S.A.)*, 73:4685–4688.
3. Basbaum, A. I., and Fields, H. L. (1978): Endogenous pain control mechanisms: review and hypothesis. *Ann. Neurol.*, 4:451–462.
4. Basbaum, A. I., and Fields, H. L. (1980): Pain control: a new role for the medullary reticular formation. In: *The Reticular Formation Revisited,* edited by J. A. Hobson and M. A. B. Brazier, pp. 329–348. Raven Press, New York.
5. Beall, J. A., Martin, R. F., Applebaum, A. E., and Willis, W. D. (1976): Inhibition of primate spinothalamic tract neurons by stimulation in the region of nucleus raphe magnus. *Brain Res.*, 114:328–333.
6. Belcher, G., Ryall, R. W., and Schaffner, R. (1978): The differential effects of 5-hydroxytryptamine, noradrenaline and raphe stimulation on nociceptive and non-nociceptive dorsal horn interneurons in the cat. *Brain Res.*, 151:307–321.
7. Besson, J. M., Catchlove, R. F. H., Feltz, P., and Le Bars, D. (1974): Further evidence for post-synaptic inhibitions on lamina V dorsal horn neurons. *Brain Res.*, 66:531–536.
8. Besson, J. M., Dickenson, A. H., Le Bars, D., and Oliveras, J. L. (1979): Opiate analgesia: the physiology and pharmacology of spinal pain systems. In: *Advances in Pharmacology and*

Therapeutics, Vol. 5. Neuropsychopharmacology, edited by C. Dumont, pp. 61–81. Pergamon Press, Oxford.

9. Besson, J. M., Guilbaud, G., Abdelmoumene, M., and Chaouch, A. (1982): Physiologie de la nociception. *J. Physiol. (Paris),* 78:7–107.

10. Besson, J. M., Oliveras, J. L., Chaouch, A., and Rivot, J. P. (1981): Role of the raphe nuclei in stimulation producing analgesia. In: *Serotonin: Current Aspects of Neurochemistry and Function,* edited by B. Haber, S. Gabay, M. R. Issidorides, and S. G. A. Alivisatos, pp. 153–176. Plenum Publishing Corporation.

11. Blair, R. W., Ammons, W. S., and Foreman, R. D. (1984): Responses of thoracic spinothalamic and stinoreticular cells to coronary artery occlusion. *J. Neurophysiol.,* 51:636–648.

12. Blair, R. W., Weber, R. N., and Foreman, R. D. (1981): Characteristics of primate spinothalamic tract neurons receiving viscerosomatic convergent inputs in T3-T5 segments. *J. Neurophysiol.,* 46:797–811.

13. Blair, R. W., Weber, R. N., and Foreman, R. D. (1982): Responses of thoracic spinothalamic neurons to intracardiac injection of bradykinin in the monkey. *Circ. Res.,* 51:83–94.

14. Bourgoin, S., Oliveras, J. L., Bruxelle, J., Hamon, M., and Besson, J. M. (1980): Electrical stimulation of the nucleus raphe magnus in the rat. Effects on 5-HT metabolism in the spinal cord. *Brain Res.,* 194:377–389.

15. Brown, A. G., Hamann, W. C., and Martin, H. R. (1973): Interactions of cutaneous myelinated (A) and non-myelinated (C) fibres on transmission through the spinocervical tract. *Brain Res.,* 53:222–226.

16. Cadden, S. W., Villanueva, L., Chitour, D., and Le Bars, D. (1983): Depression of activities of dorsal horn convergent neurons by propriospinal mechanisms triggered by noxious inputs; comparison with Diffuse Noxious Inhibitory Controls (DNIC). *Brain Res.,* 275:1–11.

17. Calvillo, O., Henry, J. L., and Neuman, R. S. (1979): Actions of narcotic analgesics and antagonists on spinal units responding to natural stimulation in the cat. *Canad. J. Physiol. Pharmacol.,* 57:652–663.

18. Calvino, B., Villanueva, L., and Le Bars, D. (1984): The heterotopic effects of visceral pain: behavioural and electrophysiological approaches in the rat. *Pain,* 20:261–271.

19. Campbell, J. N., and Taub, A. (1973): Local analgesia from percutaneous electrical stimulation. A peripheral mechanism. *Arch. Neurol. (Chicago),* 28:347–350.

20. Carstens, E., Bihl, H., Irvine, D. R. F., and Zimmermann, M. (1981): Descending inhibitions from medial and lateral midbrain of spinal dorsal horn neuronal responses to noxious and non-noxious cutaneous stimuli in the cat. *J. Neurophysiol.,* 45:1029–1042.

21. Carstens, E., Klumpp, D., and Zimmermann, M. (1980): Differential inhibitory effects of medial and lateral midbrain stimulation on spinal neuronal discharges to noxious skin heating in the cat. *J. Neurophysiol.,* 43:332–342.

22. Cervero, F., and Iggo, A. (1980): The substantia gelatinosa of the spinal cord. A critical review. *Brain,* 103:717–772.

23. Cervero, F., Iggo, A., and Ogawa, H. (1976): Nociceptor-driven dorsal horn neurons in the lumbar spinal cord of the cat. *Pain,* 2:5–24.

24. Chitour, D., Dickenson, A. H., and Le Bars, D. (1982): Pharmacological evidence for the involvement of serotonergic mechanisms in Diffuse Noxious Inhibitory Controls (DNIC). *Brain Res.,* 236:329–337.

25. Christensen, B. N., and Perl, E. R. (1970): Spinal neurons specifically excited by noxious or thermal stimuli: marginal zone of the dorsal horn. *J. Neurophysiol.,* 33:293–307.

26. Dickenson, A. H., and Le Bars, D. (1983): Diffuse Noxious Inhibitory Controls (DNIC) involve trigemino and spinothalamic convergent neurones in the rat. *Exp. Brain Res.,* 49:174–180.

27. Dickenson, A. H., Le Bars, D., and Besson, J. M. (1980): Diffuse Noxious Inhibitory Controls (DNIC). Effects on trigeminal nucleus caudalis neurones in the rat. *Brain Res.,* 200:293–305.

28. Dickenson, A. H., Le Bars, D., and Besson, J. M. (1980): An involvement of nucleus raphe magnus in Diffuse Noxious Inhibitory Controls (DNIC). *Neurosci. Lett. (Suppl.),* 5:S375.

29. Dickenson, A. H., Rivot, J. P., Chaouch, A., Besson, J. M., and Le Bars, D. (1981): Diffuse Noxious Inhibitory Controls (DNIC) in the rat with or without pCPA pretreatment. *Brain Res.,* 216:313–321.

30. Duggan, A. W., and Griersmith, B. T. (1979): Inhibition of the spinal transmission of nociceptive information by supraspinal stimulation in the cat. *Pain,* 6:149–161.

31. Fields, H. L., and Basbaum, A. I. (1978): Brain stem control of spinal pain transmission neurons. *Annu. Rev. Physiol.,* 40:193–221.

32. Fields, H. L., Basbaum, A. I., Clanton, C. H., and Anderson, S. D. (1977): Nucleus raphe magnus inhibition of spinal cord dorsal horn neurons. *Brain Res.*, 126:441–453.
33. Fields, H. L., Meyer, G. A., and Partridge, L. D. (1970): Convergence of visceral and somatic input onto cat spinal neurons. *Exp. Neurol.*, 26:36–52.
34. Fitzgerald, M. (1982): The contralateral input to the dorsal horn of the spinal cord in the decerebrate spinal rat. *Brain Res.*, 236:275–287.
35. Foreman, R. D. (1977): Viscerosomatic convergence onto spinal neurons responding to afferent fibers located in the inferior cardiac nerve. *Brain Res.*, 137:164–168.
36. Foreman, R. D., Beall, J. E., Applebaum, A. E., Coulter, J. D., and Willis, W. D. (1976): Effects of dorsal horn column stimulation on primate spinothalamic tract neurons. *J. Neurophysiol.*, 39:534–546.
37. Foreman, R. D., Blair, R. W., and Weber, R. N. (1984): Viscerosomatic convergence onto T2-T4 spinoreticular, spinoreticular-spinothalamic, and spinothalamic tract neurons in the cat. *Exp. Neurol.*, 85:597–619.
38. Foreman, R. D., Hancock, M. B., and Willis, W. D. (1981): Responses of spinothalamic tract cells in the thoracic spinal cord of the monkey to cutaneous and visceral inputs. *Pain*, 11:149–162.
39. Gerhart, K. D., Wilcox, T. K., Chung, J. M., and Willis, W. D. (1981): Inhibition of nociceptive and non-nociceptive responses of primate spinothalamic cells by stimulation in medial brain stem. *J. Neurophysiol.*, 45:121–136.
40. Gerhart, K. D., Yezierski, R. P., Giesler, G. J., Jr., and Willis, W. D. (1981): Inhibitory receptive field of primate spino-thalamic tract cells. *J. Neurophysiol.*, 46:1309–1325.
41. Ghia, J. N., Mueller, R. A., Duncan, G. H., Scott, D. S., and Mao, W. (1981): Serotonergic activity in man as a function of pain, pain mechanisms and depression. *Anesth. Analg.*, 60:854–861.
42. Giesler, G. J., Jr., Gerhart, K. D., Yezierski, R. P., Wilcox, T. K., and Willis, W. D. (1981): Postsynaptic inhibition of primate spinothalamic neurons by stimulation in nucleus raphe magnus. *Brain Res.*, 204:184–188.
43. Gokin, A. P., Kostyuk, P. G., and Preobrazhensky, N. N. (1977): Neuronal mechanisms of interactions of high threshold visceral and somatic afferent influences in spinal cord and medulla. *J. Physiol. (Paris)*, 73:319–333.
44. Gregor, M., and Zimmermann, M. (1972): Characteristics of spinal neurons responding to cutaneous myelinated and unmyelinated fibres. *J. Physiol. (Lond.)*, 221:555–576.
45. Griersmith, B. T., and Duggan, A. W. (1980): Prolonged depression of spinal transmission of nociceptive information by 5-HT administered in the substantia gelatinosa: antagonism by methysergide. *Brain Res.*, 187:231–236.
46. Guilbaud, G., Benelli, G., and Besson, J. M. (1977): Responses of thoracic dorsal horn interneurons to cutaneous stimulation and to administration of algogenic substances into the mesenteric artery in the spinal cat. *Brain Res.*, 124:437–448.
47. Guilbaud, G., Besson, J. M., Liebeskind, J. C., and Oliveras, J. L. (1972): Analgésie induite par stimulation de la substance grise périaqueducale chez le chat: données comportementales et modifications de l'activité des interneurones de la corne dorsale de la moelle. *C. R. Acad. Sci. (Paris)*, 275:1055–1057.
48. Guilbaud, G., Oliveras, J. L., Giesler, G. J., Jr., and Besson, J. M. (1977): Effects induced by stimulation of the centralis inferior nucleus of the raphe on dorsal horn interneurons in cat's spinal cord. *Brain Res.*, 126:355–360.
49. Hancock, M. B., Rigamonti, D. D., and Bryan, R. N. (1973): Convergence in the lumbar spinal cord pathways activated by splanchnic nerve and hindlimb cutaneous nerve stimulation. *Exp. Neurol.*, 38:337–348.
50. Handwerker, H. O., Iggo, A., and Zimmermann, M. (1975): Segmental and supraspinal actions on dorsal horn neurons responding to noxious and non-noxious skin stimuli. *Pain*, 1:147–165.
51. Hayes, R. L., Price, D. D., Ruda, M., and Dubner, R. (1979): Suppression of nociceptive responses in the primate by electrical stimulation of the brain or morphine administration: behavioral and electrophysiological comparisons. *Brain Res.*, 167:417–421.
52. Headley, P. M., Duggan, A. W., and Griersmith, B. T. (1978): Selective reduction by noradrenaline and 5-hydroxytryptamine of nociceptive responses of cat dorsal horn neurons. *Brain Res.*, 145:185–189.
53. Hillman, P., and Wall, P. D. (1969): Inhibitory and excitatory factors influencing the receptive fields of lamina 5 spinal cord cells. *Exp. Brain Res.*, 9:284–306.

54. Iggo, A., McMillan, J. A., and Mokha, S. S. (1981): Modulation of spinal cord multireceptive neurons from locus ceruleus and nucleus raphe magnus in the cat. *J. Physiol. (Lond.)*, 319:107–108P.

55. Johnson, S. M., and Duggan, A. W. (1981): Evidence that the opiate receptors of the substantia gelatinosa contribute to the depression, by intravenous morphine, of the spinal transmission of impulses in unmyelinated primary afferents. *Brain Res.*, 207:223–228.

56. Jordan, L. M., Kenshalo, D. R., Martin, R. F., Haber, L. H., and Willis, W. D. (1978): Depression of primate spinothalamic tract neurons by iontophoretic application of 5-hydroxytryptamine. *Pain*, 5:135–142.

57. Jordan, L. M., Kenshalo, D. R., Martin, R. F., Haber, L. H., and Willis, W. D. (1979): Two populations of spinothalamic tract neurons with opposite responses to 5-hydroxytryptamine. *Brain Res.*, 164:342–346.

58. Kitahata, L. M., Kosaka, Y., Taub, A., Bonikos, K., and Hoffert, M. (1974): Lamina specific suppression of dorsal-horn unit activity by morphine sulfate. *Anesthesiology*, 41:39–48.

59. Le Bars, D., Calvino, B., Villanueva, L., and Cadden, S. (1984): Physiological approaches to counterirritation phenomena. In: *Stress Induced Analgesia*, edited by M. D. Trickleband and C. Curzon, pp. 67–101. John Wiley Ltd.

60. Le Bars, D., and Chitour, D. (1983): Do convergent neurons in the spinal dorsal horn discriminate nociceptive from non-nociceptive information? *Pain*, 17:1–19.

61. Le Bars, D., Chitour, D., and Clot, A. M. (1981): The encoding of thermal stimuli by Diffuse Noxious Inhibitory Controls (DNIC). *Brain Res.*, 230:394–399.

62. Le Bars, D., Chitour, D., Kraus, E., Clot, A. M., Dickenson, A. H., and Besson, J. M. (1981): The effect of systemic morphine upon Diffuse Noxious Inhibitory Controls (DNIC) in the rat: evidence for a lifting of certain descending inhibitory controls of dorsal horn convergent neurones. *Brain Res.*, 215:257–274.

63. Le Bars, D., Chitour, D., Kraus, E., Dickenson, A. H., and Besson, J. M. (1981): Effects of naloxone upon Diffuse Noxious Inhibitory Controls (DNIC) in the rat. *Brain Res.*, 204:387–402.

64. Le Bars, D., Dickenson, A. H., and Besson, J. M. (1979): Diffuse Noxious Inhibitory Controls (DNIC). I. Effects on dorsal horn convergent neurones in the rat. *Pain*, 6:283–304.

65. Le Bars, D., Dickenson, A. H., and Besson, J. M. (1979): Diffuse Noxious Inhibitory Controls (DNIC). II. Lack of effect on nonconvergent neurones, supraspinal involvement and theoretical implications. *Pain*, 6:305–327.

66. Le Bars, D., Dickenson, A. H., and Besson, J. M. (1982): The triggering of bulbo-spinal serotonergic inhibitory controls by noxious peripheral inputs. In: *Brainstem Control of Spinal Mechanisms*, edited by B. Sjölund and A. Björklund, pp. 381–410. Elsevier Biomedical Press.

67. Le Bars, D., Dickenson, A. H., and Besson, J. M. (1983): Opiate analgesia and descending inhibitory controls systems. In: *Advance in Pain Research and Therapy, Vol. 5*, edited by J. J. Bonica et al., pp. 341–372. Raven Press, New York.

68. Le Bars, D., Dickenson, A. H., Besson, J. M., and Villanueva, L. (1986): Aspects of sensory processing through convergent neurons. In: *Spinal Afferent Processing*, edited by T. Yaksh, pp. 467–504. Plenum Publ. Corp.

69. Le Bars, D., Guilbaud, G., Jurna, I., and Besson, J. M. (1976): Differential effects of morphine on response of dorsal horn lamina V type cells elicited by A and C fiber stimulation in the spinal cat. *Brain Res.*, 115:518–524.

70. Le Bars, D., Ménétrey, D., and Besson, J. M. (1976): Effects of morphine upon the lamina V type cells activities in the dorsal horn of decerebrate cat. *Brain Res.*, 113:293–310.

71. Le Bars, D., Ménétrey, D., Conseiller, C., and Besson, J. M. (1975): Depressive effects of morphine upon lamina V cells activities in the dorsal horn of the spinal cat. *Brain Res.*, 98:261–277.

72. Le Bars, D., Rivot, J. P., Guilbaud, G., Ménétrey, D., and Besson, J. M. (1979): The depressive effect of morphine on the C fiber response of dorsal horn neurones in the spinal rat pretreated or not by pCPA. *Brain Res.*, 176:337–353.

73. Liebeskind, J. C., Giesler, G. J., Jr., and Urca, G. (1976): Evidence pertaining to an endogenous mechanism of pain inhibition in the central nervous system. In: *Sensory Functions of the Skin in Primates*, edited by I. Zotterman, pp. 561–573. Pergamon Press, Oxford.

74. Liebeskind, J. C., Guilbaud, G., Besson, J. M., and Oliveras, J. L. (1973): Analgesia from electrical stimulation of the periaqueductal gray matter in the cat: behavioral observations and inhibitory effects on spinal cord interneurons. *Brain Res.*, 50:441–446.

75. Lindblom, U., Tapper, D. N., and Wiesenfeld, Z. (1977): The effect of dorsal horn column stimulation on the nociceptive response of dorsal horn cells and its relevance to pain suppression. *Pain*, 4:133–144.
76. Long, D. M., and Hagfors, N. (1975): Electrical stimulation in the nervous system: the current status of electrical stimulation of the nervous system for relief of pain. *Pain*, 1:109–123.
77. McCreery, D. B., Bloedel, J. R., and Hames, E. G. (1979): Effects of stimulating in raphe nuclei and in reticular formation on response of spinothalamic neurons to mechanical stimuli. *J. Neurophysiol.*, 42:166–182.
78. Mayer, D. J. (1979): Endogenous analgesia systems: neural and behavioral mechanisms. In: *Advances in Pain Research and Therapy, Vol. 3*, edited by J. J. Bonica, J. C. Liebeskind, and D. Albe-Fessard, pp. 385–410. Raven Press, New York.
79. Mayer, D. J., and Price, D. D. (1976): Central nervous system mechanisms of analgesia. *Pain*, 2:379–404.
80. Melzack, R., and Wall, P. D. (1965): Pain mechanism: a new theory. *Science*, 150:971–979.
81. Mendell, L. M. (1966): Physiological properties of unmyelinated fiber projections to the spinal cord. *Exp. Neurol.*, 16:316–332.
82. Meyer, G. A., and Fields, H. L. (1972): Causalgia treated by selective large fiber stimulation of peripheral nerve. *Brain*, 95:163–168.
83. Milne, R. J., Foreman, R. D., Giesler, G. J., Jr., and Willis, W. D. (1981): Convergence of cutaneous and pelvic visceral nociceptive inputs onto primate spinothalamic neurons. *Pain*, 11:163–183.
84. Nashold, B. S., and Friedman, H. (1972): Dorsal column stimulation for control of pain. Preliminary report on 30 patients. *J. Neurosurg.*, 46:590–597.
85. Nathan, P. W. (1976): The gate-control theory of pain: a critical review. *Brain*, 99:123–158.
86. Nathan, P. W., and Wall, P. D. (1974): Treatment of post-herpetic neuralgia by prolonged electrical stimulation. *Br. Med. J.*, 3:645–647.
87. Nielson, K. D., Adams, J. E., and Hosobuchi, Y. (1975): Phantom limb pain. Treatment with dorsal column stimulation. *J. Neurosurg.*, 42:301–307.
88. Oliveras, J. L., Besson, J. M., Guilbaud, G., and Liebeskind, J. C. (1974): Behavioral and electrophysiological evidence of pain inhibition from midbrain stimulation in the cat. *Exp. Brain Res.*, 20:32–44.
89. Oliveras, J. L., Guilbaud, G., and Besson, J. M. (1979): A map of serotoninergic structures involved in stimulation producing analgesia in unrestrained freely moving cats. *Brain Res.*, 164:317–322.
90. Oliveras, J. L., Hosobuchi, Y., Redjemi, F., Guilbaud, G., and Besson, J. M. (1977): Opiate antagonist naloxone strongly reduces analgesia induced by stimulation of a raphe nucleus (centralis inferior). *Brain Res.*, 120:221–229.
91. Oliveras, J. L., Redjemi, F., Guilbaud, G., and Besson, J. M. (1975): Analgesia induced by electrical stimulation of the inferior centralis nucleus of the raphe in the cat. *Pain*, 1:139–145.
92. Pomeranz, B., Wall, P. D., and Weber, W. V. (1968): Cord cells responding to fine myelinated afferents from viscera, muscle and skin. *J. Physiol. (Lond.)*, 199:511–532.
93. Price, D. D., and Wagman, I. H. (1970): The physiological roles of A and C fiber inputs to the dorsal horn of M. mulatta. *Exp. Neurol.*, 29:373–390.
94. Randic, M., and Yu, H. H. (1976): Effects of 5-hydroxytryptamine and bradykinin in cat dorsal horn neurons activated by noxious stimuli. *Brain Res.*, 111:197–203.
95. Rexed, B. (1952): The cytoarchitectonic organization of the spinal cord in the cat. *J. Comp. Neurol.*, 96:415–496.
96. Rexed, B. (1954): A cytoarchitectonic atlas of the spinal cord in the cat. *J. Comp. Neurol.*, 100:297–380.
97. Rivot, J. P., Chaouch, A., and Besson, J. M. (1979): The influence of naloxone on the C-fiber response of dorsal horn neurons and their inhibitory control by raphe magnus stimulation. *Brain Res.*, 176:355–364.
98. Rivot, J. P., Chaouch, A., and Besson, J. M. (1980): Nucleus raphe magnus modulation of response of rat dorsal horn neurons to unmyelinated fiber inputs: partial involvement of serotoninergic pathways. *J. Neurophysiol.*, 44:1039–1057.
99. Rivot, J. P., Chiang, C. Y., and Besson, J. M. (1982): Increase of serotonin metabolism within the dorsal horn of the spinal cord during nucleus raphe magnus stimulation, as revealed by *in vivo* electrochemical detection. *Brain Res.*, 238:117–126.

100. Ruch, G. C. (1949): Visceral sensation and referred pain. In: *Howell's Textbook of Physiology*, edited by J. F. Fulton, pp. 360–374. Saunders, Philadelphia.
101. Satran, R., and Goldstein, M. N. (1973): Pain perception: modification of threshold of intolerance and cortical potentials by cutaneous stimulation. *Science*, 180:1201–1202.
102. Selzer, M., and Spencer, W. A. (1969): Convergence of visceral and cutaneous afferent pathways in the lumbar spinal cord. *Brain Res.*, 14:331–348.
103. Shealy, C. N., Mortimer, J. T., and Hagfors, N. R. (1970): Dorsal column electro-analgesia. *J. Neurosurg.*, 32:560–564.
104. Takahashi, M., and Yokota, T. (1983): Convergence of cardiac and cutaneous afferents onto neurons in the dorsal horn of the spinal cord in the cat. *Neurosci. Lett.*, 38:251–256.
105. Tyce, G., and Yaksh, T. (1981): Monoamine release from cat spinal cord by somatic stimuli: an intrinsic modulatory system. *J. Physiol. (Lond.)*, 314:513–529.
106. Villanueva, L., Cadden, S. W., and Le Bars, D. (1984): Evidence that Diffuse Noxious Inhibitory Controls (DNIC) are mediated by a final post-synaptic inhibitory mechanism. *Brain Res.*, 298:67–74.
107. Villanueva, L., Cadden, S. W., and Le Bars, D. (1984): Diffuse Noxious Inhibitory Controls (DNIC): evidence for post synaptic inhibition of trigeminal nucleus caudalis convergent neurons. *Brain Res.*, 321:165–168.
108. Villanueva, L., Chitour, D., and Le Bars, D. (1985): Involvement of the dorsolateral funiculus (DLF) in the descending part of the loop subserving Diffuse Noxious Inhibitory Controls (DNIC). *Neurosci. Lett. (Suppl.)*, 22:S468.
109. Villanueva, L., and Le Bars, D. (1985): The encoding of thermal stimuli applied to the tail of the rat by lowering the excitability of trigeminal convergent neurons. *Brain Res.*, 330:245–251.
110. Villanueva, L., Peschanski, M., Calvino, B., and Le Bars, D. (1986): Ascending pathways in the spinal cord involved in triggering of Diffuse Noxious Inhibitory Controls (DNIC) in the rat. *J. Neurophysiol.* 55:34–55.
111. Wagman, I. H., and Price, D. D. (1969): Responses of dorsal horn cells of M. mulatta to cutaneous and sural nerve A and C-fiber stimulation. *J. Neurophysiol.*, 32:803–817.
112. Wall, P. D. (1967): The laminar organization of dorsal horn and effects of descending impulses. *J. Physiol. (Lond.)*, 188:403–423.
113. Wall, P. D. (1978): The gate control of pain mechanisms: a re-examination and re-statement. *Brain*, 101:1–18.
114. Wall, P. D. (1980): The substantia gelatinosa. A gate control mechanism set across a sensory pathway. *Trends in Neurosci.*, 9:221–224.
115. Wall, P. D., and Sweet, W. H. (1967): Temporary abolition of pain in man. *Science*, 155:108–109.
116. Wang, J. K. (1977): Antinociceptive effect of intrathecally administered serotonin. *Anesthesiology*, 47:269–271.
117. Weil-Fugazza, J., Godefroy, F., and Le Bars, D. (1984): Increase in 5-HT synthesis in the dorsal part of the spinal cord, induced by a nociceptive stimulus: blockade by morphine. *Brain Res.*, 297:247–264.
118. Willer, J. C., Roby, A., and Le Bars, D. (1984): Psychophysical and electrophysiological approaches to the pain relieving effect of heterotopic nociceptive stimuli. *Brain*, 107:1095–1112.
119. Willis, W. D., Haber, L. H., and Martin, R. F. (1977): Inhibition of spinothalamic tract cells and interneurons by brain stem stimulation in the monkey. *J. Neurophysiol.*, 40:968–981.
120. Woolf, C. J., and Fitzgerald, M. (1981): Lamina-specific alteration of C-fiber evoked activity by morphine in the dorsal horn of the rat spinal cord. *Neurosci. Lett.*, 25:37–41.
121. Yaksh, T. L., and Wilson, P. R. (1979): Spinal serotonin terminal system mediates antinociception. *J. Pharmacol. Exp. Ther.*, 208:446–453.
122. Zorman, G., Hentall, I. D., Adams, J. E., and Fields, H. L. (1981): Naloxone-reversible analgesia produced by microstimulation in the rat medulla. *Brain Res.*, 219:137–148.
123. Zorman, G., Belcher, G., Adams, J. E., and Fields, H. L. (1982): Lumbar intrathecal naloxone blocks analgesia produced by microstimulation of ventromedial medulla in the rat brain. *Brain Res.*, 236:77–84.

Hammersmith Cardiology Workshop Series, Vol. 3,
edited by A. Maseri, B. E. Sobel, and S. Chierchia.
Raven Press, New York © 1987.

Evidence and Significance of Silent Ischemia in Patients with Angina Pectoris

Sergio Chierchia and James J. Glazier

Cardiovascular Research Unit, Royal Postgraduate Medical School, Hammersmith Hospital, London W12 OHS, England

Silent myocardial ischemia refers to episodes of transient acute myocardial ischemia occurring in the absence of angina pectoris or its usual equivalents. This concept is difficult for both patients and physicians to accept since angina has always been taken to represent the cardinal manifestation of ischemic heart disease.

Silent myocardial ischemia occurs in two general types of subjects (1). One type has never had symptoms of ischemic heart disease. These persons have never experienced angina or its equivalents or suffered a myocardial infarction. The other type of patient has known coronary artery disease, usually in the form of chronic angina or previous myocardial infarction.

A necessary part of the definition and classification of silent myocardial ischemia is the demonstration of continuing myocardial ischemia (2), and evidence for disease activity is particularly important in asymptomatic postinfarct patients. In only some of these latter patients is it possible to demonstrate active myocardial ischemia (3), suggesting that, in the others, the disease process is either temporarily inactive or "burned out."

In the totally asymptomatic patients, ischemia is detected only fortuitously, usually as a result of exercise testing performed as part of a periodic examination. Accordingly, such patients come to medical attention only by chance and are rarely seen. As a result, our investigations have mainly focused on patients who present with typical anginal attacks but also exhibit a variable and usually very large proportion of ischemic episodes that are totally asymptomatic.

THE EVIDENCE

The predominance of silent ischemic episodes in anginal patients was initially suggested by our studies (4,5) and by those of Guazzi et al. (6) in patients with the so-called variant form of angina. Subsequent reports in patients with both unstable (7) and chronic stable angina (8–10) showed a 70% prevalence of episodes of acute myocardial ischemia unaccompanied by pain. Formerly, discussion of silent ischemia was limited to isolated reports of asymptomatic myocardial infarction. Clearly, this can no longer be the case, particularly when one realizes that, in anginal patients, painless episodes occur three or four times more frequently than those with pain. Given the predominance of silent ischemic episodes, it is important to determine their significance and how they differ from those with pain.

A number of observations suggest that totally silent ST segment elevation or depression indicates severe ischemia. In patients with documented ischemic heart disease, transient ischemic ST segment changes are accompanied by an increase in left ventricular filling pressures (7), a decrease in left ventricular contractility (7), an increase in myocardial oxygen extraction (11), net lactate production (11), and an increase in left ventricular volume (12). These changes occur regardless of the presence or absence of angina, a rather late and poorly sensitive marker of ischemia. Also, the appearance of defects in thallium-201 (13) and rubidium-82 (8,14) regional myocardial uptake have been observed during episodes of transient, asymptomatic ST segment changes. Severe ventricular arrhythmias are nearly as common in prolonged episodes of silent and painful ST segment elevation (5). Antianginal treatment with calcium blockers (15), nitrates (16), and beta blockers (17) reduces the number of painful and painless episodes to the same extent, and successful coronary bypass surgery eliminates or reduces symptomatic as well as silent ischemic events (18).

THE CAUSES

A number of studies have been performed to determine the possible differences between episodes of painful and painless myocardial ischemia. Hemodynamic monitoring in patients with variant and rest angina showed that episodes of less than 3 min and those associated with an increase in left ventricular diastolic pressure of less than 7 mm Hg were invariably painless. However, above these levels a large overlap was observed, and it was practically impossible to predict whether an episode would be painful or painless (19). Furthermore, a study of patients with chronic stable angina showed a poor correlation between the occurrence of angina and the severity and duration of ST segment depression as detected during ambulatory ECG monitoring, although, on average, episodes with pain tended to be more prolonged and severe (8). Finally, the rate and extent of ventricular dilatation that occurs during ischemia appear to be similar in painful and painless episodes (12). These studies indicate that the severity and duration of myocardial ischemia are only two of the many factors determining the occurrence of angina.

A number of investigations in patients with painless myocardial infarction suggest that these subjects have an unusually reduced sensitivity to pain (20,21). Quantitative studies of pain threshold support this hypothesis (22,23). It appears that the mechanisms responsible for a diminished sensitivity to pain in these patients may be related to a reduced ability to discriminate algogenic stimuli (24). Moreover, they also exhibit a reduced tendency to complain in general; on a personality questionnaire, they have significantly lower scores on parameters of nervousness, excitability, and dominance, and a higher score on the masculinity scale (24).

However, if these results are examined more closely, it becomes apparent that, although many of the differences between patients with painful and those with painless ischemia attain statistical significance, the overlap between the two groups is so great that other important and yet unidentified factors must be responsible for the presence or absence of pain. This reasoning appears even more justified in patients alternating episodes with and without angina. For the reasons discussed earlier, it is difficult to justify the presence or absence of cardiac pain purely on the basis of the severity and duration of the ischemic stimulus. Therefore, it appears necessary to postulate that potentially painful stimuli are inhibited at the level of the spinal cord, in agreement with the gate control theory (25). Alternatively, should nociceptive stimuli reach higher centers, the perception of pain may be variable, even within the same person, at different times (26).

CLINICAL IMPLICATIONS

The incidence of silent myocardial ischemia in an unselected population of patients with chronic stable angina appears to be rather high. In a study performed in 83 consecutive patients with this syndrome, 49 (59%) had episodes of diagnostic ischemic ST segment depression during ambulatory ECG monitoring. Of these, 19 (39%) had both symptomatic and asymptomatic episodes, 6 (12%) only had episodes with pain, and 24 (49%) only exhibited episodes of silent myocardial ischemia (27).

Although, at first glance, these results could suggest that ambulatory ECG monitoring should be widely used for the clinical assessment and follow-up of patients with chronic stable angina, it should be noted that the majority of ischemic episodes with or without pain occurred in patients with a very limited exercise tolerance (less than 6 min on the modified Bruce protocol). Of the 24 patients with only silent ischemia, only 10 exhibited a high incidence of ischemic events (greater than or equal to three episodes in 24 hr) in the monitoring period; of these 10, eight had a very limited coronary reserve, as assessed by exercise testing (27).

The direct implication of these observations is that at least for patients with chronic stable angina, episodes of silent ischemia are usually fairly well correlated with the severity of impairment of coronary flow reserve. When exercise capacity is reasonably well preserved, the number of ischemic episodes, with or without angina, that occur during normal daily life can be expected to be relatively low.

The prognostic significance of silent ischemia has not yet been clarified. However, as discussed earlier, episodes of asymptomatic ST segment depression or elevation are associated with hemodynamic, biochemical, and electrophysiological changes that are indistinguishable from those observed during anginal attacks. When treated appropriately, patients exhibit disappearance or reduction of both painful and painless episodes. Finally, about 25% of all myocardial infarctions are completely asymptomatic (28). All these considerations strongly suggest that the prognostic significance of silent ischemic episodes is probably similar to that of anginal attacks and that treatment, currently titrated to anginal episodes, should be, ideally, aimed at the total elimination of both painful and painless events.

There is an increasing tendency to treat silent ischemia as a specific syndrome rather than, as it is, simply one part of the spectrum of ischemic heart disease. Such an approach may encourage the idea that certain drugs are more active in the treatment of silent ischemia. Given the present concern about the significant prevalence of totally asymptomatic ischemia in the general population, estimated to be between 2.5% and 4% (29), this reasoning has sinister tones of commercialism. There is no evidence whatsoever to suggest that the pathophysiological mechanisms of ischemia can influence the presence or absence of pain. Painless ischemia can be caused by thrombosis (as in acute myocardial infarction), by spasm (as in variant angina), or by a combination of an excessive increase in demand and decrease in blood flow (as in chronic stable angina). Thus, it seems logical that drugs that are effective in the prophylactic treatment of angina will be equally effective in preventing silent myocardial ischemia. Accordingly, treatment of the totally asymptomatic patient who presents to medical attention only by chance should be guided by the identification of the pathophysiological mechanisms that are responsible for the ischemia.

CONCLUSIONS

Physicians have, up to now, based their diagnosis and gauged their treatment of ischemic heart disease on the presence or absence of anginal pain. However, a large body of evidence suggests that angina can no longer be considered the only marker of ongoing myocardial ischemia and, indeed, suggests the possibility that angina only represents the tip of the iceberg of myocardial ischemia (30). The frequent occurrence of asymptomatic myocardial ischemia has to be considered in the clinical follow-up of anginal patients and in the evaluation of therapeutical interventions. As the mechanisms responsible for silent ischemia are not different from those causing angina, the choice of treatment in the individual patient should only be guided by pathophysiological and prognostic considerations.

REFERENCES

1. Cohn, P. F. (1983): Seminar on asymptomatic coronary artery disease. Introduction. *J. Am. Coll. Cardiol.*, 1(3):922–923.
2. Cohn, P. F., Brown, E. J., Jr., and Cohn, J. K. (1984): Detection and management of coronary artery disease in the asymptomatic population. *Am. Heart J.*, 108:1064–1067.

3. Theroux, P., Waters, D. D., Halphen, C., De Baisieux, J. C., and Mizgala, H. F. (1979): Prognostic value of exercise testing soon after myocardial infarction. *N. Engl. J. Med., 301:341–345.*

4. Maseri, A., Mimmo, R., Chierchia, S., Marchesi, C., Pesola, A., and L'Abbate, A. (1975): Coronary artery spasm as a cause of acute myocardial ischemia in man. *Chest, 68:625–633.*

5. Maseri, A., Severi, S., De Nes, M., L'Abbate, A., Chierchia, S., Marzilli, M., Ballestra, A. M., Parodi, A., Biagini, A., and Distante, A. (1978): "Variant" angina: one aspect of a continuous spectrum of vasospastic myocardial ischemia. *Am. J. Cardiol., 41:1019–1035.*

6. Guazzi, M., Magrini, F., Fiorentini, C., and Polese, A. (1970): Continuous electrocardiographic recording in Prinzmetal's variant angina pectoris. A report of four cases. *Br. Heart J., 32:611–616.*

7. Chierchia, S., Lazzari, M., Simonetti, I., Maseri, A. (1980): Hemodynamic monitoring in angina at rest. *Herz, 5:189–198.*

8. Deanfield, J. E., Maseri, A., Selwyn, A. P., Ribeiro, P., Chierchia, S., Krikler, S., and Morgan, M. (1983): Myocardial ischemia during daily life in patients with stable angina. Its relation to symptoms and heart rate changes. *Lancet, 11:753–758.*

9. Schang, S. J., and Pepine, C. J. (1977): Transient asymptomatic S-T segment depression during daily activity. *Am. J. Cardiol., 39:396–402.*

10. Chierchia, S., Gallino, A., Smith, G., Deanfield, J., Morgan, M., Croom, M., and Maseri, A. (1984): Role of heart rate in pathophysiology of chronic stable angina. *Lancet, 11:1353–1358.*

11. Chierchia, S., Brunelli, M. D., Simonetti, I., Lazzari, M., and Maseri, A. (1980): Sequence of events in angina at rest: primary reduction in coronary flow. *Circulation, 61:759–768.*

12. Davies, G. J., Chierchia, S., Bencivelli, W., Pratt, T., Crean, P. A., and Maseri, A.: Sequence and magnitude of ventricular volume changes in painful and painless myocardial ischemia assessed by a precordial probe. *Circulation (in press).*

13. Maseri, A., Parodi, O., Severi, S., and Pesola, A. (1976): Transient transmural reduction of myocardial blood flow, demonstrated by Thallium-201 scintigraphy, as a cause of variant angina. *Circulation, 54:280–288.*

14. Deanfield, J. E., Shea, M., Kensett, M., Horlock, P., Wilson, R. A., De Landsheere, C. M., and Selwyn, A. P. (1984): Silent myocardial ischemia due to mental stress. *Lancet, 11:1001–1005.*

15. Parodi, O., Maseri, A., and Simonetti, I. (1979): Management of unstable angina at rest by Verapamil. A double-blind cross-over study in coronary care unit. *Br. Heart J., 41(2):167–174.*

16. Distante, A., Maseri, A., Severi, S., Biagini, A., and Chierchia, S. (1979): Management of vasospastic angina at rest with continuous infusion of isosorbide dinitrate. A double cross-over study in a coronary care unit. *Am. J. Cardiol., 44:533.*

17. Glazier, J. J., Chierchia, S., Smith, G. C., Berkenboom, G., Crean, P. A., Gerosa, S., and Maseri, A. (1986): Beta blockers for angina pectoris: How do they really work? *Clin. Sci., 70(13):1–2p (abstract).*

18. Kaski, J. C., Sykora, J., Rodrigues-Plaza, L., Ratcliffe, D., Hackett, D., and Maseri, A. (1985): Asymptomatic episodes of ST segment depression during ambulatory ECG monitoring disappear after successful coronary by-pass. *Clin. Sci., 68(11):1–84.*

19. Chierchia, S., Lazzari, M., Freedman, B., Brunelli, C., and Maseri, A. (1983): Impairment of myocardial perfusion and function during painless myocardial ischemia. *J. Am. Coll. Cardiol., 1(3):924–930.*

20. Babey, A. M. (1939): Painless acute infarction of the heart. *N. Engl. J. Med. 220:410–412.*

21. Roseman, M. D. (1954): Painless myocardial infarction of the heart, a review of the literature and analysis of 220 cases. *Ann. Intern. Med., 41:1–8.*

22. Procacci, P., Zoppi, M., Padeletti, L., and Maresca, M. (1976): Myocardial infarction without pain. A study of the sensory function of the upper limbs. *Pain, 2:309–313.*

23. Keele, K. D. (1975): A physician looks at pain. In: *Weisenberg Med. Pain: Clinical and Experimental Perspectives,* edited by M. Weisenberg, pp. 45–52. C. V. Mosby, St. Louis.

24. Droste, C., and Roskamm, M. (1983): Experimental pain measurements in patients with asymptomatic myocardial ischemia. *J. Am. Coll. Cardiol., 1:940–945.*

25. Wall, P. D. (1978): The gate control theory of pain mechanisms. A re-examination and re-statement. *Brain, 101:1–18.*

26. Maseri, A. (1985): Mechanisms of ischemic cardiac pain and silent myocardial ischemia. *Am. J. Med., 79(3A):7–11.*

27. Romeo, F., Chierchia, S., and Maseri, A. (1986): Painless myocardial ischemia in chronic stable

angina. Its relation to exercise tolerance and coronary arteriography. *J. Am. Coll. Cardiol.*, 7(2):240 (abstract).

28. Kannel, W. B., and Abbot, R. D. (1984): Incidence and prognosis of unrecognized myocardial infarction. An update of the Framingham study. *N. Engl. J. Med.*, 311:1144–1147.
29. Cohn, P. F. (1986): Silent myocardial ischemia classification, prevalence and prognosis. *Am. J. Med*, 79(3A):2–6.
30. Parmley, W. W. (1985): Silent ischemia. Tip of the iceberg. *Am. J. Med.*, 9(3A)1.

Hammersmith Cardiology Workshop Series, Vol. 3,
edited by A. Maseri, B. E. Sobel, and S. Chierchia.
Raven Press, New York © 1987.

Précis of the Discussion: Section I

MECHANISMS OF ANGINAL PAIN AND SIGNIFICANCE OF PAINLESS MYOCARDIAL ISCHEMIA

Attilio Maseri

Anginal pain may not necessarily result only from myocardial ischemia. Michael Oliver asked whether pain could come from coronary arteries. Alberto Malliani reported that in acute but not chronic dogs, traction in coronary arteries could produce a sudden pseudoaffective reaction. Paul Hugenholtz suggested that angioplasty in patients could be an easy way to test this possibility in humans. William Grossman suggested that anginal pain in mitral valve prolapse could be caused by mechanical stretching of the papillary muscles rather than by ischemia.

Gerry Klassen raised the question of the lack of an "alarm system" in some patients, and Attilio Maseri added that for a large majority of patients, the "alarm system" was operating only sometimes, as they have both painful and painless ischemic episodes of apparent similar severity. Alberto Malliani said that the perception of pain could be modulated by a variety of mechanisms. Michael Oliver reported the observations of his group in six patients with acute infarction, not exposed to morphine, in whom naloxone caused the pain to reappear. Daniel Le Bars cautioned the interpretation of data obtained using naloxone, as this drug at low doses gives analgesia but at high doses may cause hyperalgesia.

The second part of the discussion concerned the prognostic significance of silent myocardial ischemia. Michael Oliver expressed reservations about the observation of a 20% incidence of painless infarction in the Framingham study, as the interviews were often performed months after the episodes and the recollection of symptoms is likely to have faded. He insisted that without carefully designed follow-up studies, it is difficult to know whether the prognosis of silent and painful ischemia is similar. Burton Sobel agreed with Dr. Oliver and expressed great concern at the tendency of drug companies to inculcate in the mind of the physician the idea of treating silent ischemia, with the obvious financial benefits for the companies and burden for the health care budget.

Editorial comment: A. Maseri

That totally painless myocardial ischemia exists is clearly established. The reasons for the absence of pain may be several. The significance of silent ischemia depends on its severity, duration, and associated arrhythmias. On the one hand, the presence of pain alerts the patient to stop his activities and to seek medical attention; on the other hand, it may increase sympathetic tone and heart work, cause anxiety, and favor arrhythmias. Conversely, in the absence of pain the patient has no warning to stop his activities and to seek medical attention. As is the case for painful myocardial ischemia as well as for painless ischemia, prognosis is likely to depend on the cause of ischemia itself and on the setting in which it occurs. Frequent painless ischemic episodes noted on Holter tapes, occurring at rest in a patient with a positive exercise stress test at low work load and with severe coronary disease, are likely to indicate a poor prognosis.

Hammersmith Cardiology Workshop Series, Vol. 3,
edited by A. Maseri, B. E. Sobel, and S. Chierchia.
Raven Press, New York © 1987.

Incidence and Severity of Coronary and Extracoronary Atherosclerosis in Individuals With and Without Evidence of IHD

Henry N. Neufeld and U. Goldbourt

Heart Institute, Chaim Sheba Medical Center, 52621 Tel Hashomer, Israel

The process of atherosclerosis continues to pose a puzzling dilemma (1). This chapter is based on evidence derived from pathological and angiographic studies. Although autopsy studies do not constitute prospective investigations of ischemic heart disease (IHD) incidence, they provide the best available measure on severity of atherosclerosis in different populations. Angiographic studies, on the other hand, lend themselves to prospective evaluation but are importantly limited to individuals with evidence of IHD.

THE RESEARCH

Some 30 years ago, it became clear that atherosclerosis in the coronary arteries begins long before symptoms of IHD develop. The early findings of Enos et al. (2) were supported by findings in victims of the Vietnam War. The incidence and severity of coronary and extracoronary atherosclerosis have been shown to vary in ethnic groups. It also has been shown that particular ethnic groups might be relatively immune to coronary atherosclerosis through the absence of prearteriosclerotic changes, such as thickening of the intima in the coronary arteries. In Israel, we have shown (3) that such prearteriosclerotic changes are more typical to Jewish Ashkenazi males, while males of other ethnic groups residing in Israel, and females of all ethnic groups, are less susceptible. Similar findings were provided by studies of different ethnic groups in other countries, and ethnic differences found in these studies were shown to parallel differences in the incidence or mortality of IHD in the same countries.

Coronary atherosclerosis in men without IHD has been extensively analyzed and reported in the International Atherosclerosis Project (IAP) (4). In those results, the incidence and severity of coronary atherosclerosis was exceedingly pronounced in hypertensive and diabetic persons, indicating that hypertension and diabetes accelerate the progression. Patients dying of cancer and other causes did not indicate significant atherosclerosis.

In a study of 2,700 autopsies performed on children and adults in New Orleans between 1960 and 1968, Strong et al. (5) examined the percentage of coronary arterial intimal surface involved with raised atherosclerotic lesions in persons who died of non-CHD causes. The data highlighted a predilection of white males to coronary atherosclerosis in ages above 25 as compared with white females. White males were also clearly more susceptible than black males. In blacks in the United States, no difference is found between the sexes.

Another report related to the incidence and severity of coronary atherosclerosis is the World Health Organization (WHO) study in five European cities (6). In that study, the extent of coronary atherosclerosis was increased in persons with essential hypertension and diabetes mellitus, but not in persons dying of malignant diseases. Raised coronary lesions in general and calcified lesions in particular were more prevalent in males (1.5 times higher or more) than in females, except for those in Yalta, U.S.S.R. These pathological data parallel prospective epidemiological findings with regard to the incidence of IHD.

With respect to differences in severity and frequency of coronary atherosclerosis between persons with and without IHD, the IAP investigation identified more frequent and more extensive coronary atherosclerotic lesions in subjects dying of IHD than in the group that died of other causes. Moreover, there was large variability in the amount of coronary atherosclerosis among IHD cases from different locations and race groups. Subjects dying of (or having a history of) IHD in populations that generally had a high degree of atherosclerosis had, on average, more coronary lesions than populations with low degrees of atherosclerosis. The findings of the WHO five-town study reasserted the ethnic, age, and sex differences in the extent and severity of coronary atherosclerosis in persons dying of IHD.

ANGIOGRAPHIC STUDIES

Angiographic studies in individuals with symptomatic IHD enable us to correlate findings with the presence of conditions such as hypertension, diabetes, and hypercholesterolemia, and also correlate them to behavioral type, smoking habits, and physical activity. Clearly, this kind of study is not suitable for studying atherosclerosis in individuals without IHD. Thus, it is extremely difficult to obtain estimates of the incidence of atherosclerosis. Angiographic studies have taught us about the association of coronary artery disease with several risk factors. Although prediction of serial angiographic changes is difficult, the recent National Heart, Lung, and Blood Institute Type II Coronary Intervention Study (7) has shown that cholestyramine induced a change in high-density lipoprotein (HDL) cholesterol, as the percent of total cholesterol was the best predictor of angiographically determined changes in coronary artery disease, the association being an inverse one.

There are important differences in the incidence and severity of *extracoronary* atherosclerosis in individuals with and without evidence of IHD. For example, the IAP reported that cerebral atherosclerosis was higher in persons with clinical evidence of IHD as well as cerebrovascular disease, diabetes, and hypertension than in persons without these diseases. However, the severity of cerebral atherosclerosis did not differ between persons with clinical findings of IHD, cerebrovascular disease, and hypertension. This was in contrast to coronary atherosclerosis, which was much more marked in individuals with IHD.

In the WHO five-town study, it was shown that raised lesions occupied a greater area in subjects with a fresh or recent myocardial infarction, or large myocardial scars. This held true not only in the coronary arteries but also in the aorta. Just as seen in the IAP study, little or no difference in aortic atherosclerosis between the sexes was observed in persons with or without IHD. Atherosclerosis of arterial systems other than the coronary one and the aorta was not addressed in the WHO study.

In a summary of the IAP findings with respect to atherosclerosis in different arterial systems, McGill et al. (4) concluded that in individuals, the severity of atherosclerosis in one artery did not predict the severity in another artery.

ETHNIC AND SEX DIFFERENCES

Early-life ethnic differences in prearteriosclerotic coronary arterial changes and subsequent individually varying expressions of genetically determined factors (such as decreased HDL cholesterol during puberty, abrupt rise of blood pressure, and onset of noninsulin dependent diabetes mellitus) may underlie the major individual variability in the severity of coronary atherosclerosis. Similar factors may be responsible for variability and differing male/female ratios of atherosclerosis of other arteries. The IAP authors attributed the individual variability in the severity of atherosclerosis of all systems primarily to varying genetic susceptibility.

Having compared the severity of atherosclerosis in different arterial systems, a major question is being posed: Why the different susceptibility to atherosclerosis in arterial systems of an individual exposed to a given environment and subject to an identical blood flow in terms of its physical and biochemical properties? Arteries of similar sizes show radical differences in their response to the above stimuli, as a recent observation by Sims (8) has indicated.

Sims examined the extent of intimal thickening in the anterior descending branch of the left coronary artery and in the internal mammary artery, which is of similar size. He demonstrated major differences in the extent of intimal lesions between the left anterior descending (LAD) coronary artery and the internal mammary artery in 352 necropsy examinations. With internal mammary and coronary arteries being of similar size and similar physical and chemical stimuli, it would appear that intimal thickening differences are caused by local, anatomic, and possibly genetically determined differences in receptor activity and in the structure of these arteries. Probably relevant is a recent report indicating that graft patency in patients after bypass surgery was more favorable when the internal mammary artery was used as a graft than when venous grafts were used (9). We are currently conducting electromicroscopic studies of arterial walls in an effort to expand knowledge regarding the local, anatomic factors (8) that may render some arteries more susceptible to atherosclerosis than others.

What is the source of the sex differences in coronary atherosclerosis in persons both with and without IHD evidence? Why is the male/female ratio typically decreased in populations or ethnic groups in whom IHD is less frequent? What are the properties of the arterial wall in different systems that determine which arteries will succumb to atherosclerosis? Further, in the presence of atherosclerosis, what is the mechanism responsible for production of pain in some individuals and its absence in others, and which individuals will develop MI or die suddenly, beyond the limited predictive knowledge provided by the risk factors?

CONCLUSION

These are some of the questions that we must answer in order to remove some of the mystery surrounding coronary atherosclerosis and hopefully increase our understanding, leading perhaps to improved strategies of intervention against atherosclerosis and its clinical sequelae. Research into all aspects of arterial wall physiology, particularly the role of lipoprotein receptors, their abnormalities, and their response to varying stimuli by the blood flow, appears as the most promising avenue in an effort to resolve the questions arising from the available evidence on atherosclerosis in different arterial systems and its correlation with clinically manifested disease.

REFERENCES

1. McGill, H. C., Jr. (1984): Persistent problems in the pathogenesis of atherosclerosis. *Arteriosclerosis,* 4:443–451.
2. Enos, W. F., Jr., Beyer, J. C., and Holmes, R. H. (1955): Pathogenesis of coronary disease in American soldiers killed in Korea. *J.A.M.A.,* 158:912–914.
3. Vlodaver, Z., Kahn, H. A., and Neufeld, H. N. (1969): The coronary arteries in early life in three different ethnic groups. *Circulation,* 39:541–549.
4. McGill, H. C., Jr., Arian-Stella, J., Caronell, L. M., et al. (1968): General findings of the International Atherosclerosis Project. *Lab. Invest.,* 18:498–502.
5. Strong, J. P., Restrepo, C., and Geizman, M. (1978): Coronary and aortic atherosclerosis in New Orleans. II. Comparison of lesions by age, sex and race. *Lab. Invest.,* 39:364–369.
6. Kagen, A. R., Sternby, N. H., Uemora, K., et al. (1976): Atherosclerosis of the aorta and coronary arteries in 5 towns. *Bull WHO,* 53:485–645.
7. Levy, R. I., Brensike, J. F., Epstein, S. E., et al. (1984): The influence of changes in lipid values induced by cholestyramine and diet on progression of coronary artery disease: results of the NHLBI Type II Coronary Intervention Study. *Circulation,* 69:325–337.
8. Sims, F. H. (1983): A comparison of coronary and internal mammary arteries and implications of the results in the etiology of atherosclerosis. *Am. Heart J.,* 105:560–566.
9. Tyras, D. H., Barner, H. B., Kaiser, G. C., et al. (1980): By-pass grafts to the left interior descending coronary artery. *J. Thorac. Cardiovasc. Surg.,* 80:327–333.

Hammersmith Cardiology Workshop Series, Vol. 3,
edited by A. Maseri, B. E. Sobel, and S. Chierchia.
Raven Press, New York © 1987.

Relative Importance of Lipids and Thrombus in the Genesis of Coronary Atherosclerosis

William C. Roberts

Pathology Branch, National Heart, Lung, and Blood Institute, National Institutes of Health, Bethesda, Maryland 20205

ROLE OF LIPIDS IN THE DEVELOPMENT OF ATHEROSCLEROTIC PLAQUES

Several factors indicate that cholesterol plays a major, and, in my view, *the* major role in the development of atherosclerotic plaques large enough to lead to organ ischemia. Certain animals fed a high-cholesterol diet develop atherosclerotic plaques and the plaques contain cholesterol deposits. Arterial atherosclerosis severe enough to cause organ ischemia occurs only in human populations whose average blood total cholesterol level is greater than 150 mg/dL, and symptomatic atherosclerosis, for practical purposes, is nonexistent when the average total serum cholesterol level is less than 150 mg/dL. The higher the total scrum cholesterol value (which roughly parallels the low-density lipoprotein cholesterol level), the greater the chance of developing symptomatic coronary atherosclerosis.

Among human beings with total plasma cholesterol levels greater than 265 mg/dL, the lowering of the total plasma cholesterol level decreases the frequency of development of coronary events (coronary death, acute myocardial infarction, and angina pectoris) (1,2). Thus, human animals respond to high blood cholesterol levels the same way as do nonhuman animals. Humans whose blood total cholesterol level is greater than 150 mg/dL develop atherosclerosis, while humans whose blood total cholesterol level is less than 150 mg/dL do not develop atherosclerotic plaques large enough to cause organ ischemia. Nonhuman animals raise their blood cholesterol levels by eating food and/or drinking liquids containing high levels of cholesterol and saturated fats, and human animals raise their blood cholesterol levels the same way.

Another item considered important by some in causing atherosclerosis is *genetics.* There is no question that genetics is of prime importance in patients with homozygous type II hypercholesterolemia (familial hypercholesterolemia), but this condition is found in only about one of every 1 million persons (3). The total serum cholesterol level is usually over 600 mg/dL, and without effective blood cholesterol lowering, death occurs before age 20. The amount of atherosclerosis in them is so extensive and it occurs so rapidly that it might be referred to as malignant atherosclerosis. In persons with total serum cholesterol levels under 300 mg/dL (only 5% of the U.S. population has total plasma cholesterol levels >265 mg/dL), in my view, proof of a genetic factor is lacking.

Many investigators have implicated other factors as having an importance similar to that of hypercholesterolemia in causing atherosclerosis. *Systemic hypertension,* for example, has been given the same level of importance in the development of symptomatic atherosclerosis in the Framingham studies as has hypercholesterolemia (4). The problem here involves what is considered a level of total cholesterol that can be associated with increased risk of development of symptomatic atherosclerosis. This level in the Framingham studies is a total serum cholesterol level greater than 250 mg/dL. The mean level of total serum cholesterol in patients with acute myocardial infarction in the Framingham population is about 240 mg/dL. The average plasma total cholesterol in U.S. subjects over 40 years of age is now about 215 mg/dL. To be virtually assured of not developing symptomatic coronary atherosclerosis, the blood total cholesterol level must remain below 150 mg/dL. In populations where the average total cholesterol level in adults is above 150 mg/dL, systemic hypertension clearly accelerates the development of atherosclerosis, and the higher the total cholesterol level the worse the effect of systemic hypertension (assuming equal levels of pressure elevation). In populations where the average total cholesterol blood level is less than 150 mg/dL, there is no evidence that systemic hypertension either causes atherosclerosis or accelerates it.

In the early 1970s, I visited Kampala, Uganda, and examined many circles of Willis and many epicardial coronary arteries at autopsy. Many of the hearts were enlarged and the only explanation for the enlargement was systemic hypertension. (It was known that systemic hypertension was extremely common in the population of Kampala and yet atherosclerosis was extremely uncommon.) The amount of atherosclerosis observed was minimal and consisted only of yellow streaks and dots. The average total serum cholesterol in the population was well below 150 mg/dL, and many patients had levels between 90 and 120 mg/dL. It is most reasonable to believe that systemic hypertension accelerates atherosclerosis only when the total serum cholesterol level is greater than 150 mg/dL. Systemic hypertension has its major effect on the arterial media, not the intima, which atherosclerosis affects. The major direct consequences of systemic hypertension are the rupture of a berry aneurysm (cerebral) and dissection (aorta) (5).

The same type argument can be made for *cigarette smoking.* Cigarette smoking is rampant in many parts of the world in which atherosclerosis of any significance is nearly nonexistent. Thus, cigarette smoking may accelerate atherosclerosis if the serum total cholesterol is above 150 mg/dL, but if the serum total cholesterol is below 150 mg/dL, there is no atherosclerosis to accelerate.

ROLE OF THROMBUS IN THE DEVELOPMENT OF
ATHEROSCLEROTIC PLAQUES

Although the above discussion suggests that only cholesterol is important in the genesis of atherosclerotic plaques, I would now like to propose, as have others, that thrombosis also plays an important role in the development of the plaque (6,7). Rokitansky, in 1852, was the first, to my knowledge, to propose that atherosclerotic plaques resulted from the organization of thrombi. Virchow disputed this view, and later Virchow apparently convinced Rokitansky that his thrombogenic thesis was untenable. Several observations suggest, however, that atherosclerotic plaques result, at least in part, from the organization of thrombi.

First, there is the presence of known components of thrombi, namely, fibrin and platelets, within atherosclerotic plaques. Second, there is the occurrence of known components of atherosclerotic plaques, namely, foam cells, cholesterol clefts, pultaceous debris, and calcium, in organized hematomas or known thrombi wherever they occur in the body. An example is the left atrial thrombus in the patient with mitral stenosis; organization of this thrombus may produce typical complicated atherosclerotic plaques. Third, we find the presence of multiluminal channels in vessels, a recognized consequence of the organization of pulmonary arterial thromboemboli. Multiple luminal channels commonly are found in severely atherosclerotic coronary arteries, suggesting that thrombi or emboli were at one time present and that they organized. The tissue between the channels is similar to that found in arteries with only one channel. Because the artery with multiple channels has been recognized as the hallmark of an organized thrombus and because the tissue in multi- and unichanneled arteries is similar, Duguid (8) reasoned that the causative process also was similar. Fourth, the major component of the complicated atherosclerotic plaque, i.e., the one capable of causing fatal coronary artery disease, is fibrous tissue or collagen, not lipid. This is true whether or not severe hyperlipidemia is present. Foam cells actually are infrequent in coronary arteries of patients with fatal coronary artery disease. Often the "density" of the fibrous tissue plugging a coronary artery varies in different portions of a plaque, and these subunits may be demarcated by distinct elastic lamellae. These subunits suggest that thrombus is deposited at different times and that the density of the resulting fibrous tissue may be determined by the composition of the initial thrombus, i.e., whether platelets or fibrin predominated. Fifth, experimentally induced thrombi under proper conditions may be transformed into atherosclerotic plaques closely resembling those observed in human coronary arteries. Finally, we find high levels of precursors for fibrin and platelet deposition in the plasma of patients with acute myocardial infarction and in some patients with angina pectoris.

These six factors obviously do not prove that thrombosis is the cause of atherosclerosis, but together they strongly suggest that the organization of thrombi plays a major role in the development of the complicated atherosclerotic plaque. Indeed, most serious students of the morphology of the arterial plaque currently support, in whole or in part, the thrombogenic origin of atherosclerosis.

Because the clotting factors in the blood appear to be similar in all population groups and because symptomatic atherosclerosis develops only in those population groups with serum total cholesterol levels greater than 150 mg/dL, the latter also plays a major role in the development of the plaque. Lipids may exert their effect, however, more by their ability to alter the clotting mechanism than by their ability to infiltrate the arterial wall.

FACTORS IMPLICATING LIPIDS IN THE DEVELOPMENT OF THROMBUS

At least five factors suggest that lipids play a major role in promoting thrombus formation. First, individuals on high-fat diets have increased susceptibility to both arterial and venous thrombosis. Second, in certain experimental animals, long-chain saturated fatty acids enhance blood coagulation. Third, rats maintained on a diet rich in butter are more susceptible to endotoxin-induced thrombosis than control rats on a diet rich in corn oil. The thrombosis was associated with an increased sensitivity of the platelets to thrombin. Fourth, in pigs maintained for a year on a high-fat diet rich in egg yolk, more mural thrombus formed in extracorporal shunts than in shunts connected to animals maintained on a low-fat diet. Fifth, humans given diets rich in egg yolk and butter fat have shorter platelet survivals and greater platelet turnovers than subjects maintained on a low-fat diet or a diet rich in corn oil.

REFERENCES

1. Lipid Research Clinics Program (1984): The lipid research clinics coronary primary prevention trial results. I. Reduction in incidence of coronary heart disease. *J.A.M.A.*, 251:351–364.
2. Lipid Research Clinics Program (1984): The lipid research clinics coronary primary prevention trial results. II. The relationship of reduction in incidence of coronary heart disease to cholesterol lowering. *J.A.M.A.*, 251:365–374.
3. Sprecher, D. L., Schaefer, E. J., Kent, K. M., Gregg, R. E., Zech, L. A., Hoeg, J. M., McManus, B., Roberts, W. C., and Brewer, H. B., Jr. (1984): Cardiovascular features of homozygous familial hypercholesterolemia: analysis of 16 patients. *Am. J. Cardiol.*, 54:20–30.
4. Kannel, W. B. (1976): Some lessons in cardiovascular epidemiology from Framingham. *Am. J. Cardiol.*, 37:269–282.
5. Roberts, W. C. (1975): The hypertensive diseases. Evidence that systemic hypertension is a greater risk factor to the development of other cardiovascular diseases than previously suspected. *Am. J. Med.*, 59:523–532.
6. Roberts, W. C. (1973): Does thrombosis play a major role in the development of symptom-producing atherosclerotic plaques? *Circulation*, 48:1161–1166.
7. Roberts, W. C. (1974): Coronary thrombosis and fatal myocardial ischemia. *Circulation*, 49:1–3.
8. Duguid, J. B. (1946): Thrombosis as a factor in the pathogenesis of coronary atherosclerosis. *J. Path. Bact.*, 58:207–211.

Hammersmith Cardiology Workshop Series, Vol. 3,
edited by A. Maseri, B. E. Sobel, and S. Chierchia.
Raven Press, New York © 1987.

Précis of the Discussion: Section II

ATHEROSCLEROSIS IN CORONARY AND OTHER SYSTEMIC ARTERIES

Attilio Maseri

It was argued that the risk factor concept in coronary artery disease is too simplistic and that other factors, such as genetics and coagulation, probably play a very important role. It is also naive to compare risk factors in different populations to accumulate evidence in favor of a major role of traditional risk factors; for example, the Masai in Africa have coronary atherosclerosis but they do not have myocardial infarction.

Michael Oliver also cautioned against too much interpretation of male/female ratios, particularly when an age span up to 74 years is considered: Different compounding factors cause mortality in advancing age in different communities. It would be wiser to adhere to those under the age of 55, where the male/female ratio in the United Kingdom, for example, is something on the order of 5½:1. Henry Neufeld agreed that above 65, the ratio becomes smaller. However, in Finnish men and women, blood pressure and cholesterol levels are much higher than in Israeli women, and smoking is the same. The male/female ratio in Finland is 4:1 up to age 65. In Israel, male to female mortality was 2:1 despite the fact that cholesterol levels and blood pressure were much lower in the Israeli female compared with the Finnish female. The modern Israeli smokes and is overweight, but still the male/female ratio is the same and there is still a low mortality rate. Even though their blood pressure is higher than their fathers' and the cholesterol level is a little higher, there is still low mortality.

Attilio Maseri asked about the possibility of having a risk profile of factors that control coagulation. Many plaques have fibrin, and when the plaques are ulcerated you get thrombosis; when you get thrombosis you may get occlusion. William Roberts said it is very difficult to be sure of ulcerations, particularly in coronary arteries; it is much easier in aortas, where they may be more important.

Michael Oliver said that for 25 years the epidemiological world has been dominated by the lipid hypothesis, to a large extent because there has not been very much else to measure: "If we had the same precision as we think we have for HDL and its subfractions and apoproteins for measuring thrombogenic risk, and if we had been able to establish prospective surveys 25 years ago with precision measurements of thrombogenic risk, I suspect we might have a better explanation as to why the standard risk factors explain less than half of the disease. Let us be quite clear that they explain less than half of the disease, even in young people. But I suspect that the area which we know nothing about is the thrombogenic tendency, and let us hope that in the next 25 years we will be able to get up these prospective studies.''

William Roberts commented that the average cholesterol level in America now in patients over 40 years is 215 mg/dL and that half the people in America are dying from coronary disease. Can that be considered a normal cholesterol level? Only 5% of Americans over 40 years old have a cholesterol level under 150 mg/ dL; that is common among high school students. Michael Oliver stressed that the relationship between cholesterol and coronary heart disease is a curvilinear one because the relationship between them in the lowest three quintiles is rather weak; this has been shown very recently by the huge MRFIT trial, confirming what many thought previously and confirming the results of the Israeli Civil Service study. In his estimation, the threshold value may be around 210 mg/dL.

Editorial comment: A. Maseri

The search for a unique common denominator that is responsible for the varied postmortem picture of coronary atherosclerosis may be too simplistic. This search has led to focusing on the elements that make patients look alike so they can be grouped into large syndromes, rather than on the elements that make them different and that would allow their separation into smaller, but more homogeneous, subsets with a similar etiology.

It is time to begin to reverse this trend if we wish to precisely identify specific causes and their relative role in the commonly accepted traditional clinical and pathological syndrome.

Hammersmith Cardiology Workshop Series, Vol. 3,
edited by A. Maseri, B. E. Sobel, and S. Chierchia.
Raven Press, New York © 1987.

The Endothelial Relaxant Factor

*Andrew Henderson, **Tudor M. Griffith, *David H. Edwards,
*Peter Collins, and ***Malcolm J. Lewis

*Departments of *Cardiology, **Radiology, and ***Pharmacology, University of Wales
College of Medicine, Cardiff CF4 4XN, Wales*

The phenomenon of endothelium-mediated vasodilatation was not recognized until 1980 (1,2). For those of us who are working on it, this is hard to believe, for it is so obvious once you have learned to look for it! Whether it contributes to the subject of dynamic control of the coronary lumen remains to be proved (absolute proof must await the identification of the agent responsible and the development of reliable ways to measure its contribution *in vivo*), but it is difficult to imagine that it does not. In the meantime, we already know quite a lot about the phenomenon, as well as the type of agent responsible and its mode of action: We can offer informed speculation about its possible physiological and pathological roles. The phenomenon of endothelium-mediated vasodilatation seems likely to have a major impact on our understanding of cardiovascular physiology.

It has long been recognized that *in vivo* and *in vitro* studies of vasomotor responses often gave apparently conflicting results: The anomalies had been attributed generally to the difficulty of measuring these responses in isolation from other complicating influences in the intact circulation. In particular, it was known that acetylcholine has a constrictor effect in isolated preparations, whereas *in vivo* its action is generally to vasodilate. The explanation appeared when Furchgott and Zawadski (1) reported that acetylcholine causes preconstricted rabbit aortic preparations to constrict further when they are denuded of endothelium but to relax in the presence of intact endothelium. In other words, acetylcholine causes endothelium-mediated relaxation as well as direct constriction of vascular smooth muscle.

About this time, we were developing an isolated perfused epicardial coronary artery system of the rabbit and serendipidously observed that endothelial preservation virtually abolished the constrictor responses, e.g., to 5-hydroxytryptamine, phenylephrine, histamine, and acetylcholine (3). With a bioassay system, consisting of a preconstricted denuded rabbit coronary artery (perfused at constant flow with oxygenated aqueous buffer at 37°C) as a sensor for dilator substances released from an aorta perfused in series, we demonstrated that the phenomenon was indeed due to a dilator substance (4). This is known as the endothelium-derived relaxant factor (EDRF). Its half-life is estimated at 6 sec under these conditions (4), a figure subsequently confirmed by other workers using endothelial sources from different species and, in one case, cell culture. A large number of pharmacological probes have been explored for their ability to stimulate or inhibit the phenomenon (4). It has been possible, by infusing them at different sites in bioassay systems, to determine those that act on the production of EDRF, those that interact directly with EDRF in transit, and those that influence the action of EDRF on vascular smooth muscle.

EDRF PRODUCTION

The activity and production of EDRF are continuous in the basal unstimulated state. Its production can be stimulated by acetylcholine and also by a number of other agents. These agents include the calcium ionophore, A23817, and (with some apparent variation between species and artery type) adenosine monophosphate (ATP), adenosine diphosphate (ADP), and thrombin; 5-HT, histamine, and norepinephrine (in the dog but not in the rabbit); vasopressin (in cerebral but not in other arteries); and a limited range of peptides such as VIP, substance P, and bradykinin (2). Further experiments have shown the obligatory dependence of EDRF production on both extracellular calcium and mitochondrial ATP production (5).

Endothelium-Dependent Flow-Related Dilatation

Notably, too, endothelium-dependent dilatation has been described in relation to flow rate (though not yet proved to be due to EDRF) (6). This must prompt a reevaluation of all pharmacological studies on vasomotor tone that have failed to take it into account. Indeed, it prompts a fairly fundamental reevaluation of our understanding of the physiological control of flow through the vascular tree.

Different Blood Vessels

There appear to be major differences in EDRF activity between different arteries (3). Whereas cumulative dose responses in the rabbit coronary preparation to the four constrictor agents noted were virtually abolished by the presence of endothelium, the presence of endothelium had relatively little effect in rabbit aortic preparations: Indeed, it slightly and paradoxically increased the response in this preparation unless allowance was made for the different base line that results from basal EDRF activity. Formal studies comparing one artery with another in crossover bioassay systems are awaited to confirm these apparent differences and to show whether they are due to differences in basal EDRF activity, stimulation of EDRF, EDRF half–life, or smooth muscle response. Veins exhibit the phenomenon. The preliminary evidence suggests that it is present also in small resistance arteries and arterioles.

Nature of EDRF

As to the nature of EDRF itself, it appears to be a novel type of biological compound, almost certainly a very potent vasodilator, and unstable. The evidence shows that it is not a prostanoid, free radical, lipid, protein, or peptide (4). It is inhibited by a number of agents, the two chemical properties common to which are that they are antioxidant and combine with carbonyl groups, suggesting that EDRF possesses a carbonyl group at or near its active site. There appear to be many similarities between EDRF and the (also unidentified) neurotransmitter in anococcygeus and bovine retractor penis muscles.

Mode of Action

There is now good evidence that EDRF causes relaxation of vascular smooth muscle by elevating cyclic guanosine monophosphate (GMP) levels, as do nitrovasodilators (7,8). Mechanisms of smooth muscle contraction and relaxation are inadequately understood. Dephosphorylation of myosin light chains has been shown to correlate with elevated cyclic GMP levels, and this may contribute to the mechanism of the relaxation. More recently, we have provided evidence that inhibition of norepinephrine-induced constriction, whether mediated by EDRF, nitrovasodilators, or by a cyclic GMP analogue, is associated with reduced influx and efflux of ^{45}Ca (9). This points to a probable primary influence of cyclic GMP on calcium movements within the smooth muscle cell, analogous in some ways to the multiple actions of cyclic AMP in cardiac muscle.

Inactivation

Hemoglobin blocks EDRF activity (10), probably by binding it. Plasma is also a potent and rapid inhibitor of EDRF activity. We have identified the active component as the haptoglobin/hemoglobin complex, the activity of which in normal plasma is sufficient to inhibit EDRF released into the vascular lumen and thus to prevent downstream vascular effects of EDRF (11). We may suppose, therefore, that EDRF is an autacoid, acting locally on its subjacent smooth muscle in the presence of an intact endothelium barrier.

Physiological Role?

What are the physiological implications of EDRF? It is a potent, ubiquitous vasodilator, likely to act as a very local autacoid on subjacent smooth muscle.

Its activity *in vivo* may well be tonic as it is *in vitro*. Three general types of stimulants of endothelium-dependent vasodilatation have been identified: those which will be released locally at the site of platelet aggregation or thrombosis, from which we may speculate that EDRF may tend to vasodilate at sites of potential thrombosis as a kind of negative feedback; those which could mediate neurogenic vasodilatation, perhaps particularly in small vessels where the diffusion distance between adventitial nerves and endothelium is small; and the flow-dependent phenomenon, which may be responsible for coordinating (optimizing?) changes in vessel diameter throughout the vascular tree in response to changes in flow.

Pathological Role?

It is even more speculative to consider possible pathological roles involving EDRF at the present state of knowledge. Does local lack of EDRF activity cause coronary vasospasm? Certainly, local endothelial damage in the perfused rabbit artery preparation provides a model of reproducible nonspecific and reversible localized coronary spasm (3). This has also been demonstrated by local mechanical damage to the coronary artery in the intact dog (12). In addition, ergometrine stimulates EDRF (13) so that local lack of EDRF activity could explain the efficacy of this agent in the provocation of coronary spasm in susceptible patients. It is thus a feasible proposition that the actual occurrence of clinical coronary vasospasm may require the right combination of locally impaired EDRF activity and normally reactive smooth muscle contraction in an artery unsplinted by atheromatous deposit.

Does inactivation of EDRF cause cerebral artery spasm with subarachnoid hemorrhage? The hemoglobin data suggest this as a strong possibility. The inactivating hemoglobin or haptoglobin/hemoglobin complex may be supposed not to penetrate a normal intact endothelial barrier. Is EDRF activity altered in hypertension? Experimental studies suggest that EDRF activity is indeed impaired, and preliminary evidence suggests that EDRF is indeed active in the smaller resistance vessels, though direct experimental investigations are beset with technical problems. Is EDRF activity altered at sites of atheroma? Experimental models of lipid feeding have given consistent evidence from a number of centers of reduced EDRF activity, probably due to the barrier effect of the lipid rather a reduction of EDRF production (14,15). This has been confirmed in human coronary arteries from unwanted donor hearts and shown to occur locally at the sites of atheroma (16). Does EDRF contribute in any way to the pathogenesis of atheroma? Here one can but note that arterial tone will probably influence mass transport of particles across the arterial wall so that EDRF-mediated dilatation could influence lipid deposition. Also note that flow-dependent endothelium-mediated dilatation will contribute to the control of artery caliber and thus affect mechanical factors influencing the propensity to atheroma. These are questions for the future. Although EDRF is not yet identified, what we do know about it is exciting a great deal of interest.

REFERENCES

1. Furchgott, R. F., and Zawadski, J. V. (1980): The obligatory role of endothelial cells in the relaxation of arterial smooth muscle by acetylcholine. *Nature,* 288:373–376.
2. Furchgott, R. F. (1983): Role of endothelium in responses of vascular smooth muscle. *Circ. Res.,* 53:557–563.
3. Griffith, T. M., Henderson, A. H., Hughes, Edward D., and Lewis, M. J. (1984): Isolated perfused rabbit coronary artery and aortic strip preparations: the role of endothelium-derived relaxant factor. *J. Physiol.,* 51:13–24.
4. Griffith, T. M., Edwards, D. H., Lewis, M. J., Newby, A. C., and Henderson, A. H. (1984): The nature of endothelium-derived vascular relaxant factor. *Nature,* 308:645–647.
5. Griffith, T. M., Edwards, D. H., Newby, A. C., Lewis, M. J., and Henderson, A. H. (1986): Production of endothelium-derived relaxant factor is dependent on oxidative phosphorylation and extracellular calcium. *Cardiovasc. Res.,* 20:7–12.
6. Holtz, J., Busse, R., Giesler, M. (1983): Flow-dependent dilation of canine epicardial coronary arteries *in vivo* and *in vitro:* Mediated by the endothelium. *Naunyn Schmiedebergs Arch. Pharmacol.,* 322:R44.
7. Holzmann, S. (1982): Endothelium-induced relaxation by acetylcholine associated with larger rises in cyclic GMP in coronary arterial strips. *J. Cyclic N. Res.,* 8(6):409–419.
8. Rapaport, R. M., Draznin, M. B., and Murad, F. (1983): Endothelium-dependent relaxation in rat aorta may be mediated through cyclic GMP-dependent protein phosphorylation. *Nature,* 306:174–176.
9. Collins, P., Griffith, T. M., Henderson, A. H., and Lewis, M. J. (1985): Endothelium and calcium flux in rabbit aortic preparations. *J. Physiol.,* 360:63P.
10. Martin, W., Villani, G. M., Jothianandan, D., and Furchgott, R. F. (1985): Selective blockade of endothelium-dependent and glyceryl trinitrate-induced relaxation by hemoglobin and by methylene blue in the rabbit aorta. *J. Pharmacol. Exp. Ther.,* 233(3):708–716.
11. Edwards, D. H., Griffith, T. M., Henderson, A. H., Lewis, M. J., and Ryley, H. C. (1985): Endothelium-dependent relaxation is inhibited by a high molecular weight protein fraction of whole human plasma. *Br. J. Pharmacol.,* 85:341P.
12. Brum, J. M., Sufan, Q., Lane, G., and Bove, A. A. (1984): Increased vasoconstrictor activity of proximal coronary arteries with endothelial damage in intact dogs. *Circulation,* 70:1066–1073.
13. Griffith, T. M., Hughes E. D., Lewis M. J., and Henderson, A. H. (1984): Ergometrine induced arterial dilatation: an endothelium-mediated effect. *J. Mol. Cell. Cardiol.,* 16:479–483.
14. Chappell, S. P., Griffith, T. M., Henderson, A. H., and Lewis, M. J. (1985): Influence of cholesterol feeding on endothelium-dependent vasomotor response in rabbit aortic strips. *Br. J. Pharmacol.,* 85:266P.
15. Coene, M-C, Herman, A. G., Jordaens, F., Van Hove, C., Verbeuren, T. J., and Zonnekeyn, L. (1985): Endothelium-dependent relaxations in isolated arteries of control and hypercholesterolemic rabbits. *Br. J. Pharmacol.,* 85:267P.
16. Ginsburg, R., and Zera, P. H. (1984): *Circulation (Suppl II),* 70:122.

Hammersmith Cardiology Workshop Series, Vol. 3,
edited by A. Maseri, B. E. Sobel, and S. Chierchia.
Raven Press, New York © 1987.

Vasomotion in Epicardial Coronary Arteries

G. A. Klassen and A. Y. K. Wong

*Departments of Medicine and Physiology and Biophysics, Dalhousie University and Victoria
General Hospital, Halifax, Nova Scotia B3H 2Y9*

The critical function of coronary arteries was recorded in 1698 when Chirac (1) occluded one and observed the immediate death of the animal. Physiological regulation of their function is dependent upon their vasomotion. For our purposes, coronary arterial constriction will be defined as a reduction in the internal diameter of the vessel from the resting state and dilation as an increase. This alteration in diameter is achieved by the mechanics of vascular smooth muscle in the wall of the artery. The presence of occlusive vascular disease in the endothelium will have an added effect upon the hemodynamic consequences of such vasomotion.

NORMAL VASOMOTION

Coronary epicardial arteries are muscular vessels (2). Under resting conditions there is a small pressure gradient along the vessel (3) and these vessels are only moderately compliant (4). Cox (5) has observed that the cellular content of the artery is low (20.5 + 1.8% of wet weight), the percent change (20.6 ± 2.9%) in midwall diameter in response to K^+ is small, and the force that can be developed by these vessels (387 ± 57 10^3 dyn/cm^2) is much less than other arteries. Thus, normal vasomotion of these vessels is not impressive. Under normal physiological conditions they behave as stiff-walled, slowly responsive plastic tubes. How can this description be reconciled with the intense coronary spasm that occurs in these vessels, as described by Maseri et al. (6)? The answer may lie in an understanding of their normal function and control.

THE VASCULAR SMOOTH MUSCLE CELL

These cells are located in the media between two elastic laminae, surrounded by a matrix of elastic tissue and collagen. The matrix of elastin and collagen supplies a restricting framework of fibers whose stiffness increases rapidly as dilation occurs and which, under resting conditions, when arterial distending pressure falls, promotes vessel collapse (5). Smooth muscle bundles are arranged in an inner layer of longitudinally oriented fibers surrounded by a circumferentially oriented layer (7). The presence of a longitudinal layer is atypical (8). Gross et al. (2) reported that at birth, this layer of muscle is not present and that its development coincides with thickening of the endothelium and increase in elastic tissue, particularly in those coronary vessels prone to atheroma. The longitudinal muscle layers' potential role in the genesis of coronary spasm has not been considered. Somlyo (9) has provided the structural basis for the action of smooth muscle cells, but we lack a clear understanding of the control systems for their tension development. The concentration of internal ionized calcium appears to be the trigger that initiates and controls tension development in vascular smooth muscle (10). Dilating agents that promote smooth muscle relaxation may be characterized as those substances which interfere with calcium uptake by the cell, promote its binding intracellularly, or accelerate its removal from the cell, while constricting agents do the opposite. Examples of vasodilators are hypoxia, high P_{CO_2}, adenosine, nitroglycerin, acetylcholine, PGI_2, atriopeptides, slow channel calcium blockers, and β-receptor agonists such as isoproterenol. Vasoconstrictors are hyperoxia, low P_{CO_2}, sympathetic neural stimulation (11), alpha-receptor agonists, vasopressin, ergot derivatives, histamine, serotonin, most eicosanoids, thromboxane A_2, platelet damage factors, magnesium deficiency, and smooth muscle cell membrane damage. Whether these may also be responsible for coronary spasm has been much debated (12).

NEURAL CONTROL

Those factors which alter coronary artery vasomotion through neural activity have been reviewed by Feigl (13). Sympathetic and parasympathetic fibers travel in the adventitia of the epicardial coronary arteries, with endings restricted to the outer layers of smooth muscle (14). How the signal for a response is transmitted from such fibers to the full thickness of the wall is a matter of conjecture. Under resting conditions, there is alpha-mediated constrictor tone present, which may account for the resting pressure gradient along the epicardial arteries.

MYOGENIC REFLEX

Bayliss (15) observed that arteries respond to a sudden increase in pressure by vasoconstriction. This response has been noted to occur in arteries, veins, and lymphatics (16) and, in addition, may be induced by a negative pressure applied to the outer wall. The importance of this reflex in physiological regulation is well established. The effect of a sudden increase in systemic pressure, inducing coronary arterial spasm, has not been observed (6).

EXTRAVASCULAR COMPRESSION

The role of extravascular forces in the control of the coronary circulation remains controversial. Spaan (17) maintains that coronary arterial resistance is sustained by a compliant intramyocardial blood pool and that the arterial zero flow pressure is determined by the physical characteristics of this compartment. In contrast, Klocke et al. (18) maintain that vessel closure occurs as a result of extravascular force, perhaps exerted at the level of the veins, and that this pressure is the determinant of downstream resistance. Extravascular resistance is important in determining the systolic distending pressure within the epicardial artery in the absence of significant proximal obstruction. When significant proximal obstruction exists, collateral resistance becomes an important determinant of distending pressure.

AUTOREGULATION

Autoregulation is the process by which coronary vascular resistance is matched to myocardial metabolic need, independent of perfusion pressure (19). The mechanism by which this is achieved, and the specific role of the epicardial arteries in the maintenance of perfusion pressure with varying metabolic demand, remains unknown.

VASOMOTION IN THE PRESENCE OF OBSTRUCTIVE DISEASE

MacAlpin (20) noted that coronary spasm tended to occur at the sites of obstructive disease in epicardial arteries. Brown et al. (21) noted that normal vasomotion in the presence of obstructive coronary disease could seriously limit flow. This is particularly true for eccentric lesions. Even a 20% reduction in diameter could result in effective occlusion in the presence of a 60% to 70% noncritical stenosis. Wong et al. (22) have described that eccentric lesions contribute more to obstruction than do concentric lesions and that the length of the lesion contributes to a reduction in flow. Thus, it is possible that in some instances, angina results from normal vasomotion in the presence of coronary obstruction.

CORONARY SPASM

Most arteries spasm when they are cut transversely. This is a physiological response when it occurs in a uterine arteriole during menstruation or in the umbilical artery at birth (23). The characteristics of this event are that there is damage to vascular smooth muscle, i.e., calcium enters the cell and is not removed, longitudinal smooth muscle contracts and thereby aids in reducing the lumen, and the luminal distending pressure falls, producing hypotension. Can this help us understand abnormal vasomotion as characterized by vasospastic angina (6)?

Damage to the Vessel

It has been noted that patients with coronary artery disease are prone to vasospastic angina (24). They also show evidence of adventitial neovascularization (25) and inflammation (26). Damage to the endothelium (27) or atherosclerosis (28,29) enhance the responsiveness of coronary vessels to vasoconstrictors. It is thus apparent that damage to vascular smooth muscle may be a precondition to the initiation of vasospastic angina.

Abnormality in Calcium Metabolism of Smooth Muscle

The role of calcium as a cofactor is given credibility by the success of slow channel calcium-blocking drugs in the effective treatment of the disease (30).

Hypotension

The role of hypotension in the initiation of spasm has not received much attention. Maseri et al. (6) observed that attacks of vasospastic angina occurred at night, when blood pressure is low. A decrease in systemic blood pressure or a lower blood pressure distal to a critical stenosis may have similar effects. Under conditions of low arterial distending pressure, vascular smooth muscle may contract isotonically; hence, for the same wall, tension shortening will be greater. This may explain Santamore and Bove's (31) observations concerning the dynamic nature of a stenosis when distal pressure is reduced.

In conclusion, atherosclerosis, the local damage it induces, and the hypotension resulting from proximal epicardial arterial obstruction may enhance the physiological constrictor control of vessel tone, permitting coronary arterial spasm.

ACKNOWLEDGMENT

This work was supported by a Program Grant from the Medical Research Council of Canada.

REFERENCES

1. Chirac, P. (1698): De motu cordis adversaria analytica, Monspelii.
2. Gross, L., Epstein, E. Z., and Kugel, M. A. (1934): Histology of the coronary arteries and their branches in the human heart. *Am. J. Pathol.*, 10:253–274.
3. Fam, W. M., and McGregor, M. (1969): Pressure-flow relationships in the coronary circulation. *Circ. Res.*, 25:293–301.
4. Klassen, G. A., and Wong, A. Y. K. (1982): Coronary artery compliance in the dog. *Can. J. Physiol. Pharmacol.*, 60:942–951.
5. Cox, R. H. (1984): Mechanics of blood vessels: Conduit arteries. In: *Smooth Muscle Contraction*, edited by N. L. Stephens, pp. 405–425. Marcel Dekker, New York.
6. Maseri, A., Pesola, A., Marzilli, M., Severi, S., Parodi, O., L'Abbate, A., Ballestra, A. M., Maltinti, G., De Nes, D. M., and Biagini, A. (1977): Coronary vasospasm in angina pectoris. *Lancet*, 1:713–717.
7. Greensmith, J. E., and Duling, B. R. (1984): Morphology of the constricted arteriolar wall: physiological implications. *Am. J. Physiol.*, 247:H687–H698.

8. Rhodin, J. A. G. (1980): Architecture of the vessel wall. In: *Handbook of Physiology Section 2: The Cardiovascular System, Vol. 2, Vascular Smooth Muscle,* edited by D. F. Baker, A. V. Somlyo, and H. V. Sparks, Jr., pp. 1–31. American Physiological Society, Bethesda.

9. Somlyo, A. V. (1980): Ultrastructure of vascular smooth muscle. In: *Handbook of Physiology Section 2: The Cardiovascular System, Vol. 2, Vascular Smooth Muscle,* edited by D. F. Baker, A. V. Somlyo, and H. V. Sparks, Jr., pp. 35–67. American Physiological Society, Bethesda.

10. Sperelakis, N. (1982): Electrophysiology of vascular smooth muscle of coronary artery. In: *The Coronary Artery,* edited by S. Kalsner, pp. 118–167. Croom Helm, London.

11. Vatner, S. F., and Macho, P. (1981): Regulation of large coronary vessels by adrenergic mechanisms in conscious dogs. *Basic Res. Cardiol.,* 76:408–517.

12. Kalsner, S. (1985): Coronary artery reactivity in human vessels: some questions and some answers. *Fed. Proc.,* 44:321–325.

13. Feigl, E. O. (1983): Coronary physiology. *Physiol. Rev.,* 63:1–205.

14. Gerova, M. (1982): Autonomic innervation of the coronary vasculature. In: *The Coronary Artery,* edited by S. Kalsner, pp. 189–215. Croom Helm, London.

15. Bayliss (1902): On the local reaction of the arterial wall to changes in internal pressure. *J. Physiol. (Lond.),* 28:220–231.

16. Johnson, P. C. (1980): The myogenic response. In: *Handbook of Physiology Section 2: The Cardiovascular System, Vol. 2, Vascular Smooth Muscle,* edited by X. Bohr, A. V. Somlyo, and H. V. Sparks, Jr., pp. 409–439. American Physiological Society, Bethesda.

17. Spaan, J. A. E. (1985): Coronary diastolic pressure-flow relation and zero flow pressure explained on the basis of intramyocardial compliance. *Circ. Res.,* 56:293–309.

18. Klocke, F. J., Mates, R. E., Canty, J. M., Jr., and Ellis, A. K. (1985): Coronary pressure-flow relationships. *Circ. Res.,* 56:310–323.

19. Sparks, H. V., Jr. (1980): Effect of local metabolic factors on vascular smooth muscle. In: *Handbook of Physiology Section 2: The Cardiovascular System, Vol. 2, Vascular Smooth Muscle,* edited by X. Bohr, A. V. Somlyo, and H. V. Sparks, Jr., pp. 475–513. American Physiological Society, Bethesda.

20. MacAlpin, R. N. (1980): Relation of coronary arterial spasm to sites of organic stenosis. *Am. J. Cardiol.,* 46:143–153.

21. Brown, B. G., Bolson, E. L., and Dodge, H. T. (1984): Dynamic mechanisms in coronary stenosis. *Circulation,* 70:917–922.

22. Wong, A. Y. K., Klassen, G. A., and Johnstone, D. E. (1984): Hemodynamics of coronary artery stenosis. *Can. J. Physiol. Pharmacol.,* 62:59–69.

23. Roach, M. (1972): The mechanism of closure of sheep and human umbilical arteries. In: *Vascular Smooth Muscle,* edited by E. Betz, p. 101. Springer-Verlag, Berlin.

24. Maseri, A., L'Abbate, A., Baroldi, G., et al. (1978): Coronary vasospasm as a possible cause of myocardial infarction: a conclusion derived from the study of preinfarction angina. *N. Engl. J. Med.,* 299:1271–1277.

25. Barger, A. C., Beeuwkes, R., III, Lainey, L. L., and Silverman, K. J. (1984): Hypothesis: Vasa vasorum and neovascularization of human coronary arteries. *N. Engl. J. Med.,* 310:175–177.

26. Kohchi, K., Takeboyashi, S., Hiraki, T., and Nobayoshi, X. (1985): Significance of adventitial inflammation of the coronary artery in patients with unstable angina: results of autopsy. *Circulation,* 71:709–716.

27. Brum, J. M., Sufan, Q., Lane, G., and Bove, A. A. (1984): Increased vasoconstrictor activity of proximal coronary arteries with endothelial damage in intact dogs. *Circulation,* 70:1066–1073.

28. Ginsburg, R., Bristow, M. R., Davis, K., Dibiase, A., and Billingham, M. E. (1984): Quantitative pharmacologic response of normal and atherosclerotic isolated human epicardial coronary arteries. *Circulation,* 69:430–440.

29. Kawachi, Y., Tomoike, H., Maruoka, Y., Kikuchi, Y., Araki, H., Ishii, Y., Tanaka, K., and Nakamura, M. (1984): Selective hypercontraction caused by ergonovine in the canine coronary artery under conditions of induced atherosclerosis. *Circulation,* 69:441–450.

30. Parodi, O., Maseri, A., and Simonetti, I. (1979): Management of unstable angina at rest by Verapamil. *Br. Heart J.,* 41:167–174.

31. Santamore, W. P., and Bove, A. A. (1985): A theoretical model of a compliant arterial stenosis. *Am. J. Physiol.,* 248:H274–H285.

Hammersmith Cardiology Workshop Series, Vol. 3,
edited by A. Maseri, B. E. Sobel, and S. Chierchia.
Raven Press, New York © 1987.

Mechanisms of Coronary Obstructions

G. V. R. Born

Department of Pharmacology, King's College, London WC2R 2LS, England

Obstructive coronary thrombosis is initiated, in most cases, by a plaque fissure with local hemorrhage, which induces intravascular platelet aggregation. Recent observations with novel techniques have provided evidence that platelet aggregation *in vivo* is initiated by adenosine diphosphate (ADP) and potentiated by thromboxane A_2 and thrombin, with actual contribution of exposed collagen still undetermined. These observations provide an explanation for the ineffectiveness of any single platelet-inhibiting drug (including aspirin) whenever arterial, e.g., coronary or cerebral, thrombosis is initiated by hemorrhages into atheromatous plaques. On the other hand, aspirin *is* significantly effective when myocardial infarction follows unstable angina and when strokes follow transient episodes of cerebral ischemia. This partial effectiveness can be explained through an action of aspirin on platelets by assuming that, in such cases, their thromboembolic aggregation is initiated by hemodynamic effects of atheromatous lesions.

The principal pathological facts of obstructive coronary thrombosis are as follows (3): (a) Thrombi do not form in normal arteries, but in atherosclerotic arteries; (b) atherosclerosis increases slowly, whereas thrombosis occurs rapidly and is individually unpredictable; therefore, atherosclerotic arteries must be subject to sudden, unpredictable events; (c) most occlusive thrombi are associated with fissures in underlying atheromatous plaques; (d) the central portion of occlusive thrombi consists mainly of aggregated platelets.

MECHANISM?

What is the mechanism responsible for initiating platelet aggregation in an atherosclerotic artery, as an apparently random event in time? Close serial sectioning (9,14) and reconstruction of occluded segments of coronary arteries (10,11) established that the central platelet-rich segment of an obstructive·thrombus is usually, if not invariably, associated with recent hemorrhage into an underlying atherosclerotic plaque. Such hemorrhages occur through fissures or fractures in the plaque, and it is reasonable to assume that the sudden appearance of such a fissure or fracture is the random, individually unpredictable event affecting coronary arteries that has to be assumed to account for the clinical onset of acute myocardial infarction (3). Why such a defect should develop at a particular moment is uncertain. Perhaps it is analogous to the sudden appearance of fine cracks in the wings of jet aircraft, which is ascribed to the cumulative effects of variable stresses on metal, known as fatigue failure (3).

How does hemorrhage into a ruptured plaque trigger platelet thrombogenesis? This can be regarded as part of the general question of how platelets are caused to aggregate by hemorrhage. An explanation commonly put forward is that the process is initiated by platelets adhering to collagen that is exposed where damaged vessel walls are denuded of endothelium (20). Adhering platelets then release other agents, including thromboxane A_2 and ADP, which, in turn, are responsible for the adhesion of more platelets as growing aggregates. This is unlikely, however, to be the complete explanation for the following reasons: First, hemostatic and thrombotic aggregates of platelets grow very rapidly and without delay (1,15). In contrast, platelet aggregation by collagen begins, ever under optimal conditions for rapid reactivity, only after a delay or lag of several seconds (25). Second, platelets tend to aggregate as mural thrombi when anticoagulated blood flows through plastic vessels (12), for example, in artificial organs such as oxygenators or dialyzers (22) that contain neither collagen nor anything else capable of activating platelets similarly. This implies that there are conditions under which platelets are activated in the blood by something other than, or in addition to, the collagen in the walls of living vessels.

RECENT EXPERIMENTS

Recent *in vivo* experiments on three mammalian species, one of them man, indicate that the hemostatic aggregation of platelets is initiated by ADP (26), which is released from injured cells in the blood vessels (2,6). It is reasonable to assume that cellular injury associated with the cracking of atheromatous plaques releases enough ADP locally to initiate thrombotic platelet aggregation in coronary arteries. The effect of this ADP, which is very rapid, is augmented first by thromboxane A_2 and later by much more ADP released from the platelets themselves. When a hemorrhage occurs through an atheromatous fissure into the arterial walls, the extravasated blood remains comparatively static; this condition can be presumed to favor the appearance of thrombin, which initiates fibrin formation and contributes to platelet aggregation.

In this situation, therefore, platelets are apparently exposed simultaneously to several potent aggregating agents, only some of which are produced by the platelets themselves through their release reaction, which is inhibited by aspirin. These considerations can therefore, in principle, account for the comparative ineffectiveness of aspirin in clinical trials of the secondary prevention of myocardial infarction; but they leave open the question as to why the drug is apparently effective when myocardial infarction is associated with unstable angina. Could it be that this type of angina points to a pathogenetic mechanism that differs from other antecedents of myocardial infarction and is more similar to the mechanism underlying cerebrovascular disturbances?

PROPOSED PATHOGENETIC MECHANISM

Through an unusual and interesting development, it has recently become possible to propose a pathogenetic mechanism for unstable angina as a result of a therapeutic success. Over several years there have been extensive and expensive clinical trials of drugs potentially effective against the most serious complication of atherosclerotic cardiovascular disease, namely, cerebral thrombosis which causes stroke and coronary thrombosis which causes heart attacks. In several large controlled trials of aspirin for the secondary prevention of myocardial infarction (involving a total of over 13,000 patients), the drug produced no significant benefit, although some of the trials showed a trend in that direction (19).

However, in two recently reported trials, aspirin was very significantly effective in preventing myocardial infarction and death when the selection of patients was limited to those with unstable angina (8,16). Controlled trials that used aspirin for the prevention of stroke and two other clinical disorders that commonly precede stroke, namely, transient ischemic attacks and visual disturbances, have also demonstrated aspirin's significant benefit (13). This divergence suggests differences in the pathogenesis of these diseases. These differences may become understandable after considering how thrombogenesis may differ in atherosclerotic carotid as opposed to atherosclerotic coronary arteries.

There is increasing evidence that in carotid as opposed to coronary arteries, hemodynamic disturbances alone can initiate the formation of embolizing platelet thrombi. This conclusion is based mainly on noninvasive, ultrasound techniques that can be applied to carotid arteries but not to coronary arteries (7,17,18). In over 90% of patients affected by prestroke syndromes (characteristically transient ischemic attacks and visual disturbances), two complementary imaging techniques demonstrated atherosclerotic lesions usually at the carotid bifurcation, that is, extracranially. In most of these cases the lesions constrict the arterial lumen severely, so that continuous vortices are established in the blood flow. At constant blood pressure, the flow of blood is faster through the constriction than elsewhere in the artery. Therefore, high flow and wall shear rates are no hindrance to the aggregation of platelets as thrombi (4). Indeed, the question arises of whether thrombogenic platelet aggregation can be brought about by abnormal hemodynamic conditions alone.

Evidence of increased platelet aggregation brought about by the operation of hemodynamic factors was provided by experiments in which blood was made to flow through branching channels in extracorporeal shunts (21,23). Deposits of platelets formed consistently on the shoulders of a bifurcation in the flow chamber, but nowhere else in the channels. When the chambers were perfused, not with blood, but with platelet-rich plasma, no deposit was formed, showing that red cells were also essential if deposition was to take place. The dependence that the deposition of platelets from flowing blood has on the red cells that surround and outnumber them could be caused by physical or chemical mechanisms, or by both acting together. A physical mechanism is contributed by the flow behavior of the erythrocyte, which increases the diffusion of platelets in whole blood over that in plasma by up to two orders of magnitude (24). Thus, regions of flow separation and delays are evidently capable, as seen in similar flow in artificial vessels (21), of causing platelet aggregates to form in the bloodstream that are then carried as emboli into the cerebral circulation.

The exact mechanism that induces platelets to aggregate under these conditions is still uncertain. The established therapeutic effectiveness of aspirin in a high proportion of these cases would suggest that the platelets' release reaction is essential. Release of aggregating agents from platelets has long been assumed to subserve a "chain reaction" or positive feedback mechanism (5) that could, in principle, account for platelet aggregation in hemostasis and thrombosis. This assumption was based mainly on *in vitro* experiments that left considerable uncertainty about the contribution of the release reaction to the initiation of aggregation *in vivo*. The rapidity of the process, and the presence of other tissues, make it impossible to follow the release reaction quantitatively *in vivo* by the methods that permit its observation *in vitro*. Because it is the platelet reaction that is inhibited by aspirin, we adopted a novel *in vivo* approach (2). With quantitative electron microscopy, we showed that hemostatic aggregation of platelets can get well under way without participation of the release reaction, that is, the reaction that is inhibited by aspirin in controlled clinical trials for the secondary prevention of myocardial infarction. The question remains how the release reaction may be triggered hemodynamically, e.g., through collisions with red cells or through their reversible distortion with the release of ADP (4).

Thus, in spite of suggestive experimental evidence, the question remains as to why aspirin is, to some extent, clinically effective against primary myocardial infarction in unstable angina patients. It may be that, as has also been pointed out elsewhere (16), the pathological conditions causing these cerebral and cardiac manifestations produce similar hemodynamic effects. For the present, it must be assumed further that hemodynamic disturbances suffice to induce platelet aggregation in a way that is uninhibitable by aspirin. Clearly, much work remains to be done to find out whether or not this is so. Thus, a puzzling but important question is why, in both of the recent trials, aspirin was effective in almost exactly half of the cases (8,16). Does this indicate again two different pathogenetic mechanisms, both manifesting themselves as a consequence of unstable angina, but only one of them involving the postulated hemodynamic effects? Whatever the answer, recent evidence for the clinical effectiveness of at least one drug against the commonest and most dangerous consequence of unstable angina is very encouraging.

REFERENCES

1. Born, G. V. R., and Richardson, P. D. (1980): Activation time of blood platelets. *J. Membr. Biol.*, 57:87–90.
2. Born, G. V. R., Görög, P., and Kratzer, M. A. A. (1981): Aggregation of platelets in damaged vessels. *Philos. Trans. R. Soc. Lond. (Biol.)*, 294:241–250.

3. Born, G. V. R. (1979): Arterial thrombosis and its prevention. In: *Proc. VIII World Congress Cardiology*, edited by S. Hayase and S. Murao, pp. 81–91. Excerpta Medica, Amsterdam.
4. Born, G. V. R. (1977): Fluid-mechanical and biochemical interactions in hemostasis. *Br. Med. Bull.*, 33:193–197.
5. Born, G. V. R. (1965): Platelets in thrombogenesis: mechanism and inhibition of platelet aggregation. *Ann. R. Coll. Surg. Engl.*, 36:200–206.
6. Born, G. V. R., and Kratzer, M. A. A. (1984): Source and concentration of extracellular adenosine triphosphate during hemostasis in rats, rabbits and man. *J. Physiol. (Lond.)*, 354:419–429.
7. Born, G. V. R. (1986): The carotid plaque. In: *Extracranial Cerebrovascular Disease: Diagnosis and Management*, edited by F. Robicsek. Macmillan: New York.
8. Cairns, J., Gent, M., Singer, J., Finnie, K., Froggatt, G., Holder, D., Jablonsky, G., Kostuk, W., Melendez, L., Myers, M., Sackett, D., Sealey, B. Q., and Tanser, P. (1984): A study of Aspirin (ASA) and sulfinpyrazone (S) in unstable angina. *Circulation Suppl. 2*, 70 (abstract 1659).
9. Constantinides, P. (1966): Plaque fissures in human coronary thrombosis. *J. Atheroscler. Res.*, 6:1–17.
10. Davies, M. J., and Thomas, T. (1981): The pathological basis and microanatomy of occlusive thrombus formation in human coronary arteries. *Philos. Trans. R. Soc. Lond. (Biol.)*, 294:225–229.
11. Davies, M. J., and Thomas, A. (1984): Thrombosis and acute coronary-artery lesions in sudden cardiac ischemic death. *N. Engl. J. Med.*, 310:1137–1140.
12. Didisheim, P., Pavlovsky, M., and Kobayashi, I. (1972): Factors that influence or modify platelet function. *Ann. N.Y. Acad. Sci.*, 201:307–315.
13. Fields, W. S., Lamak, R. F., and Frankowski, R. F. (1977): Controlled trials of Aspirin in cerebral ischemia. *Stroke*, 8:301–328.
14. Friedman, M., and Byers, S. O. (1965): Induction of thrombi upon preexisting arterial plaques. *Am. J. Pathol.*, 46:567–575.
15. Hugues, J. C., (1959): Agglutination précoce des plaquettes au cours de lar formation du clou hémostatique. *Thromb. Diathès. Haemorrh.*, 3:177–186.
16. Lewis, H. D., Jr., Davies, J. W., Archibald, D. G., Steinke, W. E., Smitherman, T. C., Doherty, J. E. III, Schnaper, H. W., LeWinter, M. M., Linares, E., Maurice Pouget, J., Sabharwal, S. C., Chesler, E., and Demots, H. (1983): Protective effects of Aspirin against acute myocardial infarction and death in men with unstable angina. *N. Engl. J. Med.*, 309:396–403.
17. Lusby, R. J., Ferrell, L. D., Ehrenfeld, W. K., Stoney, R. J., and Wylie, E. J. (1982): Carotid plaque hemorrhage: its role in production of cerebral ischemia. *Arch. Surg.*, 117:1479–1488.
18. Lusby, R. J., Machleder, H. I., Jeans, W., Skidmore, R., Woodcock, J. P., Clifford, P. C., and Baird, R. N. (1981): Vessel wall and blood flow dynamics in arterial diseases. *Philos. Trans. R. Soc. Lond. (Biol.)*, 294:231–239.
19. May, G. S., Eberlein, K. A., Furberg, C. D., Passamain, E. R., and DeMets, D. S. (1982): Secondary prevention after myocardial infarction: a review of long-term trials. *Prog. Cardiovasc. Dis.*, 24:331–352.
20. Mustard, J. F., Moore, S., Packham, M. A., and Kinlough Rathbone, R. L. (1977): Platelets, thrombosis and atherosclerosis. *Prog. Biochem. Pharmacol.*, 13:312–325.
21. Mustard, J. F., Murphy, E. A., Rowsell, H. C., and Downie, H. G. (1962): Factors influencing thrombus formation *in vivo*. *Am. J. Med.*, 33:621–647.
22. Richardson, P. D., Galletti, P. M., and Born, G. V. R. (1976): Regional administration of drugs to control thrombosis in artificial organs. *Trans. Am. Soc. Artif. Intern. Organ*, 22:22–29.
23. Rowntree, L. G., and Shionya, T. (1927): Studies in experimental extracorporeal thrombosis. Part I. Methods for the direct observation of extra-corporeal thrombus formation. *J. Exp. Med.*, 46:7–12.
24. Turitto, V. T., and Baumgartner, H. R. (1975): Platelet interaction with subendothelium in a perfusion system: physical role of red blood cells. *Microvasc. Res.*, 5:167–179.
25. Wilner, G. D., Nossell, H. L., and LeRoy, E. C. (1968): Aggregation of platelets by collagen. *J. Clin. Invest.*, 47:2616–2621.
26. Zawilska, K. M., Born, G. V. R., Begent, N. A. (1982): Effect of ADP-utilizing enzymes on the arterial bleeding time in rats and rabbits. *Br. J. Haematol.*, 50:317–325.

Hammersmith Cardiology Workshop Series, Vol. 3,
edited by A. Maseri, B. E. Sobel, and S. Chierchia.
Raven Press, New York © 1987.

Précis of the Discussion: Section III

THE DYNAMIC CONTROL OF CORONARY LUMEN

C. Richard Conti

Richard Conti commented that ergometrinc seemed to relax the smooth muscle of the model presented. Andrew Henderson responded that he was also surprised by this observation, which suggested that ergometrine stimulated the endothelium-dependent dilation, but he said he was not sure of the mechanism of action. Attilio Maseri asked Andrew Henderson to explain the difference in the effect of the endothelial relaxant factor on coronary arteries and the aorta. Dr. Henderson thought that the difference is likely to be due to the different dependence of different arteries on intracellular or extracellular calcium for activation. The coronary arteries appear to be largely dependent on calcium flux through the receptor-operated channels and are thus going to be more responsive than the aorta. Richard Conti pointed out that endothelial denudation occurs frequently in patients undergoing coronary angioplasty, and yet the incidence of spasm during the procedure is low. Perhaps the failure to see spasm in the overwhelming majority of patients is related to the fact that most are receiving potent vasodilators at the time of angio plasty.

Burton Sobel commented that there is a transmural gradient in alpha receptor distribution throughout the myocardium, which could theoretically prevent an endo-cardial steal from the epicardial vasculature. Perhaps the reason that alpha blockers are not very helpful in angina pectoris is that alpha blockade might counteract a basic mechanism that is needed to maintain the appropriate transmural flow distribution. Gerry Klassen said that he suspects there is a great deal of between-patients variability and that alpha tone will be an important component in some and not in others. He quoted the preliminary results of studies by Sergio Chierchia et al., which show that blockade of coronary alpha receptors can improve coronary flow reserve of some patients with effort-related angina. Dr. Klassen also emphasized that his main message is the concept that the entire coronary system, from the epicardial arteries all the way down to the small resistance vessels within the cardiac muscle itself, has the capacity to move resistance up and down. Coronary resistance is not located at a fixed point. Any of the vessels can act as a resistance vessel and probably do.

Richard Conti asked about the experiments in the operating room, i.e., whether the vessels contract or dilate when nerves are stimulated electrically. Gerry Klassen responded that most did not do anything. In some cases, if systemic pressure increased, coronary blood flow also increased. Richard Conti commented that there is some clinical experience with denervation in patients with coronary artery spasm and atherosclerosis. Michel Bertrand expanded on these comments and noted that surgeons at his institution were able to induce spasm by stimulating the nerve plexus in a few patients who had classic Prinzmetal's variant angina. In these patients, a plexectomy was performed, which resulted in total symptomatic relief. Gerry Klassen responded that the neural control of the circulation is very complicated and our understanding of it is still at an early stage.

William Grossman commented that plaque fissuring produced by angioplasty does not seem to initiate thrombosis. Gustav Born responded that it could be easily explained by the fact that, after angioplasty, the coronary artery is dilated to such an extent that even though plaque fissuring may occur and small thrombi may form, these will not be able to occlude the lumen and impair flow. Dr. Grossman also observed that pretreatment with aspirin and dipyridamole and full heparinization would prevent thrombosis. Richard Conti added that, of course, flow increases as a result of angioplasty and this probably accounts for the washout of mural thrombi.

Lawson McDonald asked if platelet emboli might be responsible for the creation of the unstable state, i.e., unstable angina pectoris. Gustav Born responded that this was the theme of Falk's paper (*Circulation* 1985; 71:699–708), that unstable angina is related to the appearance of small plaque fissures, initiating thrombus, which gets fragmented and swept away into the distal vessel. These distal emboli could be responsible for the electrical disturbances or for the small peripheral infarctions that have been observed in this syndrome.

Michael Oliver asked if aspirin relieved ischemia in patients with unstable angina. Specifically, does it revert the electrocardiogram back toward normal in a patient who is having recurrent chest pain? Attilio Maseri responded that this was a complex phenomenon and not quite similar to the classic experiments of Folts and Rowe, in which extrinsic stenoses were created in dogs and cyclic fluctuations in coronary blood flow were observed, which were prevented by aspirin. In Maseri's experience, both aspirin and prostacyclin failed to relieve ischemia in any of the patients in whom it was tested. Although Maseri was unable to explain the difference between animal experiments and his clinical observations, it must be pointed out that no carefully controlled clinical trials are available on this subject. The only two controlled studies that were performed by Sergio Chierchia et al. (*Circulation* 1982; 65:470–477 and 1982; 66:702–705) were conducted in patients with variant angina, and angiographically documented spasm of epicardial coronary arteries. The negative conclusions to which these authors came cannot be extrapolated to other subsets of patients with unstable angina.

Graham Davies reported the occasional observation of coronary reocclusion (after patency had been reestablished) during streptokinase infusion in patients with acute myocardial infarction. He was curious as to why this should happen. Burton Sobel responded that this apparent paradoxical response may be related to the consumption of plasminogen by streptokinase, preventing the conversion of plasminogen to plasmin. Michael Davies also pointed out that the recurrence of thrombosis is related to the underlying pathology, e.g., a tiny fissure in the endothelium may result in very little lipid and collagen exposure while, in other instances, plaque may be essentially destroyed and the entire endothelial top removed, thus exposing lipid, cholesterol, and collagen over a large area to the blood elements. Michael Davies thought that the vessels that did not rethrombose may have had only small fissures.

Sergio Chierchia pointed out that in some instances in which streptokinase is ineffective after a reclosure, vessels reopen with nitrate administration. He emphasized that this probably has little to do with plaque fissuring and could instead be related to coronary vasoconstriction, possibly elicited by vasoactive platelet and clotting factors.

Editorial comment: S. Chierchia

The factors controlling coronary arterial tone are still poorly understood by both clinicians and basic scientists. The term "spasm" is frequently used (and too often misused) to explain the occurrence of ischemia that is not caused by an excessive increase of myocardial metabolic demand and is likely to be due to impairment of regional myocardial perfusion. On the clinical side, an effort should be made to separate patients in whom "spasm" (i.e., an abnormal increase in coronary vasomotion) is likely to play a role, from those whose symptoms are more likely to be caused by "vasoconstriction" (i.e., an increase in vasomotor tone within the normal physiological range) or by platelet aggregation and thrombosis. The location of spasm or vasoconstriction should also be searched for in the individual patient and the role of epicardial coronary arteries should be separated from that of smaller, resistive vessels. Patients in whom a primary thrombotic or thromboembolic component appears predominant should be separated from those whose symptoms are largely explained by coronary vasoconstriction. This effort toward a pathophysiologically oriented classification of the various clinical manifestations of ischemic heart disease should provide a better basis for "individualized" treatment and help to select homogeneous patient subsets in whom different working hypotheses could be checked by appropriate clinical trials.

By a similar reasoning, basic scientists should design carefully controlled experiments, based on selective interventions, to at least separate the large conductive coronary arteries from the resistive component. The relative physiological and pathophysiological roles of the various factors controlling coronary smooth muscle tone should be assessed separately in these two compartments, whose response to different vasoactive stimuli is likely to be different.

Only close cooperation between clinicians and experimental workers, along with a process of reciprocal feedback, can provide us with the necessary tools for facing, and hopefully solving, a problem of outstanding complexity.

Hammersmith Cardiology Workshop Series, Vol. 3,
edited by A. Maseri, B. E. Sobel, and S. Chierchia.
Raven Press, New York © 1987.

Coronary Arterial Findings in Acute Myocardial Infarction

Michel E. Bertrand, Jean M. Lablanche, J. L. Fourrier,
and G. Traisnel

Hôpital Cardiologique, Lille University, 59037 Lille, France

For many years, most of our knowledge about the lesions associated with myocardial infarction derived from autopsy. Over the last 10 years, with increasing experience, the role of coronary arteriography has expanded into the realm of acute ischemic syndromes and acute myocardial infarction. More recently, recanalization of the vessels started with intracoronary administration of streptokinase. Therefore, much information concerning coronary arterial findings during the early stage of myocardial infarction is available.

This chapter will cover some aspects of coronary angiographic findings in the acute phase of myocardial infarction. It is divided into four sections: (a) the infarct-related vessels: (b) the extent of coronary artery disease; (c) collateral circulation in acute myocardial infarction; and (d) angiographic data and the mechanisms of myocardial infarction.

THE INFARCT-RELATED VESSEL

Although it is not always easy to recognize the infarct-related vessel, especially in inferior infarction, many well documented and very informative studies are available. The first study was done in 1980 by DeWood et al. (1) who, with coronary angiography, studied 322 patients admitted within 24 hr of infarction.

Total coronary occlusion was observed in 110 of 126 patients (87%) who were evaluated within 4 hr of the onset of symptoms. This proportion declined to 68.4% within 6–12 hr and to 64.9% within 12–24 hr after onset of the symptoms. With the development of intracoronary thrombolysis, many other studies have confirmed these preliminary results.

The results of 12 studies (1–13) are listed in Table 1. The rate of total occlusion of the infarct-related vessel varied from 69% in the findings of Rentrop et al. (2) to 95% in the series of Mathey et al. (3). DeWood et al. (7) recently published results of a study that included 517 patients and confirmed the frequency of total coronary occlusion (87% within the first 6 hr).

TABLE 1. *Infarct-related vessel: frequency of total occlusion*

Author			N	0–4 hr	4–6 hr	6–12 hr	12–24 hr
DeWood et al.	1980	(1)	322	87.3%	85.3%	62.4%	57%
Rentrop et al.	1981	(2)	29	—— 69% ——			
Mathey et al.	1981	(3)	41	95%			
Reduto et al.	1981	(4)	32	—— 81% ——			
Kennedy et al.	1981	(5)	250	————— 86% —————			
Letac et al.	1983	(6)	80	—— 92% ——			
Kubler et al.	1983	(X)	30	73%	76%		
DeWood et al.	1983	(7)	368	86%		68%	64%
Ferguson et al.	1984	(8)	77	—— 84% ——			
Leiboff et al.	1984	(9)	55	78%			
TIMI et al.	1985	(10)	290	—— 74% ——			
Rentrop et al.	1985	(12)	91	69%		63%	

Some differences between the studies can result from the different times of the investigations and also from the differences in operator technique; thus, the amount of pressure and the volume of dye injected, as well as the duration of imaging during cineangiocardiography, can explain the observed differences. Therefore, it is necessary to have a clear definition of the angiographic findings, and the stratification used in the TIMI study (10) seems very useful.

Table 2 shows the definition of four groups of patients, and it is clear that Group 1 is the only one with total occlusion. With this definition, the rate of total occlusion of the infarct-related vessel was 74% in the TIMI study. However, we cannot presume the mechanisms of the total occlusion that could be related to a thrombus or a spasm. Unfortunately, DeWood et al. (1) did not perform a second angiogram after administration of nitroglycerin, which can rule out the possibility of a spasm. In their second study in 1983, DeWood et al. (7) described the prevalence of coronary thrombosis during transmural myocardial infarction. The angiographic features that defined intracoronary thrombus included: (a) persistent staining of

TABLE 2. *Definitions of perfusion: Thrombolysis in myocardial infarcation (TIMI) Trial[a]*

Grade 0: No antegrade flow beyond the point of occlusion

Grade 1: Penetration without perfusion dye passes beyond the area of obstruction but "hangs up" and fails to opacify the entire coronary distal bed

Grade 2: Partial perfusion dye passes across the obstruction and opacifies the distal bed, but the clearance is slower than in other vessels

Grade 3: Complete perfusion

[a] From TIMI study group (10).

intraluminal material at the distal end of the column of injected contrast agents; (b) local retention of the contrast medium in the involved coronary artery; and (c) intracoronary filling defect. These criteria were compared with surgical findings. In the entire study population, the frequency of coronary thrombosis was 73%. This was observed in 80% of the patients studied in the first 6 hr, but the frequency fell to 59% in the 6 to 12 hr period and 54% in the 12 to 24 hr period. Overall, the decline in the frequency of coronary thrombosis was statistically significant and paralleled the fall in the prevalence of total coronary occlusion. To assess the ability of coronary angiography to detect the presence or absence of thrombus, DeWood et al. (7) assessed the surgical findings in 96 patients undergoing emergency surgical reperfusion as treatment of acute myocardial infarction.

False positive results were observed in 11% and, in opposition, a 26% false negative result was observed. The true negative rate (74%) suggests that coronary angiography was relatively accurate.

Coronary arterial spasm could be another explanation of the angiographical aspect of coronary occlusion. This was mentioned for the first time by Oliva and Breckenridge (13) in 1977. Recent study of the literature showed that before starting intracoronary streptokinase infusion, the authors injected intracoronary nitroglycerin. A reperfusion occurred in 2.5% to 10% of the cases. However, is it really evidence of coronary spasm? More likely the partial reperfusion results from the dilation of the normal portion of the wall. The natural history of total occlusion can only be addressed with a comparison of studies performed at different times after the beginning of the symptoms, since no serial series of individual patients have been done. Table 1 shows that the frequency of total coronary occlusion decreases from 86% within 6 hr to 53% at 2 weeks and 50% at 6 months (14–17). Although these findings provide no direct evidence for spontaneous recanalization, they strongly suggest that this may occur after infarction.

If total coronary occlusion is the common feature of the early stage of acute myocardial infarction, a nontotal coronary occlusion can be observed. DeWood et al. (7) observed this aspect in 13% of their patients, and 17% of the patients of the TIMI study (10) had partial or complete perfusion (grades 2 and 3). In these particular cases, one can suspect spontaneous thrombolysis before angiography or release of transient coronary spasm in an area of preexisting atherosclerosis.

TABLE 3. *Extent of vessel disease in 693 patients without prior infarction studied within the first 6 weeks after myocardial infarction*

	n	ns	Single-vessel disease	Double-vessel disease	Triple-vessel disease
Patients with anterior infarction	274	2.9%	49.3%	29.2%	18.6%
Patients with inferior infarction	419	6.3%	35.6%	27.0%	31.1%

THE EXTENT OF CORONARY ARTERY DISEASE

Very little information concerning this problem can be obtained from the recent studies with intracoronary thrombolysis. Most often the investigators focused their attention on the infarct-related vessel and most often did not inject the other vessels. Therefore, the problem can be addressed with the results of coronary angiography performed 2 to 6 weeks later. In our experience, we have studied 693 patients with a first myocardial infarction within the first 6 weeks after the onset of myocardial infarction. They were subdivided into 274 patients with anterior infarction and 419 patients with inferior infarction. Table 3 shows that there was a significant difference in the extent of vessel disease. In anterior infarction, 49.3% had single-vessel disease, while double- or triple-vessel diseases were observed in 29.2% and 18.6%, respectively. In contrast, the patients with inferior infarction are characterized by the large extent of vessel disease: 35.6% had single-vessel disease, but 27% had double-vessel disease, and 31.1% had three significant narrowings.

COLLATERAL CIRCULATION

Table 4 shows that the incidence of collateral circulation varies from 16% to 43%. The most complete study was done by Rentrop et al. (11) who observed that 32% of the patients studied within the first 6 hr had collateral circulation, and this was observed mainly in patients with total occlusion of the vessel. Recently, Saito et al. (18) found an incidence of 43% in a group of 30 patients. Moreover, the authors observed that ejection fraction was higher in the group of patients who developed collateral circulation than in the other group. In contrast, Rousseau et al. (19) observed that the presence of vessels in 126 patients studied within 2 weeks after myocardial infarction had no significant influence on left ventricular function, extent of abnormally contracting segment, and wall motion.

MYOCARDIAL INFARCTION WITH "NORMAL" CORONARY ARTERIES

The incidence of this particular problem is completely different in the studies performed within the first hours and the coronary arterial findings obtained 2 to 6

TABLE 4. *Incidence of collateral circulation*

Reduto et al.	1981	(4)	8/32	(25%)
Leiboff	1983	(3)	7/43	(16%)
Rentrop et al.	1984	(11)	22/68	(32%)
			21/42	Total OCC
			1/26	Incomplete OCC
Saito et al.	1985	(18)	13/30	(43%)

weeks later. In the early stage of acute myocardial infarction, the frequency of myocardial infarction with normal coronary arteries is very low. DeWood et al. did not mention this problem (1). In the TIMI study (10), 2.7% of patients had nonsignificant vessel disease, and Rentrop et al. observed 2.2% of cases (11) without significant narrowing.

However, the studies performed later mention an incidence of 4% to 7%. In the so-called myocardial infarction with "normal" coronary arteries one can suspect that (a) some patients had, in fact, no myocardial infarction (myocarditis?) (b) a misinterpretation of the angiogram had occurred, (c) the role of spasm has been frequently discussed, (d) some authors discussed the role of intramural arteries or, more simply, the recanalization of a thrombus or an embolus. It is very interesting to note 8 observations (20–26) characterized by total occlusion of the vessel 0.5 to 30 hr after the onset of the symptoms and completely normal vessels 4 to 17 days later. From these observations, it is more likely that the so-called myocardial infarction with normal coronary arteries results from a spontaneous thrombolysis.

FROM THE ANGIOGRAPHIC DATA TO THE MECHANISMS OF MYOCARDIAL INFARCTION

Finally, angiographic data cover a broad spectrum of findings. The studies of the last 5 years support the concept that coronary thrombosis was the final common pathway. However, does it mean that other factors cannot be involved? It is obvious that in particular cases, coronary arterial spasm can intervene. Fourteen to 34% of patients with Prinzmetal's variant angina (some of them with normal or near-normal coronary arteries) can develop myocardial infarction as a result of prolonged refractory spasm. Bertrand et al. (27) found that 20% of patients with recent (6 weeks) myocardial infarction had provoked coronary spasm, which was superimposed to the narrowing of the infarct-related vessel in one half of the cases. Maseri et al. (28) published a case of severe Prinzmetal's variant angina where the patient developed myocardial infarction during a severe episode of spasm. The patient died and at the autopsy a fresh thrombus was detected at the site of the spasm. Recent studies mention that complex atherosclerotic narrowing could result from a fissure or hemorrhage into the atherosclerotic plaque. This situation may cause mechanical slowing of the flow and can result in coronary occlusion. Finally, the precise and respective role of these factors is unclear, but their interactions can lead to total occlusion and coronary thrombosis, which is the final common pathway of the disease.

REFERENCES

1. DeWood, M., Spores, J., Notske, R., Mouser, L. T., Burroughs, R., Golden, M. S., and Lang, H. T. (1980): Prevalence of total coronary occlusion during the early hours of transmural myocardial infarction. *N. Engl. J. Med.*, 303:897.

2. Rentrop, K. P., Blanke, H., Karsch, K. R., Kaiser, H., Köstering, H., and Leitz, K. (1981): Selective intracoronary thrombolysis in acute myocardial infarction and unstable angina pectoris. *Circulation,* 63:307–317.
3. Mathey, D. G., Kuck, K. H., Tilsner, V., Krebber, H. J., and Bleifeld, W. (1981): Nonsurgical coronary artery recanalization in acute transmural myocardial infarction. *Circulation,* 63:489–497.
4. Reduto, L. A., Freund, G. C., Gaeta, J. M., et al. (1981): Coronary artery reperfusion in acute myocardial infarction: beneficial effects of intracoronary streptokinase on left ventricular salvage and performance. *Am. Heart J.,* 102:1168–1177.
5. Kennedy, J. W., Richtie, J. L., Davis, K. B., and Fritz, J. K. (1981): Western Washington randomized trial of intracoronary streptokinase in acute myocardial infarction. *N. Engl. J. Med.,* 309:1477–1482.
6. Cribier, A., Berland, J., Champoud, O., Moore, N., Behar, P., and Letac, B. (1983): Intracoronary thrombolysis in evolving myocardial infarction. Sequential angiographic analysis of left ventricular performance. *Br. Heart J.,* 50:401–410.
7. Dewood, M., Spores, J., Hensley, G. R., Simpson, C. S., Eugster, G. S., Sutherland, K. I., Grunwald, R. P., and Shields, J. P. (1983): Coronary arteriographic findings in acute transmural myocardial infarction. *Circulation,* 68:1–39.
8. Ferguson, D. W., White, C. W., Schwartz, J. L., Brayden, G. D., Kelly, K. J., Kioschos, J. M., Kirchner, P. T., and Marcus, M. L. (1984): Influence of baseline ejection fraction and success of thrombolysis on mortality and ventricular function after acute myocardial infarction. *Am. J. Cardiol.,* 54:705–711.
9. Leiboff, R., Katz, R. J., Wasserman, A. G., Bren, G. B., Schwarz, H., Varghese, J., and Ross, A. M. (1984): A randomized, angiographically controlled trial of intracoronary streptokinase in acute myocardial infarction. *Am. J. Cardiol.,* 53:404–407.
10. TIMI study group (1985): The thrombolysis in myocardial infarction (TIMI) trial Phase I findings. *N. Engl. J. Med.,* 312:932–936.
11. Rentrop, P., Fert, F., Blanke, H., Stecy, P., Schneider, R., Rey, M., Haronitz, S., Goldman, M., Karsch, K., Meihman, H., Cohen, M., Siegel, S., Sanger, J., Shoter, J., Gorlin, R., Fox, A., Fagerstrom, R., and Calhoum, W. (1984): Effects of intracoronary streptokinase and intracoronary nitroglycerin infusion on coronary angiographic patterns and mortality in patients with acute myocardial infarction. *N. Engl. J. Med.,* 311:1457–1463.
12. Rentrop, P. (1985): Thrombolytic therapy in patients with acute myocardial infarction. *Circulation,* 71:627.
13. Oliva, P. B., and Breckenridge, J. C. (1977): Acute myocardial infarction with normal and near normal coronary arteries. Documentation with coronary arteriography within 12½ hours of the onset of symptoms in two cases (Three episodes). *Am. J. Cardiol.,* 40:1000.
14. Bertrand, M. E., Lefebvre, J. M., Laisne, C. L., Rousseau, M. F., Carre, A. G., and Lekieffre, J. P. (1979): Coronary arteriography in acute transmural myocardial infarction. *Am. Heart J.,* 97:61.
15. Betriu, A., Castaner, A., Sanz, G. A., et al. (1982): Angiographic findings 1 month after myocardial infarction: a prospective study of 259 survivors. *Circulation,* 65:1099.
16. De Feyter, P. J., Van Eenige, M. J., and Van Der Wale, E. E. (1982): Prognostic value of exercise testing, coronary angiography and left ventriculography 6–8 weeks after myocardial infarction. *Circulation,* 66:527.
17. Pichard, A. D., Ziff, C., Rentrop, P., Holt, J., Blanke, H., and Smith, H. (1983): Angiographic study of infarct related coronary artery in the chronic stage of acute myocardial infarction. *Am. Heart J.,* 106:687–693.
18. Saito, Y., Yasuno, M., Ishida, M., Suzuki, K., Mataba, Y., Emura, M., and Takahoshi, M. (1985): Importance of coronary collaterals for restoration of left ventricular function after intracoronary thrombolysis. *Am. J. Cardiol.,* 55:1259–1263.
19. Rousseau, M. F., Bertrand, M. E., Detry, M. R., Decoster, P. M., and Lablanche, J. M. (1982): Coronary collaterals and left ventricular function early after acute transmural myocardial infarction. *Eur. Heart J.,* 3:223–229.
20. Monassier, J. P., Coulbois, P. M., Valeix, B., Hanssen, M., Tonhami, L., and Schaaf, R. (1982): Infarctus du myocarde par thrombose aigue coronarienne droite. *Arch. Mal. Coeur,* 75:425–430.
21. Lindsay, J., Jr., Dwyer, S., and Pusija, U. (1983): Coronary occlusion during spontaneous acute

myocardial infarction and subsequent angiographically normal coronary arteries. *Am. J. Cardiol.*, 51:1227–1228.

22. Benacceraf, A., Scholl, J. M., Achard, F., Tonnelier, M., and Lavergne, G. (1983): Coronary spasm and thrombosis associated with myocardial infarction in a patient with nearly normal coronary arteries. *Circulation,* 67:1147–1150.

23. Vincent, G. M., Anderson, J. L., and Marshale, H. W. (1983): Coronary spasm producing coronary thrombosis and myocardial infarction. *N. Engl. J. Med.,* 309:220–223.

24. Fernandez, M. S., Pichard, A. D., Marchant, A. P., and Lindsay, J., Jr. (1983): Acute myocardial infarction with normal coronary arteries. *In vivo* demonstration of coronary thrombosis during the acute episode. *Clin. Cardiol.,* 6:553–559.

25. Anderson, J. L., Marshall, H. W., White, R. S., and Datz, F. (1983): Streptokinase thrombolysis for acute myocardial infarction in young adults with normal coronary arteries. *Am. Heart J.,* 706:1437–1438.

26. Ross, R., Kay, R., Ambrose, J., and Herman, M. W. (1983): Coronary thrombosis in the absence of angiographically evident obstructive coronary disease. *Chest,* 84:758–770.

27. Bertrand, M. E., Lablanche, J. M., Tilmant, P. Y., Thieuleux, F. A., Delforge, M. G., and Chahine, R. A. (1983): The provocation of coronary arterial spasm in patients with recent transmural myocardial infarction. *Eur. Heart J.,* 4:532–535.

28. Maseri, A., L'Abbate, A., Baroldi, G., Chierchia, S., et al. (1978): Coronary vasospasm as a possible cause of myocardial infarction. A conclusion derived from the study of "pre-infarction" angina. *N. Engl. J. Med.,* 299:1271–1275.

Hammersmith Cardiology Workshop Series, Vol. 3,
edited by A. Maseri, B. E. Sobel, and S. Chierchia.
Raven Press, New York © 1987.

Plaque Fissuring and Thrombosis

Michael J. Davies

*Cardiovascular Pathology Unit, St. George's Hospital Medical School,
London SW17 ORE, England*

The raised atheromatous plaque is the starting point from which the clinical expressions of ischemic heart disease develop. The term "raised" plaque derives from visual inspection of the intimal surface of an artery that has been opened longitudinally and observing an oval hump with sloping shoulders. "Hard" plaques consist almost entirely of connective tissue and contain small amounts of lipid, which is almost entirely intracellular; at the other extreme, "soft" raised plaques contain a pool of extracellular free lipid. There is every gradation between the two extremes. It is plaques toward the lipid-rich or soft end of the spectrum that undergo complications leading to the acute clinical manifestations of ischemic heart disease, which comprises sudden death, acute infarction, and crescendo angina.

Examination of the arteries in cross section, after perfuse fixation at physiological pressures (thus, distending the lumen), shows that the plaque bulges out into the media as well as inward toward the lumen, which remains close to circular in shape. The plaque often occupies only a segment of the circumference of the intima; as a result, the lumen becomes placed eccentric to the central axis of the vessel. The segment of arterial wall opposite the plaque often retains a normal medial structure and an intact elastic lamina, although both of these may be deficient behind the plaque itself. The lipid is a crescentic-shaped mass contained within the intima and is separated from the arterial lumen by a cap of fibrous tissue that varies in thickness, but is often thinnest over the points of the crescent (Fig. 1).

In what has become known as plaque fissuring, cracking or rupture of the fibrous cap occurs, allowing blood from the lumen to dissect into the lipid pool

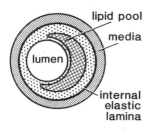

FIG. 1. Diagrammatic representation of an atheromatous plaque in cross section. The lipid pool is crescentic in shape and separated from the lumen by a fibrous cap. The outward bowing of the plaque means the lumen is circular in shape and eccentrically placed in relation to the center of the artery.

71

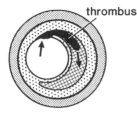

thrombus

FIG. 2. Diagrammatic representation of a fissured plaque in cross section. The cap has broken at one lateral margin, allowing a mass of thrombus to push into the plaque.

within which a platelet-rich thrombus develops. The plaque, overall, rapidly increases in size by growth of this intraintimal thrombus (Fig. 2).

The purpose of this chapter is to consider the evidence that plaque fissuring is responsible for acute infarction, sudden ischemic death, and crescendo angina.

ACUTE MYOCARDIAL INFARCTION

Many necropsy studies of patients who have died of regional myocardial infarction show that a high proportion have a major intraluminal thrombus (1–4). A number of necropsy studies have reconstructed the microanatomy of such thrombi (5,6) and have consistently shown that beneath the intraluminal thrombus, there is a fissured plaque with a large intraintimal thrombotic component (Fig. 3). A number of other morphological features of interest emerge from such reconstructions. The thrombus within the plaque, within the fissure track, and immediately adjacent to it in the lumen is rich in platelets; the thrombus filling the lumen and extending distally even into segments of normal artery is predominantly composed of fibrin. The size of the break in the fibrous cap of the plaque varies. At one extreme, it is a crack or fissure; at the other extreme, loss of the whole fibrous cap over a centimeter occurs, extruding free cholesterol into the lumen. It is not surprising that the major plaque fissures that extrude lipid should lead to major thrombosis occluding the lumen; some of the smaller fissures are to be associated with a disproportionate degree of thrombosis in response to a small exposure of lipid. Thrombus within the plaque may extend both distally and proximally far beyond the immediate point of intimal break into the lumen.

The morphological descriptions of plaque fissuring date from over 50 years

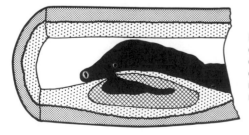

FIG. 3. Longitudinal reconstruction of occlusive coronary thrombus. The intraluminal component is in continuity with a large mass of thrombus within the plaque. The intraluminal thrombus has propagated down to lumen remote from the plaque.

ago (7,8), and it may be asked why recognition of the importance of the process had lapsed. The reason lies in a confusion between two separate phenomena: plaque fissuring and intraplaque hemorrhage. Many large atheromatous plaques, unassociated with any thrombosis in the lumen, have a leash of new small blood vessels entering the intima from across the media. The presence of some red cells lying free within the lipid pool but without platelets or fibrin is common. This process is correctly called plaque hemorrhage and is derived from rupture of the fragile new capillaries (9,10) and, while it may cause some plaque growth (11), hemorrhage must be limited by the pressure exerted from the lumen. When the atheromatous plaques beneath coronary thrombi were also seen to contain red cells, these were also considered to be derived from the transmedial vessels by hemorrhage and, consequently, ignored. What was not appreciated was that within these plaques associated with thrombosis, large numbers of platelets were present and there was free continuity of the intraluminal and intraplaque thrombus. This lack of appreciation by pathologists was both a failure to realize that fibrin may be a minor component of some thrombi, and the practice of taking random histological sections rather than reconstructing the whole arterial lesion.

The concept that plaque fissuring underlies most episodes of acute regional myocardial infarction fits well with recent data derived by angiography (12,13). In essence, clinical angiograms carried out within an hour of onset of myocardial infarction show an occluded artery in around 90% of cases. The incidence of occlusion falls with time but, if intracoronary fibrinolysis is carried out, the majority of arteries can be restored to patency. Patients who come to necropsy are of necessity selected toward those with large infarcts in whom spontaneous fibrinolysis had not restored flow before death. A high proportion of such fatal cases of infarction have developed distal propagation of thrombus from the original nidus over the plaque.

In patients who survive acute infarction and where the occluded vessel has reopened due to either spontaneous or iatrogenic fibrinolysis, a high-grade stenosis is found. The residual high-grade stenosis in these patients probably represents a plaque that has been enlarged by the intraintimal thrombotic component and, in keeping with this view, remodeling and reduction in obstruction take place over weeks (14), probably by organization and fibrosis.

The clinical work that found that radiolabeled fibrinogen was incorporated into coronary thrombi after the onset of infarction (15) can, in retrospect, be seen to demonstrate distal propagation from the proximal nidus of thrombus that had invoked the infarct. This view has been confirmed at necropsy (16) by studies which show that the proximal portion of the thrombus is not labeled, while the distal propagation thrombus is labeled by radioactive fibrin.

During the recanalization phase after arterial occlusion associated with myocardial infarction, a number of angiographic appearances (17–19) are found, which include intraluminal filling defects just distal to areas of stenosis with very ragged outlines. These would exactly coincide with what would be anticipated in fissured plaques over which luminal thrombus has developed. Clinical angiography has also demonstrated the speed at which intraluminal thrombi can change in size.

SUDDEN DEATH

A recent necropsy study (20) has concentrated on whether plaque fissuring and associated intraluminal thrombi are found in sudden ischemic death. Postmortem coronary angiograms combined with histological assessment of every 3 mm segment of the whole coronary artery were made in patients dying within 6 hr of the onset of symptoms. A blind comparison was made of two groups, one in which there was no morphological cause of death other than over 50% coronary artery stenosis (by diameter), and a control group in which there was a clear morphological cause of death outside the coronary artery tree. In the test hearts, intraluminal thrombi related to plaque fissures were found in 74% of the cases. A further 21% had plaque fissures with an intraintimal thrombus but no intraluminal component. None of the control hearts had intraluminal thrombus. A small number of control hearts did, however, have evidence of a fissured plaque in the recent past. The intraluminal thrombi present in sudden ischemic death were of varying size, ranging from less than 50% of the residual cross section of the artery (mural thrombus) to over 90% ("occlusive" thrombi). Overall, the size of the thrombi was less than that found in equivalent patients dying of acute myocardial infarction in hospitals.

Fissured plaques associated with thrombus could be readily identified in postmortem angiograms as areas of stenosis with a ragged outline and filling defects in the contrast medium. Postmortem angiography is a sensitive and reliable method of detecting thrombosis in coronary arteries.

If these plaque fissures are responsible for invoking the ventricular fibrillation that lead to sudden death, the exact mechanism can only be speculatory. A minority have intraluminal thrombi that have totally occluded the vessel. Tearing of the intima, particularly in association with large masses of thrombi which consist predominantly of platelets, may well invoke local arterial spasm. Mural thrombus may act as a source of small platelet emboli into the myocardium in a manner analogous to the ulcerated atheromatous plaques in the carotid bifurcation, which give rise to transient cerebral ischemic attacks (21,22).

UNSTABLE ANGINA

Evidence linking crescendo or unstable angina with plaque fissuring is, of necessity, less direct; however, clinical angiography has shown a high proportion of cases to have either intraluminal filling defects or areas of stenosis with very ragged outlines (23,24). These appearances have been confirmed to indicate thrombosis in postmortem angiograms (25). The similarity in appearances between the angiograms taken during life in patients with crescendo angina and postmortem angiograms in sudden ischemic death is very striking.

CONCLUSION

It seems that lipid-rich plaques may spontaneously fissure and this process may, but by no means inevitably, lead to serious sequelae. Such a fissured plaque may develop a small intraintimal thrombus, but the plaque reseals and restabilizes before an intraluminal thrombotic component develops. Such events are probably relatively common and do not invoke symptoms. The occurrence of old healed fissures in a small number of control hearts would support this view. Even though no symptoms are invoked, plaque growth will have occurred due to incorporation of a mass of thrombus within the intima, and the mechanism may well be important in the growth of plaques and the progression toward stable angina. Larger fissures exposing more lipid, or individuals who have a greater thrombotic potential, develop mural thrombus within the arterial lumen. This thrombus may grow and regress over some days before either totally lysing (allowing the plaque to reseal), or growing (to occlude the lumen). If the arterial lumen is occluded for a minimum period of 20 min (26) and collateral flow is inadequate, myocardial infarction may develop. Such arterial occlusions may subsequently reopen spontaneously or the thrombus may grow and propagate distally down the lumen. It is this latter group that particularly comes to necropsy.

Very little is known about the factors that invoke plaque fissuring. It is a complication of plaques with a large free lipid pool and thin fibrous cap. Knowledge of what processes are responsible for necrosis in the plaque and, thus, formation of free extracellular lipid is urgently needed. The site of predilection for rupture is at one lateral margin of the plaque, the resulting intimal dissection spiraling around the lumen. Local arterial spasm could put the collagen of the cap under mechanical strain; sudden rises in blood pressure may be involved. Other views invoke infiltration of the fibrous cap by lipid containing macrophages, leading to dissolution of the collagen.

REFERENCES

1. Davies, M. J., Woolf, N., and Robertson, W. B. (1976): Pathology of acute myocardial infarction with particular reference to occlusive coronary thrombi. *Br. Heart J.,* 38:659–664.
2. Chandler, A. B. (1974): Coronary thrombosis in myocardial infarction. Report of a workshop on the role of coronary thrombosis in the pathogenesis of acute myocardial infarction. *Am. J. Cardiol.,* 34:823–833.
3. Chapman, I. (1974): The cause-effect relationship between recent coronary artery occlusion and acute myocardial infarction. *Am. Heart J.,* 887:267–271.
4. Horie, T., Sekiguchi, M., and Hirosawa, K. (1978): Coronary thrombosis in pathogenesis of acute myocardial infarction. Histopathological study of coronary arteries in 108 necropsied cases using serial section. *Br. Heart J.,* 40:153–161.

5. Davies, M. J., and Thomas, T. (1981): The pathological basis and microanatomy of occlusive thrombus formation in human coronary arteries. *Philos. Trans. R. Soc. Lond. (Biol.)*, 294:225–229.
6. Falk, E. (1983): Plaque rupture with severe pre-existing stenosis precipitating coronary thrombosis: characteristics of coronary atherosclerotic plaques underlying fatal occlusive thrombi. *Br. Heart J.*, 50:127–134.
7. Benson, R. L. (1926): The present status of coronary arterial disease. *Arch. Path.*, 2:870–916.
8. Saphir, O., Priest, W. S., Hamburger, W. W., and Katz, L. N. (1935): Coronary arteriosclerosis, coronary thrombosis, and the resulting myocardial changes. An evaluation of their respective clinical pictures including the electrocardiographic records, based on the anatomical findings. *Am. Heart J.*, 10:567–595.
9. Paterson, J. C. (1936): Vascularization and hemorrhage of the intima of arteriosclerotic coronary arteries. *Arch. Path.*, 22:313–324.
10. Geiringer, E. (1951): Intimal vascularization and atherosclerosis. *J. Path. Bact.*, 63:201–211.
11. Barger, A. C., Beeuwkes, R., Lainey, L. L., and Silverman, K. J. (1983): Hypothesis: Vasa vasorum and neovascularization of human coronary arteries. A possible role in the pathophysiology of atherosclerosis. *N. Engl. J. Med.*, 310:175–177.
12. DeWood, M. A., Spores, J., Notske, R., Mouser, L. T., Burroughs, R., Golden, M. S., and Lang, H. T. (1980): Prevalence of total coronary occlusion during the early hours of transmural myocardial infarction. *N. Engl. J. Med.*, 303:897–902.
13. Brooks, N. (1983): Intracoronary thrombolysis in acute myocardial infarction. *Br. Heart J.*, 50:397–400.
14. Ganz, W., Geft, I., Shah, P. K., Lew, A. S., Rodriguez, L., Weiss, T., Maddahi, J., Berman, D. S., Charuzi, Y., and Swan, H. J. C. (1984): Intravenous streptokinase in evolving acute myocardial infarction. *Am. J. Cardiol.*, 53:1209–1216.
15. Erhardt, L. R., Lundman, T., and Mellstedt, H. (1973): Incorporation of 125 I-labelled fibrinogen into coronary arterial thrombi in acute myocardial infarction in man. *Lancet*, 1:387–390.
16. Fulton, W. F. M., and Sumner, D. J. (1976): 125 I-labelled fibrinogen, autoradiography and stero-arteriography in identification of coronary thrombotic occlusion in fatal myocardial infarction. *Br. Heart J.*, 38:880.
17. Terrosu, P., Ibba, G. V., Contini, G. M., and Franceschino, V. (1984): Angiographic features of the coronary arteries during intracoronary thrombolysis. *Br. Heart J.*, 2:154–163.
18. Ganz, W., Buchbinder, N., and Murcus, H. (1981): Intracoronary thrombolysis in evolving myocardial infarction. *Am. Heart J.*, 101:4–13.
19. Reduto, A., Smalling, R. W., Freund, G. C., and Gould, K. L. (1981): Intracoronary infusion of streptokinase in patients with acute myocardial infarction: effect of reperfusion on left ventricular performance. *Am. J. Cardiol.*, 48:403–409.
20. Davies, M. J., and Thomas, A. C. (1984): Thrombosis and acute coronary artery lesions in sudden cardiac ischemic death. *N. Engl. J. Med.*, 310:1137–1140.
21. Haerem, J. W. (1974): Mural platelet microthrombi and major acute lesions of main epicardial arteries in sudden coronary death. *Atherosclerosis*, 19:529–541.
22. El-Maraghi, N., and Genton, E. (1980): The relevance of platelet and fibrin thromboembolism of the coronary microcirculation with special reference to sudden cardiac death. *Circulation*, 62:936–944.
23. Vetrovec, G. W., Leinbach, R. C., Gold, H. K., and Cowley, M. J. (1982): Intracoronary thrombolysis in syndromes of unstable ischemia: Angiographic and clinical results. *Am. Heart J.*, 104:946–952.
24. Holmes, D. R., Hartzler, G. O., Smith, H. C., and Fuster, V. (1981): Coronary artery thrombosis in patients with unstable angina. *Br. Heart J.*, 45:411–416.
25. Levin, D. C., and Fallon, J. T. (1982): Significance of the angiographic morphology of localized coronary stenosis: histopathologic correlations. *Circulation*, 66:314–320.
26. Reimer, K. A., Lowe, J. E., Rasmussen, M. M., and Jennings, R. B. (1977): The wave-front phenomenon of ischemic cell death. 1. Myocardial infarct size vs duration of coronary occlusion in dogs. *Circulation*, 56:786–794.

Hammersmith Cardiology Workshop Series, Vol. 3,
edited by A. Maseri, B. E. Sobel, and S. Chierchia.
Raven Press, New York © 1987.

Postmortem Findings in Acute Myocardial Infarction

G. Baroldi

Institute of Biomedical Science, Institute Clinical Physiology CNR, 20162 Milan, Italy

In the present era of prevention of myocardial infarction and limitation of its size, the need is to briefly reconsider the whole postmortem pattern rather than to focus our attention on the frequency of one or a few parameters only. This seems necessary for a better understanding of the meaning of morphologic findings and pathogenesis of functional disorders and structural changes.

This review is based on 200 consecutive fatal cases (within 30 days) of clinically and histologically documented acute myocardial infarction (AMI) associated or not with hypertension. No other cardiac or noncardiac diseases were present (1,2). A distinction was made between 145 cases without (AMI, first episode) and 55 cases with extensive myocardial fibrosis (AMI, second episode). In the latter cases, monofocal and massive myocardial fibrosis involving more than 10% of the left ventricular mass has been considered as a possible morphologic hallmark of chronic ischemic heart disease (IHD).

MYOCARDIAL FINDINGS

The pathognomonic myocardial necrosis ("coagulation necrosis") of the infarct was, in general, monofocal, with a size ranging from less than 10% to more than 50% of the left ventricular mass (Table 1). The majority (72.5%) of fatal AMIs occurred as first episodes. Most (63.6%) of the AMIs with previous extensive

TABLE 1. *Percentage distribution of infarct size in 200 consecutive acute infarct cases without (AMI, first episode) and with (AMI, second episode) extensive myocardial fibrosis*

Source (cases)	Infarct size (%)					
	<10	11–20	21–30	31–40	41–50	>50
AMI, first episode (145)	22%	21%	22%	16%	10%	9%
AMI, second episode (55)	51	13	22	5	7	2
Total cases (200)	30	19	22	13	9	7

fibrosis were small infarcts (<20% size). Death following an acute infarct does not seem related to a large infarct (48.5% with an infarct size <20%; only 16% with a size >40%). A similar lack of relationship exists between infarct size and survival (Table 2).

Most of the patients (64.2%) with a small infarct (<20%) had the shortest survival (<2 days). In contrast, half of the patients (53.3%) with the longest survival (11 to 30 days) showed large infarcts (>20%). These findings (p <0.01) were similar in both AMI groups, which also showed no significant divergency in age distribution.

In not one instance was it possible to document different histological ages in the same infarcted area (e.g., the central portion in healing phase surrounded by an area of necrotic myocardium with polymorphonuclear infiltration). In humans there is no morphologic proof that expansion (or progression) of the primitive coagulation necrosis may occur when the latter is established.

Two other types of "nonischemic" myocardial necrosis were associated with infarct necrosis (3). In all AMI cases, around the infarct and in other noninfarcted regions, coagulative myocytolysis (contraction band necrosis) was demonstrated (also observed in 86% of 208 sudden coronary death cases without a history of IHD (4). This lesion is experimentally reproduced by catecholamines (5). The other nonischemic necrosis is again a primitive myofibrillar damage characteristic for low output syndrome (colliquative myocytolysis) found in 38% of AMI cases. More frequent in chronic cases (54.2% AMIs second; 31.7% AMI first) and with longer survival (28.5%, 37.8%, and 50% with 2, 3 to 11, and more than 11 days, respectively), it was mainly located in the subendocardial and perivascular myocardial layers, usually preserved by coagulation infarct necrosis.

The clear-cut structural and functional differences among the three types of myocardial necroses indicate different dysionisms and pathogenic mechanisms. Complications and death following AMI seem more related to nonischemic factors, likely linked with regional sympathetic overtone or catecholamine depletion or both. In human AMIs, the so-called "border zone" appears to be the nonischemic normal myocardium at risk of other metabolic disorders. Similarly in man, the "wavefront phenomenon" more than endocardium to epicardium progression of the infarct looks to be establishment of new metabolic damage in cases with

TABLE 2. *Percentage distribution of infarct size in relation to survival in 200 consecutive acute infarct cases*

Survival (days)	Infarct size (%)					
	<10	11–20	21–30	31–40	41–50	>50
<2 (70)	48	16	16	13	1	6
3–10 (74)	23	12	32	14	12	7
11–30 (56)	16	31	16	14	14	9
Total cases (200)	30	18	22	14	9	7

complications (e.g., malignant arrhythmias, cardiogenic failure). Accordingly, protection from the latter seems a concept more appropriate than limitation of infarct size. In the dog, ventricular fibrillation and coagulative myocytolysis following 1 hr occlusion of the left circumflex branch were prevented by beta blockers (6).

VASCULAR FINDINGS

Advanced atherosclerotic plaque with severe ($>70\%$) luminal diameter reduction of the subepicardial coronary arteries was present in 88% of AMI first episodes and in 98% of AMI second. In the latter group, there was more than 90% stenosis ($p < 0.01$), and severe stenosis in three main vessels was also significantly higher ($p < 0.05$). An identical trend was observed in sudden coronary death (Table 3).

The prevalence of small infarcts in "chronic" AMI patients, despite significantly more severe obstructive lesions; the lack of a relationship between the number of severe stenoses and the infarct size (Table 4) and extensive myocardial fibrosis; and the high frequency of severe stenosis in noncardiac patients (66%) and healthy subjects who have died by accident (39%; with 52% over 60 years) are all findings

TABLE 3. *Percentage distribution of maximal lumen reduction and number of main subepicardial vessels with severe ($>70\%$) stenosis*

Source (cases)	Maximal lumen reduction (%)				Vessels ($>70\%$)		
	<69	70	80	90	1	2	3
AMI 1st (145)	12	20	31	37	42	33	13
AMI 2nd (55)	2	14	20	64	29	40	29
SCD 1st (133)	35	16	29	20	30	25	10
SCD 2nd (75)	7	11	18	64	17	35	41
NC (100)	34	11	24	31	26	18	22
AD (97)	61	19	14	6	23	13	3

AMI, acute myocardial infarcts; SCD, sudden coronary death; NC, noncardiac patients; AD, "healthy" subjects dying from accident.
1st without and 2nd with extensive fibrosis.

TABLE 4. *Lack of relation between infarct size and number of severe stenosis ($>70\%$) in 200 consecutive total acute infarct cases*

Infarct size (%)	Lumen reduction (%)						
	<69	>70	in	1	2	3	Total
<20	7(7.2)	90(92.7)		39(40.2)	37(38.1)	14(14.4)	97(100)
>20	10(9.7)	93(90.2)		39(37.8)	34(33.0)	20(19.4)	103(100)
Total	17(8.5)	183(91.5)		78(39.0)	71(35.5)	34(17.0)	200(100)

$p > 0.05$ for trend.

that contradict a direct cause-effect relationship between atherosclerotic stenosis and ischemic heart disease, in general, and myocardial infarction, in particular. Furthermore, there is no critical point of obstruction that triggers the latter. The first episode of angina, infarction, or sudden death may occur with or without one or more severe stenoses, which preexisted months or years without manifestations despite an often stressful life-style. The sudden death of marathon runners is a good example.

All the previous facts point out the importance of the compensatory role of collaterals in the natural history of coronary atherosclerosis (7). The dramatic increase in caliber of the normal collaterals shown post-mortem is maximal with the highest number of stenoses, without relation to myocardial damage. Their existence questions the classic view that thrombus formed at the site of ruptured plaque is the cause of the infarct. In the 200 AMIs, an occlusive thrombus, when present (41%), was always found in severe (93%), concentric (90%), and long stenosis (94%) formed by an atheromatous plaque with extensive lymphoplasmacellular infiltration (92%). The frequency of the acute occlusive thrombus in relation to infarct size showed a significant trend ($p < 0.01$) toward increasing frequency of the thrombus with increasing infarct size. This may explain divergencies in literature. No evidence of lysis of the thrombus was seen. On the other hand, lysis or retraction of experimental intraluminal occlusive thrombus in normal canine coronary artery begins only after 10 days (8), being unlikely in atherosclerotic "atheromatous" plaque with diminished or abolished fibrinolytic activity (9).

Rather than frequency, the basic question is whether or not the thrombotic occlusion of a small residual lumen (often with a diameter of less than 100 μm) bypassed by numerous collaterals with a diameter greater than 500 μm may determine a total blockage of the regional nutrient flow. This finding, the occurrence of occlusive thrombus without infarction, and the experiment (in the dog, occlusion of severe stenosis lasting a few days does not determine infarction or other morphofunctional changes provided for dramatic increase of collaterals) (10) support the view that other functional mechanisms (spasm, extravascular compression of the intramyocardial system by regional impairment of contractility) may play an important role in establishing the infarct. In addition, by mechanical action or blockage of flow in plaque vessels by increased peripheral resistance, they may determine hemorrhage and/or rupture of a plaque, with possible secondary thrombus formation (highest frequency in largest infarct). A primitive rupture of the plaque is contradicted by the negative finding of cholesterol emboli, often seen in the brain, spleen, and kidney, in the infarcted region, and in the normal myocardium of ischemic patients. Finally, both mechanisms may interpret the cineangiographic imaging of coronary occlusion (11), keeping in mind that (a) a spasm may be resistant to vasodilators; (b) a thrombus, when present, may release vasoactive substances; (c) the so-called thrombus recovered at surgery according to its description (evident layering of blood elements) seems more a coagulum than a thrombus; and (d) we still are missing the view at zero time. One hour is too long a period of time to establish what is primary or secondary.

In conclusion, the degree and number of stenoses do not predict onset, complications, infarct size, and death in the natural history of IHD. The type and timing of occlusion are still a matter of investigation, and other nonischemic pathogenic mechanisms seem important in explaining the whole pattern of this disease.

In this still controversial contest, a morphopathological finding, always described but never considered, deserves further investigation in relation to the natural history of ischemic heart disease. Advanced atherosclerotic plaques frequently show an inflammatory lymphoplasmacellular reaction of unknown nature (an autoimmune process?). In a quantitative study (12), correlation of the main variables of the atherosclerotic plaque, including this inflammatory reaction, has been carried out on 3,640 selected coronary sections in different ischemic groups (acute infarcts, chronic IHD surgically bypassed, and sudden coronary death without a history of IHD) and healthy controls.

The inflammatory reaction showed (a) an increasing frequency and severity, with increasing intimal thickness and lumen reduction being already present with a low value of the latter and related to proteoglycan accumulation (Table 5); (b) a significant higher frequency and severity in ischemic patients, particularly in AMIs, with respect to controls, independent of the degree of intimal thickness and lumen reduction (Table 6); (c) in single patients, inflammatory reaction that was demonstrable in all or most of the plaques in contrast to controls; (d) inflammatory elements that showed a peculiar tropism for the pericoronary nervous structures; (e) significant topographical relation with areas undergoing coagulative myocytolysis (contraction band necrosis) or infarction (coagulation necrosis); (f) prevalence (88%)

TABLE 5. *Lymphoplasmacellular inflammatory reaction (IR), proteoglycan accumulation (PA), and atheroma (AT) in percent relation to intimal thickness and lumen reduction*

Intimal thickness (μm)	IR	PA	AT	Lumen reduction (%)	IR	PA	AT
300	2	3	2	<50	32	52	27
600	28	50	16	50–69	62	70	54
1000	54	69	43	70–79	74	71	75
2000	73	75	69	80–89	84	71	77
>2000	79	57	76	>90	82	58	74

TABLE 6. *Lymphoplasmacellular inflammatory reaction (IR) of coronary atherosclerotic plaque in different population groups*

	No. cases	IR(%)	No. stenosis	IR(%)	Mild	Moderate	Severe
Acute infarct	100	100	491	75	34	21	20
Chronic IHD	50	88	175	74	32	13	29
Sudden death	208	83	1084	55	29	16	10
Healthy controls	97	64	371	41	22	14	5

TABLE 7. *Percentage distribution of the length of atherosclerotic plaque with lumen reduction*

Stenosis	(Total section)	Length (mm)			
		<3	3–10	11–30	30
Less than 69					
Acute infarct	(264)	86	8	4	2
Chronic IHD	(77)	1	—	53	46
Sudden death	(671)	9	20	43	29
Healthy controls	(307)	14	13	17	56
Greater than 70					
Acute infarct	(227)	60	20	13	7
Chronic IHD	(98)	2	—	81	17
Sudden death	(413)	2	29	41	28
Healthy controls	(64)	3	20	23	53

of short (<10 mm), severe stenosis with inflammatory reaction in acute infarcts (Table 7).

These findings may justify, as a working hypothesis, the concept of "active" or "inactive" plaque linked with an active or inactive phase of the disease. The inflammatory reaction could be the possible trigger of spasm and/or regional impairment of the contractility and accelerated radial progression of the plaque in AMI patients by the direct release of an active substance or by irritation and/or degeneration of the pericoronary nerves. Keeping in mind that our "healthy controls" have a high probability of becoming ischemic patients, their milder inflammatory reaction may represent an early risk factor or sign of still silent ischemic heart disease.

REFERENCES

1. Baroldi, G., Radice, F., Schmid, G., and Leone, A. (1974): Morphology of acute myocardial infarction in relation to coronary thrombosis. *Am. Heart J.*, 87:65–75.
2. Silver, M. D., Baroldi, G., and Mariani, F. (1980): The relationship between acute occlusive thrombi and myocardial infarction studied in 100 consecutive patients. *Circulation* 61:219–227.
3. Baroldi, G. (1975): Different types of myocardial necrosis in coronary heart disease: a pathophysiologic review of their functional significance. *Am. Heart J.*, 89:742–752.
4. Baroldi, G., Falzi, G., and Mariani, F. (1979): Sudden coronary death. A postmortem study in 208 selected cases compared to 97 "control" subjects. *Am. Heart J.*, 98:20–31.
5. Todd, G. L., Baroldi, G., Pieper, G. M., Clayton, F., and Eliot, R. S. (1985): Experimental catecholamine-induced necrosis. I. Morphology quantification and regional distribution of acute contraction band lesions. *J. Mol. Cell. Cardiol.*, 17:220–231.
6. Baroldi, G., Silver, M. D., Lixfeld, W., and McGregor, D. C. (1977): Irreversible myocardial damage resembling catecholamine necrosis secondary to acute coronary occlusion in dog: its prevention by propranolol. *J. Mol. Cell. Cardiol.*, X:687–691.
7. Baroldi, G., and Scomazzoni, G. (1967): Coronary circulation in the normal and pathologic heart. U.S. Government Printing Office, Washington, D.C., p. 304.
8. Weisse, A. B., Lehan, P. H., Ettinger, P. O., Moschos, C. B., and Regan, T. J. (1969): The fate of experimentally induced coronary thrombosis. *Am. J. Cardiol.*, 23:229–237.
9. Myasnikov, A. L., Chazov, E. I., Koshevnikova, T. L., and Nikolaeva, L. F. (1961): Some

new data on the occurrence of coronary thrombosis in conjunction with atherosclerosis. *J. Atheroscl. Res.,* 1:401–412.

10. Khouri, E. M., Gregg, D. E., and Lowesohn, H. S. (1968): Flow in the major branches of the left coronary artery during experimental coronary insufficiency in the unanesthetized dog. *Circ. Res.,* 23:99–109.

11. DeWood, M. A., Spores, J., Notske, R., et al. (1980): Prevalence of total coronary occlusion during the early hours of transmural myocardial infarction. *N. Engl. J. Med.,* 303:897–902.

12. Baroldi, G., Silver, M. D., Mariani, F., and Giuliano, G. Variation of coronary atherosclerotic plaque morphology in relation to clinical patterns of ischemic heart disease and healthy controls (presented for publication).

Hammersmith Cardiology Workshop Series, Vol. 3,
edited by A. Maseri, B. E. Sobel, and S. Chierchia.
Raven Press, New York © 1987.

Précis of the Discussion: Section IV

MECHANISMS OF ACUTE MYOCARDIAL INFARCTION

Attilio Maseri

David Kelly commented about the anatomy in non-Q wave infarction as, in his opinion, the incidence of total obstruction in these patients is not so high. Michel Bertrand agreed.

Alberto Malliani was absolutely fascinated by Michael Davies' presentation, but he cautioned that in his beautiful presentation there was a big absence: the nervous system, as the heart is not denervated. Paul Hugenholtz asked Michael Davies whether it was possible that many patients who do well after unstable angina may do so because the thrombosed artery recanalizes. Michael Davies specified that recanalization to a pathologist means something has been occluded by thrombus and has been reopened by many new channels. However, an awful lot of thrombi over fissures almost certainly lyse: "You begin to get organization of the thrombus that is in the fissure, and so the thing is sealed off and you are back to a stable situation. One of the studies we are doing at the moment is to look for evidence of just such restabilized plaques, and you can find them very easily. You can still see the fissure track, but it is filled up with new connective tissue and it has been sealed off."

Giorgio Baroldi was asked whether the type of inflammatory perivascular reaction he showed was a secondary or primary phenomenon, which might play a role in the pathogenesis of infarction. Giorgio Baroldi said that in his opinion this was a secondary phenomenon.

Attilio Maseri attempted to find areas of consensus: "Let us see if, out of the confusion, there is some ground on which everyone agrees. It seems to me that the advent of coronary arteriography in the early phases of infarction has proven that the vast majority of infarctions in the early stages have an occluded vessel, then the vessel opens up. This is to me considerable progress compared to what I knew six years ago."

Dr. Baroldi emphasized that in his sudden coronary death series, 15% had acute occluding thrombi and about 22% had mural thrombi: "Red thrombus and true thrombus should not be confused. The true thrombus is a completely different morphological entity with fibrin and platelets in organization. The red thrombus is an aggregate of red cell and fibrin that you can see any time in the venous system."

Attilio Maseri continued: "Sudden death is a syndrome and, unfortunately, the pathological and clinical studies should be combined because you must have the clinical information of what the patient died from. If the relatives tell us that the patient had typical chest pain and within 10–50 minutes he died, then this is sudden cardiac ischemic death, no matter what we find in the coronary arteries. The coronary arteries may be clean; you can have a patient with variant angina, spasm, ST segment elevation, or VF who dies and, even though his coronary arteries are clean, this is sudden cardiac ischemic death. Therefore, I think in postmortem studies it would be important that the material is collected with a clear clinical input, or with a questionnaire so that sudden death is not something that becomes coronary or noncoronary, depending upon whether you find or you do not find a coronary plaque.''

Michael Oliver mentioned the quite extensive coronary arteriographic studies by Dr. Leonard Cobb and his group in Seattle, Washington, in individuals who have been resuscitated from ventricular fibrillation. These studies failed to show any particular occlusive pattern in any coronary arterial system, although it is impossible for angiography to detect the sort of phenomena that Michael Davies is describing.

Michael Davies clarified, ''I have never said that in sudden death there is a high incidence of total occlusion by thrombus. If there was a high incidence of total occlusion by thrombus in sudden ischemic death, you would anticipate that the incidence of infarction after resuscitation would be very high. What I think we are saying is that a patient who drops dead has fissured a plaque and what the resuscitation studies show you is that fissuring a plaque is not inevitably followed by occlusive thrombus. They show you exactly the ratio, a little more than 10%, that is the percentage that have occluded after their fissure. The rest have healed their fissure, and I would see the fact that not all patients get an infarct as being rather supportive of the views we have been expressing rather than the other way round.''

Michael Oliver replied, ''He does not answer my question. He just said that the rest, namely 90%, have healed their fissure. Now, I am sure that may well be true, but have we evidence for that?''

Robert Slama mentioned the experience of 67 patients who died during Holter monitoring, although this group of patients is not pure because they were under monitoring for some reason, either rhythm disturbances or chest pain. Of these, very few of them had ST modifications before they died, so they might have died of a primary arrhythmia (in six cases it was AV block and in 61 cases it was VF).

Michael Oliver asked about the nature of the plaque: ''What proportion of middle-aged men has florid lipid-rich lesion acting as a major obstructive lesion, and what proportion has a heavily fibrotic lesion which is also acting as an obstructive lesion, perhaps to the same degree?''

Michael Davies replied, ''The higher the grade of stenosis the more likely it is to be predominantly fibrous. The majority of lipid plaques of this sort are hovering around the 50% diameter stenosis point. A plaque at that middle order and high lipid that is undergoing change is the most likely to cause an infarct or crescendo angina or sudden death. Most people have one or two of them, some people have lots of them. There doesn't seem to be much pattern about it.''

Michael Oliver: ''That is the perspective I wanted, but now that throws in another question because it means that at coronary arteriography, we mostly ignore lesions around 50% and we pay maximal attention to those of 75% or 80%, which may provide no indication of sudden death.''

Michael Davies: ''Well, that is exactly what I was saying. You cannot expect to detect at angiography a lesion that is potentially going to cause an infarct six months later.''

Attilio Maseri added, ''If we are going to accept that plaques in the 50% region are the most dangerous, because they could become ulcerated and active and therefore develop infarction, what should we do? I am quite worried about the fact that now if one begins to pay attention also to those minor lesions, the number of patients for angioplasty or surgery will rise, the waiting lists will become longer, and the costs of medical care will escalate.''

Robert Slama: ''If you look at normal people who die by accident, a 50% type of lesion is very frequent, and they may have cholesterol, but I don't think it is a trigger point which we need to worry about because, if it were so important, everybody would die.''

Editorial comment: A. Maseri

As postmortem studies become more and more careful they reveal new information. As angiographic studies are performed earlier in infarction and unstable coronary syndromes in general, they show the dynamic nature of the occlusive process. It is natural that our attention is captured by what we see, but we should try to put it into a broader perspective before jumping to attractive conclusions. It is important to study carefully appropriate controls. In my opinion, it is important to note that Michael Davies found plaque fissures with intraintimal or mural thrombus also in about 10% of controls; that Robert Slama reminded us that 50% stenosing lipid-rich plaques are quite frequent in the population at large; and that the mechanisms that trigger ventricular fibrillation in some ischemic attacks or in some infarctions are still unknown.

Therefore, it may be wise not to commit ourselves to attractive conclusions for our research and for our daily practice. Taking due note of all new convincing findings and fitting them with an open, curious mind, into the jigsaw puzzle of ischemic heart disease remains the most fascinating aspect of research and of clinical practice.

diffuse, and occurring either spontaneously or in response to vasoconstrictor stimuli which normally only cause a minor change in vessel caliber. Other possible mechanisms, potentially responsible for a transient impairment in regional myocardial supply, include (a) a normal increase in vasomotor tone still within the physiological range at the site of a severe, eccentric plaque; (b) transient intravascular plugging by blood constituents; (c) constriction of collaterals; and (d) altered vasomotion of the small vessels.

This chapter will be limited to the discussion of mechanisms responsible for coronary vasoconstriction involving both epicardial coronary arteries as well as small, resistive vessels. The role of platelet aggregation and thrombosis are discussed elsewhere in this volume.

CORONARY VASOSPASM

Definition

As discussed earlier, we define coronary vasospasm as *an abnormal* increase in coronary vasomotor tone involving one or more epicardial coronary arteries, localized or diffuse, to a long vascular segment. It can be observed in ''angiographically normal'' coronary arteries or, more often, be superimposed on atherosclerotic narrowings of variable severity; it can occur spontaneously or be induced by various pharmacological or physical maneuvers that normally only cause the vessel to constrict to a rather small extent. By our definition, we imply that the mechanism responsible for coronary vasospasm is an abnormal, exaggerated response, well beyond the physiological range, to physiological stimuli which, under normal circumstances, only exert a moderate regulatory effect, or to pharmacological maneuvers which are otherwise ineffective. The major aim of this definition is to separate cases of frank spasm, as observed in Prinzmetal's variant angina, from other types of vasoconstriction either of lesser extent or involving different parts of the coronary circulation, which are likely to play a pathophysiological role in other clinical forms of angina pectoris. We believe that this distinction has more than a purely semantic importance, since different pathogenetic mechanisms are probably responsible for the different forms of coronary vasoconstriction, which, in turn, should require specific therapeutic interventions.

Clinical Manifestations

The most classical clinical manifestation of coronary spasm is represented by the so-called ''variant form'' of angina, originally described by Prinzmetal and associates. Clinically, these patients usually present with angina at rest, and may or may not have variable degrees of limitation or exercise capacity. Typically, anginal attacks occur in the early hours of the morning and, often, in a ''cluster'' pattern. They are usually of short duration and respond promptly to sublingual nitrates. Those patients who show an impaired effort tolerance usually exhibit a very large variability in exercise capacity, which results from variable degrees of exercise-induced coronary vasoconstriction, superimposed on fixed atheromatous lesions of different severity.

Usually, the electrocardiogram taken during an attack shows the characteristic pattern of transient ST segment elevation, which results from severe transmural myocardial ischemia; peaking or pseudonormalization of inverted or flat T waves are also often observed, as a result of lesser degrees of transmural ischemia (4). Transient subendocardial ischemia with ST segment depression is also frequently seen, especially when the flow impairment is partially compensated for by collaterals, when spasm is incomplete and nonocclusive or when it involves a small branch. Almost invariably, patients alternate different electrocardiographic patterns in the same ECG leads, depending upon the severity of the underlying ischemic process. As in acute myocardial infarction, the ECG changes are well localized and it is usually possible to identify, from the leads involved, the location of ischemia and, to a certain extent, to predict the vessel undergoing spasm.

In the large majority of patients with active disease it is possible to reproduce spasm (and its consequences) by a variety of provocative maneuvers. Ergonovine maleate, given intravenously, is by far the most effective way of reproducing the patients' symptoms, and the test is positive in more than 90% of the cases; prolonged hyperventilation and exercise yield a lesser incidence of positive results (6), about 50%. Other pharmacological agents such as metacholine, epinephrine, and histamine have also been reported to precipitate spasm in some patients. Their clinical application, however, is limited.

Several articles have reported the association between coronary spasm and acute myocardial infarction (7,8). It is certain that in some patients with variant angina, prolonged spasm occurring in both "normal" and diseased coronary arteries can result in persistent occlusion, leading eventually to vascular thrombosis and myocardial cell necrosis. Whether or not spasm plays a role in the pathogenetic events initiating other forms of acute myocardial infarction is still open to conjecture.

Pathogenetic Mechanisms

After 10 years of intense basic and clinical research, the mechanisms responsible for coronary spasm still remain obscure. On the one hand, several clinical studies aimed at investigating the role of specific mechanisms have failed; on the other, it has become increasingly apparent that there is no single trigger for spasm, as different mechanisms operate in different patients and, probably, even in the same patient at different times.

A causal role for coronary alpha as well as serotonergic receptors and acute imbalance fo the thromboxane/prostacyclin system had been proposed for the pathogenesis of spasm. Carefully conducted clinical trials, however, failed to prevent spasm by alpha blockers (phentolamine and prazosin) (9,10), serotonergic blockers (ketanserin) (11,12), prostacyclin (13), and by platelet thromboxane inhibitors (14,15).

In a group of 30 consecutive patients with active variant angina, we recently performed a study based on serial provocative testing with different stimuli acting via different receptors or mechanisms (6). In the majority of cases (82%), spasm could be reproduced by two different maneuvers and in a large proportion (40%) by three. This observation indicates that spasm is likely to result from mechanisms beyond specific agonist-receptor interactions, probably related to the transport of calcium across the cell membrane and/or its extrusion from the sarcoplasmic reticulum. The hypothesis is supported by the well-known efficacy of calcium blockers in preventing spasm and by the ability of maneuvers such as hyperventilation, which increases the availability of calcium ions for smooth muscle contraction, to induce it.

An important clinical clue to the pathogenesis of spasm is the fact that, among other powerful vasoconstrictors, ergonovine is the only one that consistently produces spasm in the vast majority of patients with active disease. The drug is active even at extremely low doses (2–10 µg) when given by the intracoronary route (16). Considering the very rapid coronary transit time, the very low dose administered, and the negligible recirculation, this observation implies that ergonovine has an extremely high affinity for the receptor(s), or whatever other mechanisms responsible for spasm.

The role of the endothelium in modulating and mediating the response of the vascular smooth muscle to various vasoactive stimuli has become increasingly apparent, and the possibility that the loss of endothelial continuity could partially account for the local coronary supersensitivity observed in vasospastic angina has been considered. The hypothesis is certainly attractive and partially supported by isolated observation showing the ability of the muscarinic agonists metacholine (17) and acetylcholine (18) to precipitate spasm in some patients. Physiologically, stimulation of muscarinic vascular receptors results in endothelium-mediated vasodilatation, which is converted to vasoconstriction when the endothelium is removed. The possible role of acetylcholine-mediated spasm is also supported by the observation that episodes of vasospastic myocardial ischemia mainly occur at night and in the early morning hours, when parasympathetic tone is at its highest level (19). However, some degree of endothelial denudation is likely to be present in most patients with coronary atheroma, while only a minority of them present with vasospastic angina. Furthermore, endothelial damage probably occurs in all patients undergoing coronary angioplasty and yet spasm is observed only rarely during the procedure.

Finally, studies conducted on isolated human coronaries suggest that, also in the presence of an intact endothelium, actylcholine, at least *in vitro,* causes human coronary arteries to constrict (20).

Unlike most other animal species, human coronary arteries exhibit, *in vitro,* spontaneous cyclical changes in tone which are exacerbated by vasoconstrictors, such as norepinephrine, and abolished by nitroglycerin, calcium blockers, and lignocaine (20). This spontaneous, intrinsic activity is probably suppressed or reduced, *in vivo,* by several yet unidentified, negative feedbacks. Lack or failure of one or more of these could result in paroxysmal bursts of coronary vasoconstrictor activity. Such an interpretation could explain the cyclical nature of episodes of vasospastic angina and their regular periodicity so often observed in patients going through a very active phase of the disease.

Whichever the underlying mechanisms, the final common pathway to spasm is likely to be related to an increased conductance of the cell membrane to calcium ions, which can be mobilized by a variety of mechanisms and agonist-receptor interactions.

"PHYSIOLOGICAL" CHANGES IN CORONARY VASOMOTOR TONE

The definition of coronary atherosclerosis as "a hardening of the arteries" has led to the belief that coronary stenoses are unbedded in a "fixed," immobile shell of fibrotic, calcified atheroma. In fact, stenoses morphology is quite variable, and although some arterial segments involved by the atherosclerotic process are indeed fixed, others exhibit an eccentric residual lumen, partially circumscribed by an arc of normal arterial wall which still retains the capability of undergoing dynamic changes in smooth muscle tone. This observation prompted McAlpin to formulate a theory according to which a normal increase in vasomotor tone, still within the physiological range and occurring at the level of severe eccentric epicardial strictures, could be responsible for spasm. This author proposed a distinction between "normal" and "abnormal" coronary vasoconstriction, the two mechanisms being, respectively, responsible for spasm in stenosed and in normal coronary arteries (21). His view has been contradicted by objective measurements obtained, at angiography, in patients with different degrees of coronary atheroma in whom spasm was induced by ergonovine (22). Furthermore, should this theory be correct, one would expect spasm to occur much more frequently than actually observed in patients with severe coronary artery disease.

Physiological changes in coronary vasomotor tone at the site of eccentric lesions are likely to be important in the pathophysiology of other forms of angina pectoris, in particular, in patients with chronic effort angina exhibiting frequent ischemic episodes occurring without any obvious precipitating cause and in those reporting a large variability in exercise capacity.

Indeed, a series of studies based on ambulatory ECG and arterial pressure monitoring have shown that, also in patients presenting with the most typical forms of effort angina, the majority of episodes is ischemia occurring during unrestricted activity are not preceded by an increase in the major determinants of myocardial oxygen consumption. These episodes most often occur for levels of heart rate or rate pressure product well below those observed at the beginning of exercise-induced ST depression. The level of rate-pressure product at which ischemia occurs is widely variable, and the patient can often sustain prolonged periods of tachycardia and hypertension, sometimes exceeding those observed during exercise testing, without exhibiting significant ST segment changes (23). These findings clearly indicate that, for these patients too, angina is likely to result also from transient impairment of coronary blood supply rather than only from an excessive increase in myocardial demand in the presence of a limited, "fixed" coronary flow reserve.

The causes of transient impairment in myocardial perfusion responsible for acute ischemia in these patients are, once more, probably multiple. Spasm, as defined above, is unlikely to play a significant role for a series of reasons, which are listed below.

First of all, the diurnal distribution of episodes of acute ischemia is completely different in patients with variant angina and in those with effort angina. In the former, ischemic events prevail in the period between 12 and 6 A.M., with a peak incidence at 4–5 A.M.; in the latter, attacks predominantly occur in the daytime and peak between 12 and 3 P.M. (19). In effort angina, the incidence of ischemic episodes parallels the circadian variation of heart rate and blood pressure: The higher the levels of heart rate and blood pressure, the more frequent ischemia. In variant angina, the opposite applies. Finally, the response to vasoconstrictor stimuli is also different. Ergonovine is positive practically in all patients with "active" variant angina. Its administration usually results in occlusive spasm of the epicardial coronary arteries and ST segment elevation on the electrocardiogram. By contrast, only 30% of patients with effort angina respond to ergonovine (24). The doses required to elicit a positive response are higher than in variant angina; the electrocardiogram invariably shows ST segment depression (and never elevation), and diffuse constriction is observed at angiography, with some increase in severity of epicardial coronary lesions. Unlike variant angina, it is usually difficult to predict the vessel(s) responsible for ischemia from the location of the ST segment depression on the ECG. Hyperventilation, often positive in variant angina, is never positive in effort angina.

The possibility for physiological changes in stenoses severity to play a role in the pathophysiology of effort angina is suggested by clinical angiographic and anatomical observations. Physiological stimuli, such as isometric (25) and dynamic (26) exercise, can result in constriction of severe coronary stenoses, which is prevented or reversed by nitroglycerin. Postmortem studies have shown that a large proportion of coronary lesions are eccentric and retain the capacity of underlying changes in cross-sectional area since the lumen is partially surrounded by an area of normal medial smooth muscle (27). Finally, a marked improvement in exercise tolerance is observed in about 30% of patients with effort angina following sublingual nitrates. The improvement in exercise time, symptoms, and ST segment changes occurs despite the fact that higher levels of rate-pressure product are achieved (28). This suggests that the mechanism by which nitrates are beneficial in these patients is not just an effect on myocardial metabolic demand related to a decreased venous return, but also an improvement in coronary blood supply. It is worth noting that the calcium antagonist verapamil, which has only minor effects on peripheral veins, produces, in the same patients, a similar improvement in effort tolerance.

Apart from the effect on epicardial coronary arteries, nitrates can improve coronary perfusion by dilatation of collaterals and, possibly, by preventing or relieving constriction of smaller vessels. The established belief that the vascular territory distal to a "critical" lesion is, by definition, "maximally vasodilated" probably only applies to some animal models. There is evidence to suggest that, also in the presence of hemodynamically significant strictures, the distal, resistive component still retains the capability of vasodilating (and of vasoconstricting). In an elegant animal experiment, Heusch and Deutz (29) showed that cardiac sympathetic stimulation can elicit an increase in distal coronary resistance, which is inversely related to the severity of the stenosis applied to the epicardial coronary artery. The more the reactive hyperemic response (a physiological index of stenosis severity) is impaired, the more distal constriction is observed following sympathetic stimulation. The response is partially abolished by phentolamine but not by prazosin, suggesting that the effect is mediated by postsynaptic alpha receptors of the 2 subtype. Recent data from our institution also indicate that, in patients with severe disease, alpha-mediated constriction of distal coronary arteries could contribute to the development of ischemia induced by dynamic exercise (30).

Persistence of an ischemic response to exercise testing is not uncommon after successful angioplasty. Although this observation is often attributed to angiographic underestimation of diffuse disease or to distal embolization, the possibility that "small vessel" constriction could still limit adequate supply despite removal of the epicardial lesion should be kept in mind. Finally, the contribution of distal coronary arteries in limiting flow reserve is more than a hypothesis in patients with "syndrome X," who present with typical angina, usually related to physical activity or emotions, a positive exercise test, and normal epicardial coronary arteries. Coronary vasodilatory reserve, as assessed by dipyridamole administration, has been shown to be markedly impaired in these patients (31). The mechanisms responsible for this impairment are not known.

Pathogenetic Mechanisms

As discussed earlier, there is evidence to indicate that stimulation of the sympathetic outflow to the heart can produce coronary vasoconstriction, especially when severe atheromatous lesions are present. The effect can involve epicardial coronary arteries and increase the severity of pliable lesions as well as cause an increase in distal resistance secondary to constriction of smaller vessels. Accordingly, all physiological stimuli that result in cardiovascular sympathetic overactivity have the potential for causing coronary vasoconstriction and for impairing regional myocardial perfusion in the presence of severe atheromatous lesions. As a consequence, conditions such as isometric and dynamic exercise, emotions, exposure to cold, heavy meals, and cigarette smoking, which have been long known to precipitate or facilitate transient acute ischemia, are likely to operate not only by increasing myocardial metabolic requirements, but also by decreasing myocardial perfusion or by limiting its adequate increase.

Observations obtained in patients with effort angina undergoing ambulatory ECG and blood pressure monitoring have shown that episodes of ischemia that occur during normal daily life are not necessarily preceded, but are invariably accompanied, by an increase in both heart rate and arterial pressure (23). The increase is not related to the presence or absence of angina, and it progresses, in a parallel fashion, with the development of the ST segment depression. There are at least two possible explanations for this observation. The first is that tachycardia and hypertension are caused by reflex activation of the sympathetic outflow to the heart, resulting from ischemia. This interpretation is supported by experimental data showing the existence of a "cardio-cardiac" sympathetic reflex elicited by a variety of stimuli, including ischemia (32). The second, and more appealing, is that primary sympathetic activation of the cardiovascular system causes, on the one hand, the blood pressure and heart rate to increase and, on the other, the coronary arteries to constrict. In this context, different degrees of background sympathetic activity, as well as a variable responsiveness of the coronary circulation to sympathetic stimuli, could account for the wide variation in both exercise capacity and levels of myocardial oxygen consumption at which "spontaneous" episodes occur in these patients.

The role of other mechanisms potentially capable of inducing coronary vasoconstriction severe enough to cause ischemia is yet to be established. The factors regulating coronary smooth muscle tone are multiple and still poorly understood, and even sympathetically mediated vasoconstriction probably results from the complex interplay of multiple mediators and feedback mechanisms.

However, the preliminary observation that exercise-induced ischemia can, in some patients, be improved by intracoronary alpha blockers (30) supports the hypothesis that the sympathetic nervous system could play an important role in the pathophysiology of this syndrome.

REFERENCES

1. Chierchia, S., Lazzari, M., Simonetti, I., and Maseri, A. (1980): Hemodynamic monitoring in angina at rest. *Herz*, 5:189–198.
2. Maseri, A., L'Abbate, A., and Ballestra, A. M. (1977): Coronary vasospasm in angina pectoris. *Lancet*, 1:713–171.
3. Maseri, A., Parodi, O., Severi, S., and Pesola, A. (1976): Transient transmural reduction of myocardial blood flow, demonstrated by thallium-201 scintigraphy: a cause of variant angina. *Circulation*, 54:280–288.
4. Chierchia, S., Brunelli, C., Simonetti, I., Lazzari, M., and Maseri, A. (1980): Sequence of events in angina at rest: primary reduction in coronary flow. *Circulation*, 61:759–768.
5. Maseri, A. (1980): Pathogenetic mechanisms of angina pectoris: expanding views. *Br. Heart J.*, 43(6):648–660.
6. Kaski, J. C., Crea, F., Meran, D., Rodriguez, L., Araujo, L., Chierchia, S., Davies, G. J., and Maseri, A. (1986). Local coronary supersensitivity to diverse vasoconstrictive stimuli in patients with variant angina. *Circulation*, 74:1255–1265.

7. Maseri, A., L'Abbate, A., Baroldi, G., Chierchia, S., Marzilli, M., Ballestra, A. M., Severi, S., Parodi, O., Biagini, A., Distante, A., and Pesola, A. (1978): Coronary vasospasm as a possible cause of myocardial infarction. A conclusion derived from the study of "pre-infarction" angina. *N. Engl. J. Med., 299:*1271–1277.

8. Davies, G. J., Chierchia, S., and Maseri, A.: Prevention of myocardial infarction by very early treatment with intracoronary streptokinase: some clinical observations. *N. Eng. J. Med., 311:*1488–1492.

9. Chierchia, S., Davies, G. J., Berkenboom, G., Crea, F., Crean, P., and Maseri, A. (1984): Alpha-adrenergic receptors and coronary spasm: an elusive link. *Circulation, 69:*8–14.

10. Winniford, M. D., Filipchuck, M., and Hillis, D. (1983): Alpha-adrenergic blockade for variant angina: a long-term double-blind, randomized trial. *Circulation, 67:*1185–1189.

11. Freedman, S. B., Chierchia, S., Rodriguez-Plaza, L., Bugiardini, R., Smith, G., and Maseri, A. (1984): Ergonovine-induced myocardial ischemia: no role for serotonergic receptors? *Circulation,* 69:178–183.

12. De Caterina, R., Carpeggiani, C., and L'Abbate, A. (1984): A double-blind, placebo-controlled study of ketanserin in patients with Prinzmetal's angina: evidence against a role for serotonin in the genesis of coronary vasospasm. *Circulation,* 69: 889–894.

13. Chierchia, S., Patrono, C., Crea, F., Ciabattoni, G., De Caterina, R., Cinotti, G. A., Distante, A., and Maseri, A.: Effects of intravenous prostacyclin in variant angina. *Circulation,* 65:470–474.

14. Chierchia, S., De Caterina, R., Crea, F., Patrono, C., and Maseri, A. (1982): Failure of TXA$_2$ blockade to prevent attacks of vasospastic angina. *Circulation,* 66:702–705.

15. Robertson, R. M., Robertson, D., Roberts L. J., Maas, R. L., FitzGerald, G. A., Friesinger, G. C., and Oates, J. A. (1981): Thromboxane A$_2$ in vasotonic angina pectoris: evidence from direct measurements and inhibitory trials. *N. Engl. J. Med.,* 304:998.

16. Hackett, D., Larkin, S., Chierchia, S., Davies, G., Kaski, J. C., and Maseri, A. (1987): Introduction of coronary artery spasm by a direct local action of ergonovine. *Circulation (in press).*

17. Yasue, H., Touyama, M., Shimamoto, M., Kato, H., Tanaka, S., and Akiyama, F. (1974): Role of autonomic nervous system in the pathogenesis of Prinzmetal's variant form of angina. *Circulation,* 50:534–540.

18. Yasue, H., Horio, Y., Makamura, M., Fujii, H., Imoto, H., Sonoda, R., Kugiyama, K., Obata, K., Morikami, Y., and Kimura, T. (1986): Induction of coronary artery spasm by acetylcholine in patients with variant angina: possible role of the parasympathetic nervous system in the pathogenesis of coronary artery spasm. *Circulation,* 74:955–963.

19. Chicrchia, S., Berkenboom, G., Deanfield, J., Morgan, M., and Maseri, A. (1982): Holter monitoring in classical and variant angina: a clue to different pathogenetic mechanisms (abstract). *Clin. Sci.,* 63:39.

20. Ginsburg, R., Bristow, M. R., Harrison, D. C., and Stimson, E. B. (1980): Studies with isolated human coronary arteries. Some general observations, potential mediators of spasm, role of calcium antagonists. *Chest,* 78(suppl. 1):180–186.

21. McAlpin, R. (1980): Contribution of dynamic vascular wall thickening to luminal narrowing during coronary arterial constriction. *Circulation,* 61:296–301.

22. Freedman, B., Richmond, D. R., and Kelly, D. T. (1982): Pathophysiology of coronary artery spasm. *Circulation,* 66:705–709.

23. Chierchia, S., Gallino, A., Smith, G., Deanfield, J. E., Morgan, M., Croom, M., and Maseri, A. (1984): Role of heart rate in pathophysiology of chronic stable angina. *Lancet,* 2:1353–1357.

24. Crea, F., Davies, G., Romeo, F., Chierchia, S., Bugiardini, R., Kaski, J. C., Freedman, B., and Maseri, A. (1984): Myocardial ischemia during ergonovine testing: different susceptibility to coronary vasoconstriction in patients with exertional and variant angina. *Circulation,* 69:690–695.

25. Brown, B. G. (1981): Coronary vasospasm: observations linking the clinical spectrum of ischemic heart disease to the dynamic pathology of coronary artherosclerosis. *Arch. Int. Med.,* 141:716–722.

26. Gage, J. E., Hess, O. M., Murakami, T., Grimm, J., and Krayenbuehl, H. P. (1985): Mechanism of coronary artery stenosis narrowing during dynamic exercise (abstract). *Circulation,* 72(3):386.

27. Vlodaver, Z., and Edwards, J. E. (1971): Pathology of coronary atherosclerosis. *Prog. Cardiovas. Dis.,* 14:256–259.

28. Kaski, J. C., Plaza, R. L., Meran, D. O., Araujo, L., Chierchia, S., and Maseri, A. (1985): Improved coronary supply: prevailing mechanism of action of nitrates in chronic stable angina. *Am. Heart J.,* 110:238–245.
29. Heusch, G., and Deussem, A. (1983): The effects of cardiac sympathetic nerve stimulation of perfusion of stenotic coronary arteries in the dog. *Circ. Res.,* 53(1):8–15.
30. Chierchia, S., Pratt, T., De Coster, P., and Maseri, A. (1985): Alpha-adrenergic control of collateral flow: another determinant of coronary flow reserve (abstract). *Circulation,* 72(3):190.
31. Cannon, R. O., Leon, M. B., Watson, R. M., Rosing, D. R., and Epstein, S. E. (1985): Chest pain and "normal" coronary arteries—role of small coronary arteries. *Am. J. Cardiol.,* 55:50B–60B.

Hammersmith Cardiology Workshop Series, Vol. 3,
edited by A. Maseri, B. E. Sobel, and S. Chierchia.
Raven Press, New York © 1987.

Syndrome X: Diagnostic Criteria and Long-Term Prognosis

Wolfgang Kübler, Dieter Opherk, and Harald Tillmanns

Abteilung Innere Medizin III (Kardiologie), Medizinische Universitätsklinik, 69 Heidelberg, Federal Republic of Germany

Angina with normal coronary arteries is not an uncommon symptom in patients with valvular heart disease, such as severe pulmonic stenosis or aortic valve disease, or in patients with either hypertrophic or congestive cardiomyopathy. In these groups of patients, the anginal symptoms can generally be explained by the impairment of coronary circulation due to the underlying heart disease.

The problem of angina with normal coronary arteries is predominantly related to a subgroup of patients without detectable heart disease, normal left ventricular function at rest, and a normal coronary angiogram. This condition is referred to in English language publications as "syndrome X." Patients suffering from this disease give a rather clear history of stress-induced angina, promptly relieved by nitroglycerin.

CHARACTERISTICS

The majority of these patients have a normal resting ECG, but on exercise, either horizontal or descending ST segment depression (>0.15 mV), the development of left bundle branch block (LBBB) has been observed. In some patients, LBBB was already present under resting conditions. This group of patients with syndrome X is characterized by the following findings. (1,2)

First, there is a reduced dilatory capacity of the coronary vessels. Whereas resting myocardial blood flow is normal, after giving dipyridamole (0.5 mg/kg), the maximal coronary blood flow in patients with syndrome X was apparently reduced to less than 150 ml/100 g/min, i.e., to less than 50% of that obtained in normal people. From these data it follows that in patients with syndrome X, minimal coronary resistance is augmented and coronary reserve is, therefore, considerably reduced. This reduction in coronary reserve is in the same magnitude as patients with obstructive coronary artery disease with and without previous myocardial infarction.

Second, as in patients with obstructive coronary artery disease, in patients with syndrome X, myocardial lactate uptake is observed under resting conditions, and lactate production during atrial pacing stress test.

Biopsy specimens taken from left ventricular myocardium in patients with syndrome X show no changes in arterioles, capillaries, and venules. In contrast to the vessels of the heart, the myocardial cells in patients with syndrome X, except one, showed distinct alterations, such as swollen mitochondria, being associated with small myelin figures. These alterations are similar to those seen in patients with congestive cardiomyopathy but are less pronounced.

Finally, in patients with syndrome X, left ventricular function is, by definition, normal under resting conditions. During isometric work by handgrip, however, patients with syndrome X showed a significant decrease in left ventricular ejection fraction and in mean velocity of circumferential fiber shortening. During dynamic exercise on a bicycle, a rise in the ejection fraction by at least 5% was observed in the control group, whereas in patients with syndrome X, pronounced reduction in the ejection fraction was observed.

DIAGNOSTIC CRITERIA

Apart from the history of rather typical stress-induced angina and apart from ECG alterations either at rest and/or during exercise, the diagnosis of syndrome X is based on normal coronary and left ventricular angiograms. Left or right ventricular catheter biopsy reveals no alterations of intramyocardial vessels, i.e., no signs of small vessel disease. The diagnosis is predominantly based on the determination of a significantly reduced coronary reserve. In addition, during stress test, myocardial lactate uptake is reversed to lactate release, which might be interpreted as a sign of myocardial ischemia.

The diagnosis may be further based on scintigraphic studies, such as myocardial T1-201 scintigraphy, using either static images or, what is more informative, measuring regional myocardial T1-201 washout kinetics. Furthermore, myocardial N-13-glutamate uptake and turnover rates have been determined. Static images using T1-210 scintigraphy after ergometric stress test may reveal reversible perfusion defects mainly in the septal area. This finding, however, cannot be observed in all patients. The contribution of static images to the diagnosis of syndrome X is limited.

Regional T1 washout kinetics can be expressed by the quotient of the regional T1-201 count rate ratio determined after 30 and 240 min. The minimal values of this count rate ratio are significantly reduced in patients with syndrome X. This indicates reduced or delayed T1 washout in this patient group. Similar results were obtained in patients with three-vessel disease and in patients with congestive cardiomyopathy. As these patients, too, exhibit a marked reduction in coronary reserve, like patients with syndrome X, reduced T1 washout kinetics are observed in all patient groups with reduced coronary reserve, i.e., coronary artery disease, congestive cardiomyopathy, and syndrome X (3).

Compared with a control group, myocardial glutamate uptake at the end of bicycle ergometry reveals only a trend toward higher values in patients with syndrome X. Myocardial glutamate elimination rates, however, are significantly increased in patients with syndrome X, indicating higher turnover rates in this patient group. According to the preliminary data of our group, similar findings can be obtained in patients with coronary artery disease (4).

PATIENTS REINVESTIGATED

To our knowledge, no follow-up study has been performed in patients with syndrome X. Therefore, 27 patients with this disorder were reinvestigated after a period of 47 ± 14 months. The pulmonary artery pressure, as an index of left ventricular filling pressure, was measured using a Swan-Ganz catheter. Left ventricular function was evaluated by the gated blood pool technique. The data were obtained at rest and during bicycle exercise. The same work load as during the first ergometry was tried to be achieved during the second investigation. In some patients, however, this could not be accomplished, so that during the second ergometry a tendency toward a slightly lower work load was observed with 126 ± 40 W versus 133 ± 30 W during the first study.

During the first ergometry, only a few patients with syndrome X revealed an increase in mean pulmonary arterial (PA) pressure above 30 mm Hg. During the second ergometry, almost four years later, a clear tendency toward higher PA pressures during exercise could be found. This was predominantly the case in patients with LBBB, either at rest and/or during exercise. Hence, for the follow-up study, patients with syndrome X were allocated to two groups. Group A patients had syndrome X but no LBBB (n = 14); and group B patients had syndrome X and LBBB, either at rest and/or during exercise (n = 13). No new LBBB was encountered during the observation period.

The Results

In group A (without LBBB) no increase in mean PA pressure was found between the first and second ergometry. Also, left ventricular ejection fraction remained slightly depressed during exercise, but did not change from the first to the second ergometry.

In contrast to group A, patients of group B, i.e., those with LBBB, revealed a significant increase in mean PA pressure between the first and the second study. In this group, already the first ergometry showed significantly increased PA pressures. Furthermore, already the first ergometry led to a significant reduction in the ejection fraction of patients in group B. This exercise-induced decline was markedly increased during the second ergometry. Also at this time, the ejection fraction at rest was significantly reduced, indicating progressive deterioration of left ventricular function in this group of patients.

As may be expected from the hemodynamic data, only two of 25 patients in group A deteriorated by one NYHA class. In group B, however, seven of 15 patients got worse during the observation period. At the second study, six patients now belonged to class III and one to class IV. These patients are now clearly suffering from congestive cardiomyopathy. In congestive cardiomyopathy, myocardial cells shows distinct alterations, e.g., of the mitochondria. These alterations, although more pronounced, are similar to those seen in syndrome X. Furthermore, like patients with syndrome X, patients with congestive cardiomyopathy reveal a marked reduction of coronary reserve. The subgroup of patients with syndrome X and LBBB may, therefore, be considered as suffering from early or latent congestive cardiomyopathy.

In conclusion, the hemodynamic data and the long-term observations in patients with syndrome X suggest some heterogeneity of the patients studied. The common pathophysiological mechanism and the main diagnostic criterium of syndrome X is a reduced dilatory capacity of coronary vessels, which produces anginal pain on exertion and other signs of myocardial ischemia.

REFERENCES

1. Opherk, D., Zebe, H., Weihe, E., et al. (1981): Reduced coronary dilatory capacity and ultrastructural changes in the myocardium in patients with angina pectoris but normal coronary arteriograms. *Circulation,* 63:817–825.
2. Kübler, W., and Opherk, D. (1982): Unusual causes of angina pectoris: the syndrome X. In: *What is Angina?,* edited by D. G. Julian, K. I. Lie, and L. Wilhelmsen, pp. 21–26. Gotenburg, Hässle.
3. Tillmanns, H., Knapp, W. H., Opherk, D., Rauch, B., Schuler, G., and Kübler, W. (1982): Myocardial N-13-glutamate and Thallium-201 kinetics in patients with syndrome X. *Circulation (Suppl. II),* 66:352.
4. Tillmanns H., Knapp, H. W., Zimmermann, R., Rauch, B., Möller, P., and Neumann, F. J. (1984): Myokardiale N-13-Glutamat- und Thallium-201-Kinetik bei Patienten mit schwerer koronarer Drei-Gefäßerkrankung. *Z. Kardiol. (Suppl. 1),* 73:74.

Hammersmith Cardiology Workshop Series, Vol. 3,
edited by A. Maseri, B. E. Sobel, and S. Chierchia.
Raven Press, New York © 1987.

Précis of the Discussion: Section V

DYNAMIC MECHANISMS OF ACUTE TRANSIENT ISCHEMIA

Sergio Chierchia

Attilio Maseri was intrigued by the concept that some patients with syndrome X may, in fact, be suffering from an early form of dilated cardiomyopathy, and he insisted that this group of patients was likely to be a very heterogeneous group. William Grossman asked Wolfgang Kübler if any of his patients had clinical or pathological evidence to suggest viral myocarditis. Wolfgang Kübler replied that, in general, it is very difficult to trace a convincing history of previous viral myocarditis. Certainly, none of his patients had evidence of acute myocarditis when they were admitted. Lionel Opie wondered if these patients' chest pains could not be consequent to impaired ventricular relaxation; he asked if the diastolic mechanical properties of the myocardium had been assessed. Dr. Kübler answered that investigations had been performed in some patients in resting conditions and turned out to be normal. However, he did not have any follow-up data in patients of group B, whose ventricular function had deteriorated. He stressed that the mechanism responsible for reduction of coronary flow reserve in patients with syndrome X was likely to be different from that operating in congestive cardiomyopathy.

It was noted that the key question is really whether these patients have myocardial ischemia or not. Wolfgang Kübler agreed on this point and commented that the fact that some have positive thallium scans may not be taken as definite evidence for ischemia. Thallium has a poor specificity and interpretation of the results is often difficult. Burton Sobel agreed on this point and said that relying on thallium scintigraphy for assessing perfusion may lead to gross misinterpretations. William Strauss, however, commented that thallium's initial distribution mainly reflects flow distribution. Lawson McDonald wondered if electrophysiological or pathological information is available on patients of group B with left bundle branch block. Was the conduction disturbance related to some specific lesion or purely a reflection of a myocardial disorder? Dr. Kübler said that he had no information on this point: Two patients in group B died suddenly but no autopsy data were available. He did not feel that the cause of these deaths was ischemic.

Another question arose: How many patients with a history of typical chest pain turned out to have syndrome X? Wolfgang Kübler could not answer since his data were obtained in a selected population of nonconsecutive patients. Alberto Malliani questioned the value of subjective symptoms, such as chest pain, when objective evidence for cardiac pathology was elusive. Dr. Kübler answered that something had to be wrong, at least in patients in group B who have a definite tendency toward impairment of left ventricular function. As far as patients in group A were concerned, more than 80% of them have an abnormal exercise test, with evidence of transient impairment of left ventricular function, and all have a marked reduction of coronary flow reserve.

Robert Slama commented that the majority of patients with chronic stable effort angina often show large variability in anginal symptoms and effort tolerance, and the data presented by Sergio Chierchia provided objective evidence for the mechanisms responsible for this observation. He agreed that classic spasm, as observed in "variant angina," was unlikely to be responsible for this. Sergio Chierchia said that the objective demonstration of coronary spasm had contributed considerably to establish the notion that coronary arteries are not just rigid tubes, and factors other than excessive increase of myocardial demand can be responsible for acute ischemia. In his opinion, however, the pendulum had gone too far in the opposite direction, and the spasm of epicardial coronary arteries was used too often to explain dynamic changes in coronary flow reserve. He said that an attempt should be made to separate in individual patients spasm from a normal increase in tone around an eccentric lesion, constriction of small vessels, and transient impairment of collateral flow, among others.

Robert Slama questioned the possible role of "passive collapse" in causing episodes of transient acute ischemia. Sergio Chierchia replied that no clinical evidence was available to support the hypothesis. He commented that, also in the experimental setting, the likelihood of a passive collapse to occur depended upon the type of experimental stenosis applied. If occlusion was produced by an intravascular balloon, a model geometrically close to coronary atheroma than a perivascular snare, passive collapse would be more unlikely to occur. Gerry Klassen asked Sergio Chierchia why he thought that changes in vasomotor tone at the level of smaller coronary vessels were important. These vessels should be mainly controlled by metabolic regulation and, in the presence of hemodynamically significant lesions, maximal vasodilatation should prevail downstream. Sergio Chierchia answered that the reasons behind his thoughts were several. First of all, he had observed patients exhibiting a large variability in exercise tolerance despite the fact that the ischemia-related vessel was totally blocked. He said he could not find a better explanation for the variability in coronary reserve observed in these patients than the occurrence of dynamic changes in the resistance of the distal or collateral vessels. Second, he quoted the experimental observation by Heusch that the increase in distal coronary resistance observed during cardiac sympathetic stimulation was proportional to the severity of the experimental stenoses produced in the epicardial coronary artery. The more critical the stenosis, the larger the increase in distal coronary resistance. This observation could perhaps indicate that, also in the presence of extremely severe coronary lesions, distal vessels are not necessarily and invariably maximally vasodilated and are still able to constrict, in response to certain stimuli.

Alberto Malliani was intrigued by the consistent observation that heart rate and blood pressure both increased during episodes of ischemia in chronic stable angina. He thought that this type of hemodynamic response was likely to be consequent to a sympathetic excitatory reflex elicited by subendocardial ischemia while a depressor reflex was usually observed during transmural ischemia. Sergio Chierchia answered that this was certainly a possible explanation. However, he thought that the possibility that the same stimulus could account for both the systemic response (i.e., tachycardia and hypertension) and for coronary vasoconstriction should also be considered.

Sergio Chierchia said that with three exceptions, all the patients studied improved when given beta blockers. The three patients who apparently did not were probably not sufficiently beta blocked, since, when treated, they only showed minimal changes in heart rate and blood pressure.

Richard Conti was impressed by the similarity between the diurnal distribution of episodes of transient acute ischemia observed by Sergio Chierchia in unrestricted anginal patients and that reported by Dr. Muller (*N. Engl. J. Med.,* 1985) for acute myocardial infarction. He asked Sergio Chierchia if he had any thoughts about this observation, especially with regard to certain changes in platelet and clotting activity. Sergio Chierchia said that the peak incidence of ischemic episodes observed between 7 and 8 A.M. was likely to be due to increased sympathetic activity, known to be higher in that particular time of day. Whether or not the increase in sympathetic tone could also be responsible for an enhanced platelet aggregability and clotting tendency was an open question. He also observed that patients with variant angina usually exhibited an earlier peak of ischemic episodes (between 4 and 6 A.M.). If one allows a 2 to 3 hr time lag for spasm to produce a persistent coronary occlusion, then the distribution of episodes of transient ischemia and that of acute myocardial infarction would become very similar. He thought this observation was worth exploring further.

Lionel Opie stated that, despite all limitations on the interpretation of myocardial lactate studies, he could not think of any better explanation than ischemia for the occurrence of ST segment changes, chest pain, and lactate release observed in patients with syndrome X. Sergio Chierchia commented on the same point by saying that, to his knowledge, there were no systematic studies based on two-dimensional echocardiography to show the occurrence of transient regional wall motion abnormalities in this condition. In his opinion, the documentation of ST segment changes, lactate release, and regional impairment of myocardial function would probably prove the point beyond any reasonable doubt.

Attilio Maseri asked the contributors to give their views on the clinical relevance of this syndrome, that is, its incidence, prognosis, and treatment. Robert Slama said that, as far as treatment was considered, the answer was simple: These patients should only be given nitroglycerin for pain relief and nothing else. Michel Bertrand argued that if objective evidence for ischemia was obtained during exercise or pacing by coronary sinus lactates, impairment of ejection fraction, or increase in

LV end-diastolic pressure, beta blockers should be indicated. Attilio Maseri concluded that the approach should be empirical and different drugs should be used, depending upon the individual patient response.

Editorial comment: S. Chierchia

Growing evidence suggests that mechanisms other than coronary spasm (i.e., an abnormal increase in vasomotor tone at the level of epicardial coronary arteries) can be responsible for acute myocardial ischemia due to transient impairment of coronary myocardial perfusion. The occurrence of spasm, however, is almost invariably advocated to explain episodes of angina that occur in the absence of an increase in myocardial oxygen demand and to justify the variability in exercise tolerance, so often observed in patients with chronic stable angina. In other words, the term "spasm" is used interchangeably to encompass all possible forms of coronary vasoconstriction that may operate in the pathophysiological setting of various forms of angina pectoris.

As a direct consequence, nitrates and calcium blockers are widely (and sometimes wildly) used, on the assumption that (a) transient constriction of epicardial coronary arteries plays a major pathophysiological role in most patients with angina pectoris, and (b) all forms of coronary vasoconstriction, regardless of the cause, location, and severity, will respond to the same drugs.

So far spasm, as observed in Prinzmetal's variant angina, is the only mechanism capable of impairing regional myocardial perfusion, which has been convincingly demonstrated, in man. Undoubtedly, its discovery produced a major change in our clinical, diagnostic, and therapeutical approach to patients with angina pectoris. It had a major role in accelerating our understanding of the various clinical manifestations of ischemic heart disease and in conditioning the direction of our research lines. The fact that epicardial coronary arteries are not anymore considered "rigid tubes," important and yet immobile components of the plumbing system of the heart, is an invaluable physiological byproduct of the objective demonstration of spasm.

The reborn interest in the study of coronary receptors, nerves, endothelium, and all factors potentially involved in the regulation of coronary smooth muscle tone is also a consequence of this observation. However, as it is often the case in human history, the pendulum has swung too far in the opposite direction. Driven by the cultural inertia of the media, by our mental laziness, and by the hammering advertising campaigns of some drug companies, we tend to generalize and to use the same explanations, definitions, and interpretations for different phenomena. Twenty years ago the term "spasm" was carefully avoided, if not categorically banned, from the cardiology textbooks: Now it is used, misused, and abused to explain everything.

The mechanisms capable of producing a transient impairment of regional myocardial perfusion, severe enough to cause acute myocardial ischemia, are likely to be multiple. Their causes are likely to be varied and the relative role they can play in different clinical situations is probably also different. The term ''spasm'' is too general to allow an even tentative classification of coronary vasoconstriction and, in our opinion, it should be used only when an exaggerated vasoconstriction response, well beyond the physiological range, is observed.

An attempt should be made, in the individual patient, to define whether vasoconstriction is still within the normal physiological range or if it is frankly abnormal. Its localization (proximal, distal, collateral vessels) and extent (localized, segmental, diffuse) should also be established. Furthermore, the pharmacological agents routinely used to induce coronary vasoconstriction (i.e., ergonovine) have probably little resemblance to the mechanisms actually involved in the pathophysiology of most patients' symptoms. Other stimuli, more physiological and more likely to play a significant role in the causation of acute myocardial ischemia, should be identified.

Most of the ongoing research on coronary vasomotion has concentrated on the study of large epicardial coronary arteries, and little attention has been given to the role of smaller vessels. However, preliminary observations indicate that, in a sizable proportion of patients with coronary artery disease, coronary flow reserve can remain severely impaired despite the removal of epicardial coronary stenoses by successful angioplasty. This observation, and the fact that patients with ''syndrome X'' exhibit a significantly impaired coronary flow reserve, indicates that an increase in distal coronary resistance could be an important factor, preventing regional myocardial blood flow from increasing in response to metabolically active stimuli. As pointed out by Dr. Klassen, resistance is probably not set at a fixed level of the coronary circulation. The contribution of different vascular sections to coronary vascular resistance is likely to be different in different clinical situations and, possibly, to vary within the same patient at different times.

Hammersmith Cardiology Workshop Series, Vol. 3,
edited by A. Maseri, B. E. Sobel, and S. Chierchia.
Raven Press, New York © 1987.

Correlation Between Exercise Stress Testing and Coronary Angiography

Raphael Balcon

London Chest Hospital, London E2 9JX, England

One of the most persistent and challenging problems in cardiology is how to help community physicians decide which patients with ischemic disease should be considered for surgery or angioplasty apart from those whose symptoms demand it. The need for such a decision implies that these therapeutic methods improve prognosis in addition to relieving symptoms. This will be accepted for the purposes of this review on the value of exercise testing, although it is not yet proved, especially in the case of angioplasty.

ANGIOGRAPHIC FINDINGS AND PROGNOSIS

There is a good general correlation between angiographic findings and prognosis. Many studies have demonstrated that survival is related to the number of diseased vessels (1,2), and the stricter the criteria that are used the better the relationship (3). This is confirmed by data from my institution. The survival curves for groups, patients with 75% or more stenosis of the proximal segments in one, two, or three main coronary trunks, are significantly different from each other (Wilcoxson's log rank test). The eight-year survival was 82.5% for the 902 patients with single-vessel disease, 69.6% for the 344 with double, and 51.5% for the 144 with triple-vessel disease.

There is also a good general relationship between prognosis and left ventricular angiographic abnormality, which is also seen in our data. As with the coronary lesions, the effect is most marked for severe degrees of abnormality. The eight-year survival for these patients was 53%. In particular, the group of patients with a normal left ventricular angiogram has a good survival rate (85% at eight years), despite including patients with multivessel disease.

The prognosis value of the coronary angiogram can be improved if it is examined in more detail. We have calculated an index of severity of distal disease beyond the proximal segments and have shown that it divides patients into different prognostic groups. This distal index is derived by analyzing all of the lesions beyond the main coronary trunks. Both their site and severity are accounted for. The index is expressed as a percentage; low figures indicate severe disease. For instance, the 470 patients with a single proximal stenosis and relatively mild distal disease (index 75–100) had an eight-year survival rate of 87.2%, significantly better than the 243 with more distal disease (index 50–75). Further subdivision would be possible if the state of the left ventricle is taken into account. In summary, angiographic findings give a reasonable indication of likely prognosis and, in particular, the patients with the very worst prognosis can be easily predicted. Unfortunately, these are not very suitable for treatment and their prognosis may not be improvable by it.

EXERCISE TEST RESULTS AND SENSITIVITY

The questions that will now be addressed are whether symptoms and exercise testing can be used to predict these findings and, perhaps more importantly, whether exercise test results independently add to the sensitivity of the prediction of survival. The fact that patients without symptoms who have severe triple-vessel disease and are not discovered until they have a routine exercise test or become the victims of sudden death are frequently quoted as examples of the poor correlation between symptoms and the degree of coronary disease. However, there is a good general relationship between the two. In our series, there is a significant correlation between severity of effort angina and prevalence of multivessel disease. This tendency is partially reversed for patients with angina at rest. These patients, however, are almost certainly a more heterogeneous subgroup with a more complex pathogenesis. The degree of effort angina is not generally thought to be related to prognosis. In our series, however, the 82 patients with severe effort angina (Canadian Heart Association grade 3) had significantly worse survival (61.1% at 9 years) compared with 78.3% to 85.7% for the patients with lesser degrees of effort angina.

Considerable controversy exists concerning the ability to predict angiographic findings from exercise test results. There are a number of reports from one group (3) that the number of main coronary arteries affected by 75% or more stenosis can be accurately assessed from the heart rate/ST segment slope calculated from a usually submaximal bicycle ergometer exercise test. Most other workers have not been able to reproduce the results. Amiesen et al. (5) found the slope to be a better predictor of the presence of coronary disease in patients without previous infarction, but they were unable to predict its severity. We also were unable to find a correlation between the slope and the number of diseased vessels using the methods and criteria described by the original authors (6). In addition, values were found between the slope ranges for one-, two-, and three-vessel disease which were not found by the original workers in a large number of studies. This inability to reproduce the results outside the original centers renders this method unsuitable for general use.

We found a good general correlation between maximum exercise load achieved on a bicycle ergometer and a general index of coronary disease in a group of 551 patients. However, there is no correlation between maximum load on the treadmill and distribution of coronary disease in another group of patients. It may be necessary to further subdivide the patients according to symptomatic level to find such a correlation. Similarly, the amount of ST segment depression during the treadmill exercise did not correlate with the amount of coronary disease.

Exercise test variables do, however, seem to be reasonable indicators of prognosis in various groups. Bruce et al. (7) showed, in a group of 2,000 apparently normal men, that future coronary events were significantly associated with chest pain, a low maximum work load, failure to reach 90% of predicted maximum heart rate, or "ischemic" ST segment change during a maximal exercise test. However, in a larger group followed for 10 years rather than five they found that the prediction from exercise test variables was not as good but was improved by including risk factors in the analysis (8).

Postinfarction ST depression during early submaximal exercise tests was shown to be an indicator of poor prognosis in a study without angiographic control (9), but later studies with angiography have demonstrated that those factors which reflect left ventricular damage, such as fall in blood pressure or failure to complete the test, correlate best with prognosis (10,11).

It is possible that the clinical and exercise test data merely reflect what the angiograms would have shown and have no independent value, but there is evidence that this is not so. Single stenoses of the descending coronary artery have been intensively studied, particularly because of their suitability for angioplasty, and provide a good clinical model for study. Apparently similar lesions have very different physiological effects, as demonstrated by exercise testing, radioisotope perfusion scanning, and various forms of stress imaging to evaluate their effect on regional left ventricular wall motion. This variability has been attributed to a number of different influences, which include the degree of collateral supply, the amount of variability of the lesion itself, either due to vasospasm or platelet aggregation and dissolution and, indeed, the accuracy of the assessment of its severity. This latter difficulty is, to a certain extent, overcome by the use of quantitative angiography.

Little is known about the relationship between physiological effect and prognosis. Repeat angiography has demonstrated that minor lesions can be the cause of future major events, such as infarction, and presumably with or without plaque rupture. Whether or not lesions with demonstrable major effects on myocardial function have a sinister prognostic influence has not been elucidated. It is likely that prognosis will best be assessed by a consideration of all the factors, both physiological and angiographic. Multiple regression analyses can be confusing, and division of patients in subgroups according to a large number of variables leads to very small groups of patients unless the data base is very large. The largest data bases are inevitably multicenter, which introduces new confounding problems. In any event, these large accumulations of data usually do not have the detailed physiological information to form the subgroups. There is, thus, no obvious solution to the problem, but it is hoped that the newer, noninvasive techniques will provide better methods of assessing patients.

It is unrealistic to suggest that all patients with known or suspected, or even unsuspected, coronary disease must undergo angiography. Thus, at present, the advice must be that patients with important symptoms, or those with exercise test findings that suggest reduced survival or severe disease, should be studied.

REFERENCES

1. Brushke, A. V. G., Proudfit, W. L., and Sones, F. M. (1973): Progress study of 590 consecutive non-surgical cases of coronary disease followed 5–9 years. I. Cine arteriographic correlations. *Circulation,* 47:1147–1153.
2. Mock, M. B., Ringquist, I., Fisher, L. D., et al. (1982): Survival of medically treated patients in the Coronary Artery Surgery Study (CASS) registry. *Circulation,* 66:562–568.
3. Harris, P. J., Behar, V. S., Conley, M. J., et al. (1980): The prognostic significance of 50% coronary stenosis in medically treated patients with coronary artery disease. *Circulation,* 62:240–248.
4. Elamin, M. S., Boyle, R., Kardash, M. M., et al. (1982): Accurate detection of coronary disease of new exercise test. *Br. Heart J.,* 48:311–320.
5. Amiesen, O., Okin, P. M., Devereux, R. B., et al. (1985): Predictive value and limitations of ST/HR slope. *Br. Heart J.,* 53:547–551.
6. Balcon, R., Brooks, N., and Layton, C. (1984): Correlation of heart rate/ST slope and coronary angiographic findings. *Br. Heart J.,* 71:118–135.
7. Bruce, R. A., De Rouen, T. A., and Hossack, K. F. (1980): Value of maximal exercise tests in risk assessment of primary coronary heart disease events in healthy men. Five years' experience of the Seattle heart watch study. *Am. J. Cardiol.,* 46:371–378.
8. Bruce, R. A., Hossack, K. F., De Rouen, T. A., and Hofer, V. (1973): Enhanced risk assessment for primary coronary heart disease events by maximal exercise testing: 10 years' experience of Seattle heart watch. *J.A.C.C.,* 2:565–573.
9. Theroux, P., Waters, D. D., Halphen, C., De Baisieux, J., and Mizgala, H. F. (1979): Prognostic value of exercise testing soon after myocardial infarction. *N. Engl. J. Med.,* 301:341–345.
10. Jennings, K., Reid, D. S., and Julian, D. G. (1983): Role of early postinfarction exercise test in identifying candidates for early coronary surgery. *Br. Heart J.,* 48:289.
11. Sullivan, I. D., Davies, D. W., and Sowton, E. (1985): Submaximal exercise testing early after myocardial infarction. Difficulty of predicting coronary anatomy and left ventricular performance. *Br. Heart J.,* 53:180–185.

Hammersmith Cardiology Workshop Series, Vol. 3,
edited by A. Maseri, B. E. Sobel, and S. Chierchia.
Raven Press, New York © 1987.

Exercise Testing and the Assessment of the Severity of Coronary Artery Disease

K. M. Fox

National Heart Hospital, London W1M 8BA, England

Exercise testing has long been used in the diagnosis of ischemic heart disease using the coronary arteriogram as the "gold" standard. Variable success has been reported, with some studies showing sensitivities and specificities of even greater than 90%. Others have been unable to obtain such good results. The differences in these findings are probably related to the patients being studied. Patients with a good history of chest pain, in whom there is a high likelihood of coronary artery disease, are more likely to be correctly diagnosed than patients with atypical chest pain, in whom the prevalence of coronary artery disease is much lower.

The finding that three-vessel coronary disease has a better prognosis when treated surgically than medically stimulated the search for techniques that may be used to identify such patients noninvasively (1). The exercise test seemed the logical solution, and refinements in techniques have been directed toward this goal.

12-LEAD EXERCISE TEST

It was quite clear from early on that using a single lead for exercise testing was going to be inadequate, particularly if an attempt was to be made to try to identify the site and extent of coronary disease on the basis of the test result. Mason and Likar, therefore, adapted the 12-lead ECG to exercise testing so that the different regions, i.e., anterior, inferior, and posterior of the myocardium, may be examined (2). Some early success was reported using the 12-lead exercise test to identify multivessel disease (3), but it is now generally held that the overlap is so large that multivessel disease and single-vessel disease cannot be readily distinguished using the 12-lead exercise test.

PRECORDIAL ST SEGMENT MAPPING

To obtain more accurate localization of alteration in ST segment changes, a precordial mapping technique was developed (4). The simplest and most readily applicable technique employed the use of 16 electrodes arranged over the left hemithorax. In this way, it was possible to identify regional alterations in the ST segment that occurred on exercise. Using this technique, contour maps were drawn and ST segment changes occurring in the anterior, lateral, and inferior portions of the myocardium could be identified. Initial results showed that patients with isolated left anterior descending coronary artery disease had changes that were confined to a large anterior area, while circumflex patients had changes confined to a lateral area, and right coronary disease had changes confined to the lower portions of the precordial map. Patients with three-vessel disease had changes involving all these areas. Using this technique it was possible to identify single-vessel disease with a sensitivity of 65% and a specificity of 89%. Three-vessel disease was identified with a sensitivity of 64% and a specificity of 100%. More recent use of this technique has shown that, although superior to the 12-lead exercise test, the overlap between single-vessel disease and multivessel disease is again too large to make useful differentiation possible.

THE ST/HEART RATE SLOPE

Recently, a new technique has been described which, using exercise testing, can, it is claimed, identify with complete accuracy coronary artery disease into one-, two-, and three-vessel narrowing (5). This technique makes use of the relationship between heart rate, as an index of myocardial oxygen consumption, and ST segment depression, as an index of myocardial ischemia. The rate of increase of heart rate with the development of ST segment depression was shown in an initial study of 64 patients to correlate with the severity of the disease.

The technique involves the use of a bicycle ergometer, and submaximal exercise is performed. There are 3 min increases in work load to achieve heart rate increases of 10 beats/min, and the 12-lead electrocardiogram with CM5 replacing lead aVR is recorded. The heart rate and ST segment displacement is measured in each lead, with the ST segment displacement measured to an accuracy of 0.1 mm. The maximum rate of development of ST segment depression with increasing heart rate is determined in each lead, and the maximum ST segment heart rate slope of all the leads provides an index of the severity of coronary artery disease. This work has found that this slope could accurately predict the severity of coronary disease with absolutely no overlap between the different severities of disease.

We have attempted to reproduce these results in a study of 84 patients and have found that while there is indeed a rough correlation between the steepness of the ST/heart rate slope and the extent of coronary disease, there is a wide overlap (6). Furthermore, when compared to the exercise test using the 12-lead electrocardiogram and the Bruce protocol, the ST/heart rate slope gave an improved sensitivity at the expense of an unacceptable fall in specificity.

The place of the ST/heart rate slope, therefore, is still in the balance. Other workers such as ourselves have been unable to confirm the initial findings, while one group in the United States has found that the ST/heart rate slope can be used with some degree of accuracy in the prediction of patients with three-vessel disease (7). Further studies are necessary before the final place for this technique can be determined, but at present, in light of this debate and also in light of the fact that the ST/heart rate slope does take a considerable period of time to calculate, it probably still remains a research tool.

CONCLUSIONS

At present, there is no satisfactory technique that can noninvasively assess the severity of coronary artery disease. However, the results of the recent CASS study, in which patients with three-vessel disease did no better when treated surgically than medically, perhaps obviates this need to a large extent (8). What is clearly needed is not so much an assessment of the severity of coronary artery disease by exercise testing, but an assessment of coronary vascular reserve. This is likely to be much more important in terms of identifying patients at risk and at assessing the suitability of surgery than a simple anatomical evaluation. It remains to be seen whether the heart rate to the onset of ST segment depression, exercise duration, or even the ST/heart rate slope provide the best assessments of coronary vascular reserve.

REFERENCES

1. European Coronary Surgery Study Group (1982): Long-term results of prospective randomized study of coronary artery bypass surgery in stable angina pectoris. *Lancet,* II:1173–1180.
2. Mason, R. E., and Likar, I. (1966): A new system of multiple lead exercise electrocardiography. *Am. Heart J.,* 71:196–205.
3. Robertson, D., Kostuk, W. J., and Aliuja, S. P. (1976): The localization of coronary artery stenosis by 12 lead ECG response to graded exercise test: support for intercoronary steal. *Am. Heart J.,* 91:437–444.
4. Fox, K. M., Selwyn, A., Dabley, D., and Shillingford, J. P. (1979): Relation between the precordial projection of ST segment changes after exercise and coronary angiographic findings. *Am. J. Cardiol.,* 44:1068–1075.
5. Elamin, M. S., Mary, D. A. S. G., Smith, D. R., and Linden, R. J. (1980): Prediction of the severity of coronary artery disease using slope of submaximal ST segment/heart rate relationship. *Cardiovasc. Res.,* 14:681–691.
6. Quyyumi, A. A., Raphael, M. J., Wright, C., Bealing, L., and Fox, K. M. (1984): Inability of the ST segment/heart rate slope to predict accurately the severity of coronary artery disease. *Br. Heart J.,* 52:304–307.
7. Ameisen, O., Okin, P. M., Devereux, R. B., Hochrciter, C., Miller, D. H., Zullo, M. A., Borer, J. S., and Kligfield, P. (1985): Predictive value and limitations of the ST/HR slope. *Br. Heart J.,* 53:547–555.
8. CASS Principal Investigations and Their Associates (1983): Coronary artery surgery study (CASS). A randomized trial of coronary artery bypass surgery. Survival data. *Circulation,* 68:951–960.

Hammersmith Cardiology Workshop Series, Vol. 3,
edited by A. Maseri, B. E. Sobel, and S. Chierchia.
Raven Press, New York © 1987.

Practical Assessment of the Role of Dynamic Coronary Stenoses in Patients with Stable Exertional Angina

Juan Carlos Kaski and Filippo Crea

Cardiovascular Research Unit, Royal Postgraduate Medical School, Hammersmith Hospital, London W12 OHS, England

It is now generally accepted that in patients with chronic stable angina, transient impairment of coronary blood flow may play a role in the genesis of ischemic episodes during daily life (1–6). Growing evidence indicates that this impairment in coronary supply may be mediated by dynamic changes in the severity of coronary stenoses (dynamic stenosis) (3,4,7).

Rational management of patients with coronary artery disease requires an understanding of the mechanisms and cause of their ischemic attacks. Therefore, it is essential to assess the extent to which dynamic events that transiently interfere with coronary supply are responsible for spontaneous variability of angina threshold and symptoms in general.

Useful clues to the relative role of "fixed" and dynamic stenosis in causing ischemic episodes can be gathered directly from an accurate clinical history and from a series of appropriate investigations (Fig. 1).

The aim of this chapter is to present our current strategy to assess the role of dynamic stenosis in the genesis of ischemic episodes in patients with stable exertional angina.

ASSESSMENT OF ANGINA DURING DAILY LIFE: CLINICAL HISTORY AND AMBULATORY ECG MONITORING

A careful clinical history may reveal that although most anginal attacks are effort-related, the level of exercise that causes angina is often variable: Angina may occur with little activity early in the morning despite a good exercise capacity later during the day. Day-to-day, week-to-week, and seasonal variations in anginal threshold are commonly reported. Angina at rest is also a frequent feature of patients with chronic stable angina, as indicated by the results of a standardized angina questionnaire that we routinely administer to all patients (Fig. 2). Reports

Patients with Stable Angina:
Transient impairment
in coronary flow

- Clinical

  Angina at rest

  Variability in angina threshold

- Ambulatory ECG monitoring

  Transient ST ↓ with no increase in

  MVO_2 determinants

- Stress−Testing

  Variability

  Improvement with coronary dilators

- Tests of vasoconstriction

  Ergonovine - induced ST depression

FIG. 1. In patients with chronic stable angina, dynamic stenoses may modulate the response to exercise and induce angina during daily life by reducing coronary supply. Evidence for the presence of transient impairment of coronary blood flow can be obtained from the clinical history of the patient and from a series of investigations.

of ambulatory monitoring of the ST segment showed that in patients with coronary artery disease, approximately 70% of episodes of ST depression are not preceded by an increase of heart rate or heart rate-blood pressure product (5,6), thus indicating that transient impairment in coronary supply may be at least as important as excessive increase in demand in the genesis of episodes of myocardial ischemia during daily life in these patients.

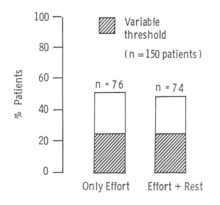

FIG. 2. Results on 150 consecutive patients with chronic stable angina, positive exercise test, and proven coronary artery disease, who completed a standardized angina questionnaire.

ASSESSMENT OF CORONARY RESERVE: EXERCISE STRESS TESTING

We submit all patients to a maximal, symptom-limited, treadmill exercise test on no therapy in order to assess their coronary reserve at the time of the test The exercise capacity is expressed as both the maximal work load and blood pressure-heart rate product that can be tolerated without developing ischemia, and as the work load at 0.1 mV of ST segment depression. External work is expressed in METS and is compared with the maximal effort the patient can do during his or her usual activities to ascertain possible mechanisms of ischemia during daily life.

ASSESSMENT OF VARIABILITY IN ISCHEMIC THRESHOLD: REPEAT EXERCISE TEST ON NO MEDICATION

Whenever possible, we perform a second exercise test *off* all antianginal medication within a week of the initial exercise in order to assess spontaneous changes in exercise capacity. We and others (8,9) have shown that individual patients often exhibit considerable variability in exercise capacity during repeated testing, although when large groups are considered, the results, expressed as mean values, are reproducible (since some patients perform better and others perform worse on different occasions).

When differences in exercise performance in the same patient are very large, the possible role of dynamic stenoses should be considered. We arbitrarily assume that dynamic stenoses may be present when individual variability exceeds 2 min in exercise duration, 2 min in time to 1 mm ST depression and/or 15 beats per min in heart rate to 1 mm ST depression, and 25×10^2 in rate-pressure product at 1 mm ST depression. This assumption is supported by the observation that variability of exercise tolerance in patients with stable angina is higher in those with ergonovine-induced ST depression than in patients with negative ergonovine tests.

ASSESSMENT OF MAXIMAL RESIDUAL CORONARY RESERVE: EXERCISE TEST FOLLOWING ACUTE SUBLINGUAL NITRATES

When ST segment depression is greater than or equal to 0.1 mV and angina develops during either the first or second exercise test, patients are asked to exercise following the administration of 10 mg of sublingual isosorbide dinitrate (or eventually 10 mg of i.v. verapamil) to determine whether angina threshold can be influenced by coronary vasodilators (Fig. 3). In a recent study we have shown that following exercise testing on isosorbide dinitrate, of 217 patients, 65 (30%) either had a negative test or increased time to 0.1 mV ST depression while also achieving a

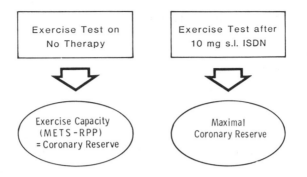

FIG. 3. In patients with a positive exercise test, repeat stress testing on sublingual nitrates allows the characterization of maximal residual coronary reserve.

significantly higher RPP, thus suggesting an increase in coronary supply; 21% did not improve exercise capacity (fixed coronary reserve <1 min increase of time to 0.1 mV ST depression in the presence of a similar or lower RPP), and 49% had an intermediate response (10). In a further study of these patients, we observed that 70% of responders to nitrates were also responders to verapamil, a calcium antagonist with little (if any) action on preload. Changes in preload (reduction of left ventricular volumes) were not found to be responsible for the improvement in exercise capacity following nitrates and verapamil. Moreover, changes in the severity of coronary stenoses were documented in these patients (but not in the nonresponders to nitrates) after the administration of intravenous ergonovine and intracoronary nitrates at angiography (10).

The fact that ergonovine and nitrates were able to induce dynamic changes at the level of the stenoses only in patients with marked improvement in exercise capacity following nitrates and calcium antagonists is an indication of the potential for dynamic stenoses in this type of patient, as well as the ability of the exercise testing to detect this subset of patients.

PRACTICAL IMPLICATIONS

In patients known to have ischemic heart disease, the clinical history and exercise testing on sublingual nitrates are probably the interventions that provide the most useful information about possible mechanisms of ischemic and therapeutic management at a very low risk and cost.

Stress testing on acute nitrates (or calcium antagonists) is an essential step in our strategy to assess dynamic stenoses because it (a) indicates the *maximal residual coronary reserve* of the patient, which we classify as low (5 METS), intermediate (5–10 METS), and high (>10 METS); (b) provides clues on mechanisms underlying ischemic attacks during daily life by comparing maximal exercise capacity with the maximum level of effort the patient is able to perform during his daily activities;

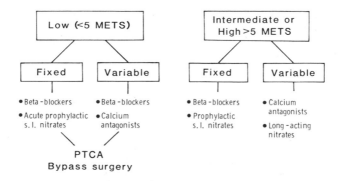

FIG. 4. Therapeutic strategy based on the level of maximal residual coronary reserve.

and (c) suggest the choice of the first line of therapy based on the pathogenetic mechanisms of ischemia acting in the individual patient (Fig. 4).

In patients with low exercise capacity despite the administration of nitrates (3–5 METS), whether it is fixed or variable, the therapeutic goal will be to allow the heart to work more economically by using beta blockers and long-acting nitrates (and to prevent dynamic stenoses, if present). However, coronary angioplasty or bypass surgery should be considered even in those patients in whom dynamic stenoses are responsible for episodes of angina, because the impairment of their exercise tolerance imposed by organic lesions is so severe that even on maximal therapy capable of abolishing dynamic mechanisms, the maximum effort those patients would be able to perform will be too little to allow a normal life-style.

Conversely, when residual coronary reserve is preserved so that the patient can tolerate efforts greater than 10 METS without signs of ischemia, the main therapeutic goal will be the prevention of episodes resulting from transient impairment of coronary flow. If this goal can be achieved, with calcium antagonists and long-acting nitrates, the patient will be angina free, except for unusually intense efforts, in which case prophylactic sublingual nitrates and eventually beta blockers can be added.

ACKNOWLEDGMENT

This research was supported by a grant from the British Heart Foundation.

REFERENCES

1. Maseri, A., Severi, S., DeNes, M., L'Abbate, A., Chierchia, S., Marzilli, M., Ballestra, A. M., Parodi, O., Biagini, A., and Distante, A. (1978): Variant angina. One aspect of a continuous spectrum of vasospastic myocardial ischemia: pathogenic mechanisms, estimated incidence, clinical and coronary arteriographic findings in 138 patients. *Am. J. Cardiol.*, 42:1019–1035.

2. Maseri, A. (1980): Pathogenetic mechanisms of angina pectoris: expanding views. *Br. Heart J.,* 43:648–660.
3. Epstein, S. E., and Talbot, T. L. (1981): Dynamic coronary tone in precipitation, exacerbation and relief of angina pectoris. *Am. J. Cardiol.,* 48:797–803.
4. Brown, B. G., Bolson, E., Petersen, R. B., Pierce, C. D., and Dodge, H. T. (1981): The mechanisms of nitroglycerin action: Stenosis vasodilatation as a major component of the drug response. *Circulation,* 64:1089–1097.
5. Deanfield, J. E., Maseri, A., Selwyn, A. P., Ribeiro, P., Chierchia, S., Krikler, S., and Morgan, M. (1983): Myocardial ischemia during daily life in patients with stable angina: its relation to symptoms and heart rate changes. *Lancet,* II:753–758.
6. Chierchia, S., Muiesan, L., Balasubramanian, V., Raftery, J., and Maseri, A. (1984): Ambulatory ECG and blood pressure monitoring in patients with chronic stable angina. Relationship between myocardial demand and acute ischemia. *Circulation,* 70:II-452.
7. MacAlpin, R. N. (1980): Contribution of dynamic vascular wall thickening to luminal narrowing during coronary arterial constriction. *Circulation,* 61:296–301.
8. Rodriguez, L., Kaski, J. C., Freedman, B., and Maseri, A. (1984): Daily individual variability of exertional ischemic threshold in stable angina pectoris. *Eur. Heart J.,* 5:205.
9. Starling, M. R., Moody, M., Crawford, M. H., Levi, B., and O'Rourke, R. A. (1984): Repeat treadmill exercise testing: variability of results in patients with angina pectoris. *Am. Heart J.,* 107:298–303.
10. Kaski, J. C., Rodriguez-Plaza, L., Meran, D. O., Araujo, L., Chierchia, S., and Maseri, A. (1985): Improved coronary supply: Prevailing mechanism of action of nitrates in chronic stable angina. *Am. Heart J.,* 110:238–245.

Hammersmith Cardiology Workshop Series, Vol. 3,
edited by A. Maseri, B. E. Sobel, and S. Chierchia.
Raven Press, New York © 1987.

Précis of the Discussion: Section VI

ELECTROCARDIOGRAPHIC DIAGNOSIS OF TRANSIENT ISCHEMIA

David T. Kelly

The initial question was whether a clinical diagnosis of angina pectoris in an individual patient was sufficient for management, or whether some objective confirmation of coronary disease should be obtained. It was agreed that some confirmation should be obtained in *all* patients, as clinical diagnosis of angina even by experienced clinicians may be inaccurate in 10% of patients.

The type of testing recommended would depend on the clinical presentation of the individual patient. Attilio Maseri would exercise all patients with suspected coronary disease and, if the test were positive at low levels of cardiac work, would probably recommend arteriography. When positive at higher levels, the test should be repeated after a possible vasospastic component has been eliminated with nitrates. He emphasized that a patient should not be characterized on the basis of a single factor but the clinical history, exercise test, and coronary arteriography together are valuable in determining prognosis.

Douglas Chamberlain questioned the value of exercise testing because of the low sensitivity and how this is affected by the patient's age, sex, and clinical symptoms. If a patient has severe symptoms, coronary arteriography should be done without prior exercise testing but, overall, 90% of patients with clinical angina, especially if mild, would have exercise testing.

Michel Bertrand would exercise all patients with angina unless it is very severe, and would perform coronary arteriography in all patients except in a few with a high coronary flow reserve. Raphael Balcon stressed again the importance of the patient's clinical presentation in determining what tests should be done, but felt all patients should have coronary arteriography.

In patients with angina pectoris, exercise testing and/or coronary arteriography should be recommended. When unstable angina or severe symptoms are present, the consensus is that arteriography should be done without exercise testing. When chronic stable angina is present, exercise testing preferably before and after nitrate therapy should be done to assess coronary flow reserve: When this is poor, coronary arteriography must be advised. It is important to emphasize that the patient's clinical presentation determines management, but all patients should undergo further diagnostic testing.

How should a patient with typical anginal pain at rest but with no electrocardiographic changes of ischemia present during pain be managed? Although some would investigate this patient by arteriography, Robert Slama said he would not investigate this type of patient, as the probability of coronary artery disease is very low, about 1 in 100. This clinical problem emphasizes that a physician may have to and should make a clinical judgment without further investigation when the probability of disease is very low.

The indications for Holter monitoring in patients with angina pectoris were discussed by Kim Fox. The clinical history is important: when angina was typical and an exercise test positive, Holter monitoring would not be indicated for diagnosis. When atypical pain is present, Holter monitoring must be interpreted very carefully, as not all of the ST segment changes are due to ischemia. Holter monitoring may help in understanding the pathophysiology of ischemic events and identify "silent" ischemia in some patients, but its exact role in helping diagnosis has not been defined. The reviews of Attilio Maseri and Juan Carlos Kaski emphasized the importance and potential prognostic significance of assessing coronary flow reserve by exercise testing before and after nitrates, which may help deter coronary angiography when resources to do such testing are limited. Although the preliminary data presented by Juan Carlos Kaski were interesting, further experience is required to establish how precisely this approach identifies the patient's prognosis or the need for revascularization.

Although exercise testing is widely used in the diagnosis of coronary artery disease and is helpful overall, there are reservations about its use because of the relatively poor sensitivity and specificity in various patient groups. This is reflected in the increasing advocacy of coronary arteriography in all patients thought to have angina pectoris unless they are old or there are other medical or social contraindications. Whenever possible, the combination of exercise testing with a knowledge of coronary anatomy, along with a careful assessment of the patient's history, offers the best guide to the patient's management.

Editorial comment: S. Chierchia

The controversy over which test should be best for diagnosing coronary artery disease, how a given technique compares to others in terms of "sensitivity and specificity," and prognostic power seems to continue. The discussion on the electro-cardiographic diagnosis of transient acute ischemia, either spontaneous or induced by various provocative maneuvers, was yet another obvious demonstration. Every so often, in the course of our day-to-day clinical practice, we find ourselves asking the same question: Should we perform exercise testing in all patients with suspected coronary artery disease? Should we obtain in everyone information from ambulatory ECG monitoring and ergonovine testing? Should all our patients undergo coronary arteriography? The answers to these questions lie in two simple, basic principles: the importance of clinical judgment in the patient's management, and the knowledge of the indications and limitations of a given diagnostic test. This might sound very obvious but, in fact, it is not.

Everyone feels attracted by the prospect of identifying the "100% specificity/

sensitivity test,'' with no false positives or negatives and no gray areas of overlap. Unfortunately, medical practice makes no exception to the general rules governing biological variability. Moreover, the simple principle that right questions should be asked of the right persons is often forgotten. In other words, it is not correct and, more importantly, it is not realistic to try to derive precise anatomical information from exercise testing. Likewise, it is equally incorrect and unrealistic to try to obtain physiological information from coronary arteriography. Exercise testing is meant to provide us with a simple, relatively inexpensive, noninvasive means of assessing a patient's coronary flow reserve. When appropriate, angiography should allow us to interpret the results of exercise testing, in light of morphological information. As discussed at length in this section, there is usually a reasonably good correlation between the results of these two investigations, although exceptions are certainly not rare. Clinical judgment and the results of individualized medical treatment should help in clarifying some apparent discrepancies.

The role of ambulatory ECG monitoring in the clinical management of patients with ischemic disease was also discussed. As pointed out by Kim Fox, the diagnostic power of this technique is, overall, quite limited, as most patients with significant coronary artery disease can be usually spotted by exercise stress testing and coronary angiography. Holter monitoring, however, has definite applications for the evaluation and treatment of patients whose symptoms are suspected or proven to be largely due to transient coronary vasoconstriction. Furthermore, it seems to have an enormous potential for documenting episodes of painless myocardial ischemia which, in our and others' experience, represent the vast majority (about 70%) of transient ischemic events. It is certainly true that the prognostic significance of painless ischemia is not completely clear. However, the results of the Framingham study show that about 20% of myocardial infarctions go totally unnoticed. Furthermore, we have seen patients who developed an infarct or died suddenly while on ambulatory ECG monitoring. In these patients, acute events were almost invariably preceded by increased frequency and severity of asymptomatic ischemia, not necessarily paralleled by deterioration of their symptoms.

In conclusion, in the majority of cases, clinical assessment, exercise testing, arteriography, and any other test should all be regarded as part of an integrated approach to a patient's diagnosis, prognosis, and management. For all techniques, priorities and indications should be dictated, again, by clinical judgment and by a great deal of common sense.

Hammersmith Cardiology Workshop Series, Vol. 3,
edited by A. Maseri, B. E. Sobel, and S. Chierchia.
Raven Press, New York © 1987.

Nuclear Cardiology: A Decade of Clinical Use for the Detection of Coronary Artery Disease

H. William Strauss

Nuclear Medicine Division, Massachusetts General Hospital, Boston, Massachusetts 02114

From 1958 to 1977 the clinical techniques of blood pool imaging and myocardial perfusion imaging were described for the detection of coronary disease. The technology grew from the rectilinear scanner, used for the detection of pericardial effusion in 1958 (1), to the multicrystal camera for first-pass radionuclide ventriculography in 1963 (2), to the Anger camera for determination of ejection fraction (3,4), and to exercise radionuclide ventriculography (5), to define ventricular function reserve. Exercise injected myocardial perfusion imaging evolved in parallel, from the use of K-43 and the rectilinear scanner in 1972 (6) to the use of thallium-201 and the scintillation camera in 1975 (7). From 1975 to 1985, a vast clinical experience has been amassed with these techniques using, essentially, stable radiopharmaceutical and imaging technology.

TECHNIQUES

The detection of coronary disease with either myocardial or blood pool imaging is indirect, since neither technique provides a direct evaluation of the degree of atheromatous disease in the coronary vessel. An abnormal ejection fraction response to exercise requires a sufficient mass of myocardium to develop ischemia that the remainder of the ventricle cannot compensate, resulting in a decrease in global contractile function. The incidence of regional wall motion abnormalities in the absence of global changes is unusual, suggesting that the spatial resolution of the technique for identifying the site of ischemia is limited. Myocardial perfusion imaging, on the other hand, can detect limited perfusion to a zone of myocardium, and indirectly identify changes in global function (through lung uptake). Since the usual goal of the imaging procecures is to define the amount and location of myocardium at risk, myocardial perfusion imaging offers a more direct approach to the problem than exercise radionuclide ventriculography. Myocardial perfusion imaging, even with the best radiopharmaceutical, cannot achieve a sensitivity greater than about 90% for the detection of coronary artery disease: A patient may have one or more severe coronary narrowings, adequate collaterals to maintain normal myocardial perfusion reserve, and a normal myocardial perfusion scan with injection at exercise.

Recent studies suggest the specificity of exercise radionuclide ventriculography is not as high as that of myocardial perfusion imaging for the detection of coronary disease. Both techniques, however, provide better sensitivity than exercise electrocardiography for the detection of coronary disease. These observations suggest that the radionuclide study of choice in the patient with an uninterpretable ECG is T1-201 (8,9).

Perhaps more important than the immediate correlation of an abnormal scan to the presence of atherosclerosis on the arteriogram is the long-term prognostic information gleaned from the examination. A recent study by Liu et al. (10) described an average of five years of follow-up of patients with a negative thallium scan. The incidence of coronary events in the population, 0.9%/year, correlated well with the expected incidence in a general population. At the other end of the spectrum, following myocardial infarction the single most powerful predictor of future coronary events is the detection of ischemia on a thallium scan. This observation was more important than the ejection fraction, or even the coronary anatomy.

Although myocardial perfusion imaging is a valuable technique, it is likely that it will be substantially enhanced by the addition of metabolic information. The recent description of radiolabeled glucose concentration in zones of myocardial

TABLE 1. *Radionuclide procedures for evaluation of coronary artery disease*
(Circa 1990)

Radiopharmaceutical	Indication
In–111 LDL	Detection of metabolically active atheromatous disease.
Tc–99m—Antifibrin	Detection of accelerated atheromatous disease. Most useful in unstable angina.
Tc–99m—Hexakis analog	Determination of first pass ventricular function and myocardial perfusion reserve with injection at exercise.
Tc–99m—Branched chain fatty acid	Evaluation of regional myocardial substrate utilization. Best used in comparison with Tc–99m in patients with severe left ventricular hypertrophy.
I–123—Monoiodobenzylguanidine	Determination of adrenergic receptor occupancy. Particularly useful in patients with atypical chest pain and anxiety.
I–123—Anti-ANF	Detect sites of production of antinatriuretic hormone. Useful in hypertensive subjects.
Ir–191m	Sequential determination of ventricular function.
F–18 Deoxyglucose	Detection of the site and extent of myocardial ischemia.

ischemia offers the potential of a direct means of defining the site and extent of injured, but viable, areas of myocardium with positron emission tomographic imaging. The direct identification of the atheromatous process, with either radiolabeled lipoproteins such as those recently described by Lees and colleagues with Tc-99m-labeled LDL, or antibodies directed against the damaged endothelium covering the plaque, is another approach under intensive investigation. In the foreseeable future, the radionuclide techniques may be the procedures of choice for the initial characterization of the patient with suspected coronary disease. A possible scheme for evaluation is presented in Table 1.

The radionuclide approach will permit the direct determination of metabolic changes in the myocardium, perfusion at the tissue level, receptor occupancy, and the metabolic activity of the atheromatous plaques. Should this evolve, it is likely that invasive procedures would primarily be employed for therapy, such as laser angioplasty, among others.

REFERENCES

1. Rejali, A. M., MacIntyre, W. J., and Friedell, H. L. (1958): A radioisotope method of visualization of blood pools. *Am. J. Roent.,* 79:129.
2. Bender, M. A., and Blau, M. (1963): The autofluoroscope. *Nucleonics,* 21:52.
3. Ashburn, W. L., Harbert, J. C., Whitehouse, W. C., and Mason, D. T. (1968): A video system for recording dynamic radioisotope studies with the Anger scintillation camera. *J. Nucl. Med.,* 9:554.
4. Strauss, H. W., Zaret, B. L., Hurley, P. J., Natarajan, T. K. N., and Pitt, B. (1971): A scintiphotographic method for measuring left ventricular ejection fraction in man without cardiac catheterization. *Am. J. Cardiol.,* 28:575.
5. Borer, J. S., Bachrach, S. L., Green, M. V., et al. (1977): Real-time radionuclide cineangiography in the non-invasive evaluation of global and regional left ventricular function at rest and during exercise in patients with coronary artery disease. *N. Eng. J. Med.,* 296:839.
6. Zaret, B. L., Strauss, H. W., Martin, N. D., Wells, H. P., and Flamm, M. D. (1973): Noninvasive determination of regional myocardial perfusion with radioactive potassium: study of patients at rest, with exercise and during angina pectoris. *N. Eng. J. Med.,* 288:809.
7. Strauss, H. W., Harrison, K., Langan, J., Lebowitz, E., and Pitt, B. (1975): Thallium-201 for myocardial imaging: relation of thallium-201 to regional myocardial perfusion. *Circulation,* 51:641.
8. Bailey, I. K., Griffith, L. S. C., Rouleau, J., et al. (1976): Thallium-201 myocardial perfusion at rest and during exercise. *Circulation,* 55:79.
9. Leppo, J. A., Scheurer, J., Pohost, G. M., Freeman, L. M., and Strauss, H. W. (1980): The evaulation of ischemic heart disease Thallium-201 with comments on radionuclide angiography. *Semin. Nucl. Med.,* 10:115.
10. Liu, P., Boucher, C. A., Kowalker, W., Strauss, H. W., and Okada, R. D. (1985): Long-term prognosis in patients with normal exercise thallium-201 scans: A five-year follow-up study. *J. Nucl. Med.,* 26(5):29 (abstract).

Hammersmith Cardiology Workshop Series, Vol. 3,
edited by A. Maseri, B. E. Sobel, and S. Chierchia.
Raven Press, New York © 1987.

Précis of the Discussion: Section VII

ROUTINE TECHNIQUES FOR THE DETECTION OF TRANSIENT ISCHEMIA

Burton E. Sobel

This session addressed noninvasive detection of transient myocardial ischemia. William Strauss emphasized the potential value of myocardial scintigraphy with thallium, particularly when stress testing is needed for a patient with left bundle branch block, resting ST/T-wave abnormalities, previous transmural infarction, or other electrocardiographic changes that obscure interpretation if the only endpoint is electrocardiographic monitoring. In addition, to facilitate detection of reversible ischemia, thallium scintigraphy in this setting provides estimates of the mass of myocardium involved. Insights may be enhanced by tomographic as opposed to conventional imaging.

A promising approach to myocardial scintigraphic assessment of ischemia involves the use of dipyridamole. For a subject unable to exercise because of noncardiac limitations (e.g., arthritis, peripheral vascular disease, or pulmonary disease), dipyridamole testing may provide information analogous to that otherwise available with exercise stress. However, dipyridamole may elicit unpleasant side effects, limiting its universal applicability.

Nuclear ventriculography has been used widely in patients with cardiac disease for assessment of regional wall motion as well as global function. It is particularly helpful for stratifying patients with respect to prognosis after acute myocardial infarction.

Rodney Foale discussed cross-sectional echocardiography in the assessment of regional wall motion in patients with ischemic heart disease. Ultrasonic techniques are evolving rapidly. The addition of Doppler approaches will undoubtedly enhance their value. Methods employing ultrasonic contrast media (often sonicated substances) may permit echocardiographic assessment of myocardial perfusion. Changes in echocardiographic density of myocardium after injection of such contrast media appear to reflect changes in myocardial perfusion.

The frequent need for invasive studies as an initial diagnostic procedure after clinical assessment was discussed. Although exercise stress testing, echocardiography, or myocardial scintigraphy may be bypassed under such circumstances, noninvasive modalities often offer considerable value for identifying subgroups that do require or do not require invasive investigation when clinical assessments are not prognostically definitive by themselves. The promise of developing digital angiographic techniques may make follow-up evaluations less invasive in the near future, although technical constraints currently require intracoronary injections for visualization of coronary arteries.

Editorial comment: B. E. Sobel

The reviews and discussions underscore the diverse nature of judgments regarding interpretation of results of diagnostic procedures. The definition of coronary artery angiographic anatomy is obviously of considerable importance. In addition, the extent of reversible ischemia induced with physiologic or pharmacologic stress must be identified to stratify appropriately patients who may benefit from invasive diagnostic testing. The clinical implications of ischemia of a given severity or definable distribution have yet to be fully elucidated. Research directed toward clarifying these issues requires tools that are intrinsically more quantitative than those that may be quite useful in diagnostic clinical applications. Insights gained with such tools should strengthen the foundation for interpretation of noninvasive tests more widely applicable to clinical decision making for the large majority of patients with coronary artery disease.

Hammersmith Cardiology Workshop Series, Vol. 3,
edited by A. Maseri, B. E. Sobel, and S. Chierchia.
Raven Press, New York © 1987.

Myocardial Ischemia and Arrhythmias

Desmond J. Sheridan

Department of Cardiology, St. Mary's Hospital, London W2 1NY, England

Sudden death due to ventricular fibrillation (VF) is the most frequent terminal event in patients with coronary artery disease. By the time most patients who suffer myocardial infarction reach the hospital, the most critical electrophysiological disturbances are likely to have taken place and the risk of developing VF is diminishing. Effective intervention, therefore, needs to be instituted very rapidly or prophylactically, which can only be achieved on the basis of a clear understanding of the mechanisms of arrhythmogenesis associated with myocardial ischemia. During the past decade, electrophysiological and metabolic disturbances associated with myocardial ischemia have been extensively studied (9), and several products that accumulate during ischemic metabolism (Table 1) have been suggested to contribute to, or cause, the electrophysiological events that lead to VF. Establishing proof that any particular metabolic change is causally related to the genesis of VF is difficult, and it requires the demonstration that specific inhibition or accentuation of the event being investigated produces an appropriate change in the incidence of VF.

ARRHYTHMOGENIC EFFECTS OF CATECHOLAMINES IN ISCHEMIC MYOCARDIUM

The growing body of evidence implicating catecholamines in the genesis of ventricular arrhythmias associated with myocardial ischemia is increasingly difficult to refute. Elevated plasma catecholamines in clinical (19) and experimental (11) myocardial ischemia provide circumstantial evidence of enhanced sympathetic activity during myocardial ischemia. Further evidence is provided by the finding that chronic surgical denervation (6) or myocardial catecholamine depletion (15,16)

TABLE 1. *Products of ischemic metabolism*

1. K^+ and H^+	4. Free fatty acids
2. Cyclic AMP	5. Phospholipids
3. Catecholamines	6. Prostanoids

significantly reduces the incidence of VF during experimental myocardial ischemia. Release of norepinephrine from sympathetic nerve endings during myocardial ischemia could result from enhanced efferent sympathetic neurotransmission or from local metabolic disturbances. There is evidence of enhanced efferent sympathetic activity soon after the onset of myocardial ischemia (1), and sympathetic stimulation increases the incidence of ventricular arrhythmias during myocardial ischemia (13).

Other reports suggest that local release of norepinephrine may be more important. Ebert et al. (6) observed that acute surgical denervation failed to reduce VF during ischemia while chronic denervation was effective. The relative importance of neuronal and locally mediated release remains unclear; however, the occurrence of VF during ischemia in hearts devoid of central connections suggests that enhanced neural activation may not be essential. Obtaining direct evidence of catecholamine release during myocardial ischemia is complicated by the reduced washout associated with ischemia. Studies in which myocardial norepinephrine content has been measured have demonstrated a reduction following coronary occlusion (8,14), but the time course of this is slower than would be expected were it to be an important arrhythmogenic factor. Such experiments, however, do not address the possibility of enhanced release and re-uptake during early ischemia, and although there is circumstantial evidence to suggest that this may occur, direct evidence is lacking.

ANTIARRHYTHMIC ACTION OF ADRENERGIC BLOCKADE

There are numerous reports on the effects of beta adrenoceptor blockade on arrhythmias associated with myocardial ischemia. Results are often difficult to explain but appear to depend on the drug being used, the animal studied, and the model of myocardial ischemia employed (7). Thus, cardioselective beta blockade seems to be most effective and propranolol, when effective, is more likely to be so in lower concentrations. These findings are generally applicable to the dog and cat while the situation is unclear in the pig (7). It is now generally accepted that chronic beta adrenoceptor blockade is effective in reducing mortality following myocardial infarction. Its effectiveness in reducing sudden cardiac death suggests that at least part of this effect involves reducing the risk of ventricular fibrillation. There is also evidence that acute beta blockade reduces ventricular arrhythmia in the early stages of myocardial infarction (12). This has not yet been shown to significantly reduce mortality and, as a result, is not routine clinical practice.

The actions of catecholamines in the heart were originally thought to be mediated solely by beta adrenoceptors. Since 1966, however, several studies have demonstrated alpha adrenoceptor-mediated prolongation in action potential duration and refractory period and positive inotropism (17). More recently, alpha adrenoceptor activity has been implicated in the genesis of ventricular arrhythmias during myocardial ischemia and reperfusion. Thus, alpha adrenoceptor blockade significantly reduces the incidence of VF during experimental myocardial ischemia and reperfusion (16,18). This effect is generally more consistent and effective than beta blockade (16) and has been demonstrated for several alpha-blocking agents (10,16).

These findings would not have been expected from the previously described electrophysiological effects of alpha adrenoceptor stimulation, which suggests that these drugs act either through a nonadrenergic mechanism or, alternatively, that ischemia increases myocardial sensitivity to alpha-mediated effects. Recent evidence suggests that the latter is the most likely explanation. There is direct evidence of enhanced myocardial sensitivity to alpha adrenoceptor stimulation during reperfusion (16). Alpha-blocking agents do have direct myocardial effects on isolated superfused myocardium (4); however, the antiarrhythmic action during myocardial ischemia occurs with substantially lower concentrations (10) and appears to be mediated by an adrenergic mechanism (10). More importantly, however, there is evidence that alpha adrenoceptor stimulation is arrhythmogenic during myocardial ischemia. In experiments using isolated perfused hearts, depletion of myocardial catecholamines to 5% of control significantly reduces the incidence of VF during myocardial ischemia and reperfusion (4).

This antiarrhythmic effect and the associated electrophysiological changes are reversed by perfusion with an alpha adrenoceptor agonist (3). Furthermore, these actions are achieved at concentrations that have little effect on normally perfused myocardium. Thus, alpha adrenoceptor stimulation appears to contribute to the arrhythmogenic effects of myocardial ischemia.

It remains to be established whether these experimental findings will be translated into a useful clinical role. Preliminary evidence suggests that alpha adrenoceptor blockade has beneficial hemodynamic effects in patients with chronic stable angina, prolonging treadmill time (2) and atrial pacing time (5) to angina. These effects are associated with a reduction in systemic and coronary vascular resistance (5). The latter appears to be the most prominent effect and is relatively greater with increasing myocardial energy demands. It may now be appropriate, therefore, to examine more critically the potential clinical value of alpha adrenoceptor blockade in the management of patients with acute myocardial ischemia.

REFERENCES

1. Brown, A. M., and Malliani, A. (1971): Spinal sympathetic reflexes initiated by coronary receptors. *J. Physiol.*, 212:685–705.
2. Collins, P., and Sheridan, D. J. (1985): Improvement in angina pectoris with alpha adrenoceptor blockade. *Brit. Heart J.*, 53:488–492.
3. Culling, W., Penny, W. J., Cunliffe, G., and Sheridan, D. J. (1983): Arrhythmogenic and electrophysiological actions of alpha adrenoceptor stimulation during myocardial ischaemia and reperfusion. *Circulation*, 68:111–154.
4. Culling, W., Penny, W. J., Lewis, M. J., Middleton, K., and Sheridan, D. J. (1984): Effects of myocardial catecholamine depletion on electrophysiology and arrhythmias during ischaemia and reperfusion. *Cardiovasc. Res.*, 18:675–682.
5. Culling, W., Sheridan, D. J., and Thomas, P. (1985): Systemic and coronary haemodynamic

effects of alpha adrenoceptor blockade in patients with coronary artery disease. *Brit. J. Clin. Pharmacol. (in press).*

6. Ebert, P. A., Vanderbeck, R. B., Allgood, R. J., and Sabiston, D. C. (1970): Effect of chronic cardiac denervation on arrhythmias after coronary artery ligation. *Cardiovasc. Res.*, 4:141–147.

7. Fitzgerald, J. D. (1982): The effects of beta adrenoceptor blocking drugs on early arrhythmias in experimental and clinical myocardial ischaemia. In: *Early Arrhythmias Resulting from Myocardial Ischaemia*, edited by J. R. Parratt, pp. 295–315. Macmillan Press, London.

8. Mathes, P., and Gudbjarnason, S. (1971): Changes in norepinephrine stores in the canine heart following experimental myocardial infarction. *Am. Heart J.*, 81:211–219.

9. Parratt, J. R. (editor) (1982): *Early Arrhythmias Resulting from Myocardial Ischaemia*. Macmillan Press, London.

10. Penny, W. J., Culling, W., Lewis, M. J., and Sheridan, D. J. (1985): Antiarrhythmic and electrophysiological effects of alpha adrenoceptor blockade during myocardial ischaemia and reperfusion in isolated guinea pig heart. *J. Mol. Cell. Cardiol.*, 17:399–409.

11. Riemersma, R. A. (1982): Myocardial catecholamine release in acute myocardial ischemia; relationship to cardiac arrhythmias. In: *Early Arrhythmias Resulting from Myocardial Ischaemia*, edited by J. R. Parratt, pp. 125–138. Macmillan Press, London.

12. Rossi, P. R., Yusef, S., Ramsdale, D., Furze, L., and Sleight, P. (1983): Reduction of ventricular arrhythmias by early intravenous Atenolol in suspected acute myocardial infarction. *Br. Med. J.*, 286:506–510.

13. Schwartz, P. J., and Vanoli, E. (1981): Cardiac arrhythmias elicited by interaction between acute myocardial ischaemia and sympathetic hyperactivity: a new experimental model for the study of antiarrhythmic drugs. *J. Cardiovasc. Pharmacol.*, 3:1251.

14. Serrano, P. A., Chavaz-Lara, B., Bisteni, A., and Sodi-Pallares, D. (1971): Effect of propranolol on catecholamine content of injured cardiac tissue. *J. Mol. Cell. Cardiol.*, 2:91–97.

15. Sethi, V., Haider, B., Ahmed, S., Oldewurtel, H. A., and Regan, T. J. (1973): Influence of beta blockade and chemical sympathectomy on myocardial function and arrhythmias in acute ischaemia. *Cardiovasc. Res.*, 7:740–747.

16. Sheridan, D. J., Penkoske, P. A., Sobel, B. E., and Corr, P. B. (1980): Alpha adrenergic contributions to dysrhythmia during myocardial ischemia and reperfusion in cats. *J. Clin. Invest.*, 65:161–171.

17. Sheridan, D. J. (1982): Myocardial alpha adrenoceptors and arrhythmias induced by myocardial ischemia. In: *Early Arrhythmias Resulting from Myocardial Ischaemia*, edited by J. R. Parratt, pp. 317–328. Macmillan Press, London.

18. Stewart, J. R., Burmeister, W. E., Burmeister, J., and Lucchesi, B. R. (1980): Electrophysiologic and antiarrhythmic effects of phentolamine in experimental coronary occlusion and reperfusion in the dog. *J. Cardiovasc. Pharmacol.*, 2:77–91.

19. Strange, R. C., Vetter, N., Rowe, M. J., and Oliver, M. F. (1974); Plasma cyclic AMP and total catecholamines during acute myocardial infarction in man. *Euro. J. Clin. Invest.*, 4:115–119.

Hammersmith Cardiology Workshop Series, Vol. 3,
edited by A. Maseri, B. E. Sobel, and S. Chierchia.
Raven Press, New York © 1987.

Characterization of Ischemic Myocardium with Positron Emission Tomography

Burton E. Sobel

Cardiovascular Unit, Washington University School of Medicine, St. Louis, Missouri 63110

Metabolic imaging with positron emission tomography (PET) is performed generally with intravenous administration of positron-emitting radionuclides incorporated into counterparts of physiologic, metabolic substrates (1,2). The biochemical behavior of such tracers is identical to that of the physiologic metabolite being traced. However, metabolism of the tracers gives rise to labeled intermediates that may confound interpretations of tomograms (3,4). Thus, tomographic information may be unambiguous only during the first few minutes after administration of the tracer. Alternatively, results can be interpreted in the context of verified mathematical models of the kinetics of appearance and deposition of the tracer under defined physiologic or pathologic conditions (5–8).

Metabolic imaging has been performed also with radiolabeled substrate analogs that are not transported in a fashion similar to that of their physiologic counterparts. Analogs containing relatively longer-lived, positron-emitting radionuclides, such as fluorine-18 (^{18}F), are trapped within the tissue rather than metabolized and can be visualized with prolonged imaging intervals. However, numerous assumptions are required to account for the disparities between the behavior of the analogs compared with that of natural substrates.

FATTY ACIDS

Under physiologic conditions, the preferred substrate of myocardium is circulating free fatty acid (FFA), which accounts for 40% to 80% of myocardial energy production. Uptake of FFA by the heart depends on the arterial concentration of FFA, the albumin fatty acid ratio, and the specific chain length and saturation of the FFA (9–11).

Uptake into myocytes involves transfer of FFA from vascular to extravascular fluid, transmembrane transport to intracellular binding proteins, intracellular activation and thioesterification, transport into mitochondria, and beta-oxidation after interconversion to acyl carnitine moieties or incorporation into triglycerides or phospholipids. Some FFA initially extracted back-diffuses to the extracellular fluid without being metabolized. Diet, endocrine status, the presence or absence of diabetes mellitus, ingestion of ethanol, cardiomyopathy, and ischemic heart disease, among numerous other factors, alter myocardial fatty acid metabolism in a fashion demonstrable by PET.

We have extensively characterized the metabolic fate of palmitate labeled with carbon-11 (^{11}C-palmitate) in normal and ischemic myocardium. Although the rate of oxidation of initially extracted ^{11}C-palmitate is diminished in ischemic myocardium, externally detectable clearance reflects not only decreased oxidation but also increased back-diffusion. Interpretation of tomograms must take into account not only effects of transitory changes in the metabolic status of the tissue, but also deviations from the conditions in which the quantitative relationships between tracer kinetics and regional biochemistry were delineated. For example, changes in the proportions of fatty acid flux through triglycerides compared with beta-oxidation might be tomographically indistinguishable from changes attributable to altered ratios of fatty acid to carbohydrate utilization.

Regional myocardial metabolism is, of course, dependent on regional work, which may vary because of an altered neurohumoral environment, among numerous other factors. Determinants of the transport of the traced substrate, including the permeability surface, are products that may vary as well. Thus, tomographic estimates of regional myocardial metabolism are unlikely to be quantitative even if the spatial and temporal resolution of the deposition of the tracer are optimal, the precursor pool size is defined, and perfusion is delineated independently.

Utilization of palmitate *in vitro* remains virtually constant despite ischemia and, hence, decreased rate of delivery of the substrate when cardiac work is maintained constant. Thus, the hypoperfused heart can increase the extraction fraction of FFA from the arterial blood. Ischemia decreases cardiac work *in vivo* and, consequently, metabolic demand. However, judging from the results *in vitro,* the impaired extraction of substrate typical of myocardium subjected to low flow *in vivo* is indicative of impaired intermediary metabolism rather than simply the decreased delivery of the tracer.

PHYSICAL CONSIDERATIONS

Cardiac positron tomography is limited quantitatively by the effects of cardiac and respiratory motion, spillover of radioactivity, and partial volume effects (8,11). Ideally, data acquisition should be accomplished under conditions of respiratory synchronization and gating with respect to the cardiac cycle. Correction for spillover (the influence of radioactivity in a region adjacent to a region of interest) and for partial volume effects (phenomena encountered when the dimensions of an imaged object are less than at least twice the absolute spatial resolution of the instrument employed) is essential.

Spatial resolution achievable with PET is limited compared with that obtainable with modalities such as X-ray computed tomography (CT) or magnetic resonance imaging (MRI). Thus, it cannot rival their anatomic delineation. However, PET can delineate the locus and temporal evolution of regional biochemical phenomena *in vivo* with a tracer of virtually any physiological substrate participating in intermediary metabolism.

CLINICAL OBSERVATIONS

Accumulation of ^{11}C-palmitate is homogeneous in normal, left ventricular myocardium. Among patients with transmural infarction, dense, homogeneous defects of accumulation of ^{11}C-palmitate are seen consistently, with loci corresponding to electrocardiographic loci of infarction and to regional wall motion abnormalities. Thus, PET permits detection and localization of jeopardized, ischemic myocardium and zones of infarction. With non-Q-wave infarction ("subendocardial" infarction), defects of accumulation of ^{11}C-palmitate are not transmural. The pattern of diminished accumulation of tracer associated with myocardial ischemia is consistent from 12 hr to as long as several weeks after the onset of symptoms in the absence of extension of infarction.

CORONARY THROMBOLYSIS

Cardiac PET with ^{11}C-palmitate has documented the efficacy of coronary thrombolysis under defined conditions. After thrombolysis induced in dogs within 2 to 4 hr following the onset of ischemia, accumulation of ^{11}C-palmitate is restored. In contrast, when thrombolysis is initiated later, defects of accumulation of ^{11}C-palmitate persist despite angiographically documented recanalization (5). Thus, PET characterizes metabolic responsivity of previously ischemic myocardium and defines the temporal limits during which reperfusion can favorably affect jeopardized myocardium.

Analogous results have been obtained in patients in whom thrombolysis was induced with streptokinase or human tissue-type plasminogen activator (t-PA), a clot-selective agent with high affinity for fibrin and low affinity for circulating plasminogen (9). Cardiac PET with $H_2^{15}O$ was used to assess myocardial perfusion and with ^{11}C-palmitate to assess the metabolic response. Successful thrombolysis restored myocardial accumulation of ^{11}C-palmitate toward normal in zones within the region of supply of the initially occluded vessel (11). Thus, despite its limitations for absolute quantification of fluxes through specific metabolic pathways, PET with tracers of metabolism has proved useful for determining whether or not coronary thrombolysis benefits compromised myocardium.

Examples of the clinical research utility of metabolic imaging of the heart with positron tomography include (a) demonstrable salvage of jeopardized myocardium by coronary thrombolysis; (b) delineation of the locus of myocardial infarction in progress, manifested by impaired accumulation of tracers of metabolism such as

[11]C-palmitate; (c) delineation of the extent and distribution of threatened or completed infarction; (d) detection of spatially heterogeneous metabolism, indicative of cardiomyopathy; (e) potential delineation of pathogenetic biochemical determinants of cardiomyopathy; and (f) documentation of concordant and dichotomous patterns of accumulation of tracers of metabolism compared with tracers of flow, indicative of viability or irreversible injury of zones of the heart subjected to transient or persistent ischemia.

CONCLUSIONS AND SPECULATIONS

Positron emission tomography delineates abnormal regional myocardial metabolism and perfusion in patients with overt and covert coronary artery disease. High-resolution, fast-scanning, multislice, time-of-flight tomographic instruments now available provide improved spatial and temporal resolution. Continued elucidation of the determinants of tracer kinetics with mathematical models developed and tested in rigorously controlled systems should place clinical tomographic interpretations on an even firmer foundation. Positron emission tomography is perhaps uniquely capable of delineating pathogenetic biochemical derangements underlying cardiac function. Thus, it is likely to be particularly useful in objectively characterizing the response of hearts compromised by ischemia to potentially therapeutic interventions, such as angioplasty or coronary thrombolysis, with or without adjunctive, pharmacologic therapy.

REFERENCES

1. Ter-Pogossian, M. M., Klein, M. S., Markham, J., Roberts, R., and Sobel, B. E. (1980): Regional assessment of myocardial metabolic integrity *in vivo* by positron-emission tomography with ^{11}C-labeled palmitate. *Circulation*, 61:242.
2. Ter-Pogossian, M. M., Raichle, M. E., and Sobel, B. E. (1980): Positron-emission tomography. *Sci. Am.*, 243:170.
3. Lerch, R. A., Ambos, H. D., Bergmann, S. R., Welch, M. J., Ter-Pogossian, M. M., and Sobel, B. E. (1981): Localization of viable, ischemic myocardium by positron-emission tomography with ^{11}C-palmitate. *Circulation*, 64:689.
4. Geltman, E. M., Biello, D., Welch, M. J., Ter-Pogossian, M. M., Roberts, R., and Sobel, B. E. (1982): Characterization of nontransmural myocardial infarction by positron emission tomography. *Circulation*, 65:747.
5. Bergmann, S. R., Lerch, R. A., Fox, K. A. A., Ludbrook, P. A., Welch, M. J., Ter-Pogossian, M. M., and Sobel, B. E. (1982): Temporal dependence of beneficial effects of coronary thrombolysis characterized by positron tomography. *Am. J. Med.*, 73:573.
6. Geltman, E. M., Smith, J. L., Beecher, D., Ludbrook, P. A., Ter-Pogossian, M. M., and Sobel, B. E. (1983): Altered regional myocardial metabolism in congestive cardiomyopathy detected by positron tomography. *Am. J. Med.*, 74:773.
7. Fox, K. A. A., Nomura, H., Sobel, B. E., and Bergmann, S. R. (1983): Consistent substrate utilization despite reduced flow in hearts with maintained work. *Am. J. Physiol.*, 13:H799.
8. Geltman, E. M., Bergmann, S. R., and Sobel, B. E.: PET studies of the heart. In: *Positron Emission Tomography*, edited by Martin Reivich. Alan R. Liss, Inc., New York (*in press*).
9. Sobel, B. E., Geltman, E. M., Tiefenbrunn, A. J., Jaffe, A. S., Spadaro, J. J., Jr., Ter-Pogossian,

M. M., Collen, D., and Ludbrook, P. A. (1984): Improvement of regional myocardial metabolism after coronary thrombolysis induced with tissue-type plasminogen activator or streptokinase. *Circulation*, 69:983.

10. Bergmann, S. R., Fox, K. A. A., Rand, A. L., McElvany, K. D., Welch, M. J., Markham, J., and Sobel, B. E. (1984): Quantification of regional myocardial blood flow *in vivo* with $H_2^{15}O$. *Circulation*, 70:724.

11. Bergmann, S. R., Fox, K. A. A., Geltman, E. M., and Sobel, B. E. (1985): Positron emission tomography of the heart. *Prog. Cardiovasc. Dis.*

Hammersmith Cardiology Workshop Series, Vol. 3,
edited by A. Maseri, B. E. Sobel, and S. Chierchia.
Raven Press, New York © 1987.

Regional Abnormalities of Myocardial Glucose Metabolism in Patients with Ischemic Heart Disease

*Paolo Camici, **Luis Araujo, **Terry Spinks,
**Adriaan A. Lammertsma, and **T. Jones

*CNR Institute of Clinical Physiology and Istituto di Patologia Speciale Medica I, University
of Pisa, 56100 Pisa, Italy; **MRC Cyclotron Unit and Cardiovascular Unit,
Hammersmith Hospital, London W12 OHS, England*

In a normal fasting subject at rest, 70% to 80% of myocardial energy needs are met by the oxidation of free fatty acids. Under these circumstances, only a small percentage of the energy is produced through the oxidation of glucose. Following a carbohydrate-rich meal, myocardial glucose utilization increases as a consequence of the enhanced insulin secretion. Myocardial glucose utilization is also increased during high work load conditions independently of insulin action. Furthermore, myocardial glucose consumption can be enhanced during conditions of reduced oxygen supply (1).

Most of our knowledge about myocardial glucose metabolism, either in the normal or oxygen-deprived heart, derives from animal experiments in which biochemical assays were performed in bioptic material. At present, regional myocardial glucose utilization can be assessed noninvasively in man with ^{18}F-2-fluoro-2-deoxy-glucose (FDG) and positron emission tomography (PET) (2,3). In this chapter, we report the preliminary observations made with FDG and PET in patients with different clinical forms of ischemic heart disease.

STABLE EXERTIONAL ANGINA

In patients with stable angina inducible by exercise, studied at rest after overnight fasting, the uptake of glucose is comparable to that found in healthy volunteers studied under the same conditions (i.e., glucose uptake is very low and regionally homogeneous). In these patients during exercise, myocardial glucose utilization is increased as compared to that measured at rest. However, the increase is not homogeneous: Glucose utilization in the nonischemic regions is increased more than in the regions where myocardial perfusion (assessed with 82-rubidium and PET) (4) is abnormal.

By contrast, in the recovery from exercise, when all the parameters that were abnormal during the stress test, including myocardial perfusion, had returned to basal values, a significantly greater glucose utilization can be demonstrated in the regions of previous ischemia (5). This persistently high glucose utilization in the postischemic myocardium could indicate a greater flux through glycolysis and/ or an increased rate of glycogen synthesis, as suggested from preliminary experiments in the isolated rat heart (6).

UNSTABLE ANGINA

Myocardial glucose utilization was assessed, with FDG and PET, in patients with severe coronary artery disease and repeated episodes of spontaneous ST depression without evidence of myocardial necrosis. Patients were studied at rest following overnight fasting, off therapy, and in the absence of symptoms or ECG signs of acute ischemia. Under these circumstances, myocardial glucose utilization in these patients is significantly different from normals and patients with stable angina studied at rest. In fact, in patients with unstable angina, glucose consumption in the myocardium is regionally or globally increased already at rest. This occurs in the absence of symptoms and ECG signs of ischemia, and most often without detectable perfusion abnormalities (7).

A significant reduction of myocardial glucose uptake, which, however, remained higher than in normals and stables, was observed when these patients were restudied during i.v. infusion of nitrates. Finally, glucose consumption was normalized in those patients who underwent a successful bypass operation.

MYOCARDIAL INFARCTION

In a recent study by Marshall et al. (8), regional myocardial perfusion and exogenous glucose utilization were assessed in patients with a recent infarction with N-13 ammonia and FDG, respectively, and PET. Two different patterns of myocardial N-13 ammonia and FDG distribution were detected in these patients. On the one hand, in some cases, both myocardial perfusion and glucose utilization were concordantly reduced in infarcted myocardium. On the other hand, in some other myocardial regions, exogenous glucose utilization was disproportionately increased relative to perfusion. This was interpreted by the authors as an index of increased extraction of glucose in ischemic but still viable myocardium. Finally, these authors report that a positive correlation was found in these patients between the increased glucose utilization demonstrable with FDG and PET and the subsequent functional recovery of the infarcted areas.

REFERENCES

1. Neely, J. R., and Morgan, H. E. (1974): Substrate and energy metabolism of heart. *Annu. Rev. Physiol.,* 35:413–459.
2. Gallagher, B. M., Ansari, A., Atkins, H., Casella, V., Christman, D. R., Fowler, J. S., Ido, T., MacGregor, R. R., Sorn, P., Wan, C. N., Wolf, A. P., Kuhl, D. E., and Reivich, M. (1977): Radiopharmaceuticals XXVII, ^{18}F labelled 2-deoxy-2-fluoro-D-glucose for measuring regional myocardial glucose *in vivo:* tissue distribution and imaging studies in animals. *J. Nucl. Med.,* 18:990–996.
3. Phelps, M. E., Hoffman, E. J., Huang, S. C., and Kuhl, D. E. (1978): ECAT: a new computerized tomographic imaging system for positron emitting radiopharmaceuticals. *J. Nucl. Med.,* 19:635–641.
4. Selwyn, A. P., Allan, R. M., L'Abbate, A., Horlock, P., Camici, P., Clark, J., O'Brien, H. A., and Grant, P. M. (1982): Relation between regional myocardial uptake of rubidium-82 and perfusion: absolute reduction of cation uptake in ischemia. *Am. J. Cardiol.,* 50:112–121.
5. Camici, P., Kaski, J. C., Shea, M. J., Lammertsma, A. A., Araujo, L., and Jones, T. (1985): Selective increase of glucose utilization in the postischemic myocardium of patients with stable angina. In: *Hammersmith Cardiology Workshop Series, Vol. 2,* edited by A. Maseri, pp. 81–85. Raven Press, New York.
6. Camici, P., and Bailey, I. (1984): Time course of myocardial glycogen repletion following myocardial ischemia. *Circulation,* 70:II–85.
7. Camici, P., Araujo, L., Spinks, T., Kaski, J. C., and Maseri, A. (1984): Persistent chronic metabolic abnormalities in patients with unstable angina pectoris. *Circulation,* 70:II–249.
8. Marshall, R. C., Tillish, J. H., Phelps, M. E., Huang, S. C., Carson, R., Henze, E., and Schelbert, H. R. (1983): Identification and differentiation of resting myocardial ischemia and infarction in man with positron computed tomography. *Circulation,* 67:766–778.

Hammersmith Cardiology Workshop Series, Vol. 3,
edited by A. Maseri, B. E. Sobel, and S. Chierchia.
Raven Press, New York © 1987.

Précis of the Discussion: Section VIII

REGIONAL MYOCARDIAL METABOLIC ABNORMALITIES

Burton E. Sobel

This session focused on methods for characterizing myocardial metabolism and perfusion *in vivo*. Much of the discussion addressed applications in clinical investigation, results of which should help clarify the interpretation of more conventionally available diagnostic modalities, including myocardial scintigraphy and single-photon tomography with labeled fatty acid analogs. Positron emission tomography was discussed by Burton Sobel, with particular reference to the use of carbon-11 (^{11}C)-labeled fatty acid for evaluation of myocardial metabolic integrity and viability. Intravenous administration of carbon-11-labeled palmitate (with the label produced by a cyclotron on site) provides data permitting assessment of myocardial metabolism by the analysis of rates of accumulation and clearance of the tracer from selected regions of interest within myocardium. Clearance generally conforms to three phases, including vascular washout, beta-oxidation of intracellular fatty acids, and slow turnover of labeled fatty acid incorporated initially into neutral and phospholipids. Interpretation of time-activity curves must take into account contributions such as back-diffusion of nontrapped fatty acid, particularly under conditions such as ischemia, in which back-diffusion is augmented. At constant cardiac work, net utilization of labeled fatty acid is constant over a wide range of flow. This consistency reflects the inverse relationship between extraction fraction and perfusion when metabolic demand is held constant.

Tomographic imaging with ^{11}C-labeled palmitate delineates the extent of infarction in dogs subjected to coronary occlusion. Results correlate with those obtained by direct analysis of myocardium. In patients with evolving myocardial infarction in whom reperfusion is initiated with activators of the fibrinolytic system, serial tomographic imaging delineates the extent of myocardium in jeopardy initially, the extent to which salvage is achieved, and the relationship between augmentation of nutritional perfusion and a salutary response of metabolic function of myocardium in the initially jeopardized zone.

Clinically, tomographic imaging has clarified the nature of "reciprocal" electrocardiographic changes. In approximately 40% of the patients evaluated, such changes are indicative of ischemia at a distance rather than true electrophysiological reciprocity.

Paolo Camici discussed the use of a glucose analog, 2-fluoro-deoxyglucose (FDG), for tomographic imaging of myocardium in patients with myocardial ischemia. Among 120 patients evaluated in this fashion, regional perfusion was assessed first after intravenous administration of ribidium-82 (^{82}Rb). The distribution of FDG conformed to the distribution of ^{82}Rb when the FDG was administered under conditions of ischemia. When FDG was administered after the ischemia had resolved at a time when the distribution of ^{82}Rb resembled that seen under control conditions, augmented accumulation of FDG was evident in the zone previously ischemic. The paradoxically enhanced uptake appears to be a reflection of altered intermediary metabolism, including augmented glycolytic flux after cessation of ischemia in association with repletion of glycogen stores. Enhanced uptake was evident as late as 180 min after cessation of ischemia, however, raising the possibility that less obvious mechanisms may contribute as well.

Relationships between metabolic changes and electrophysiological abnormalities, including surface ECG manifestations, were considered. Lionel Opie, Philip Poole-Wilson, and Burton Sobel agreed that the electrocardiographic changes seen early after the onset of ischemia may reflect release of potassium from the cell and, hence, may well precede some of the alterations in intermediary metabolism visualizable tomographically. In addition, both the electrocardiographic and metabolic changes would be anticipated to precede substantial release of macromolecules from jeopardized myocardium, including creatine kinase. Although it is not entirely clear whether or not transient ischemia in man is associated with sufficient injury to myocyte cell membranes to permit the egress of macromolecules such as creatine kinase, it seems unlikely that such egress is prominent in the clinical setting. The bulk of evidence obtained from experimental animals indicates that, except under anomalous circumstances such as perfusion of myocardium with calcium-free medium, macromolecular release is tantamount to irreversible injury.

Editorial comment: B. E. Sobel

The promise of positron emission tomography is striking for the delineation of specific metabolic defects underlying pathophysiological processes that ultimately manifest themselves as impairments of myocardial function, electrophysiological derangements, or degeneration of myocardium. The potential for this modality to provide at least semiquantitative measurements of regional myocardial perfusion is considerable. Cardiac positron emission tomography should provide information necessary for delineation of the effects of interventions designed to salvage jeopardized ischemic myocardium, enhance nutritional perfusion, maintain myocardial metabolic integrity, and ultimately maintain the functional capacity of tissue in jeopardy. Results obtained from applications of positron tomography in research settings should help provide a firm foundation for improved therapeutics and a quantitative framework for improved interpretation of conventionally available diagnostic modalities, such as single-photon scintigraphy.

Hammersmith Cardiology Workshop Series, Vol. 3,
edited by A. Maseri, B. E. Sobel, and S. Chierchia.
Raven Press, New York © 1987.

Revascularization as a Means of Sudden Death Reduction

Paul G. Hugenholtz, Patrick W. Serruys, K. Laird-Meeter, and
J. R. T. C. Roelandt

*Thoraxcenter, Erasmus University, Academic Hospital,
3000 Rotterdam DR, The Netherlands*

Arguments have been detailed as to why the most likely cause for sudden cardiac death in coronary artery disease is related to bouts of severe ischemia. It has also been suggested that since recent major trials with antiarrhythmic agents have not shown any reduction in subsequent death rates (while ventricular arrhythmias had, in most cases, been markedly reduced), the original tenet that ventricular arrhythmias are the predictors of subsequent cardiac sudden death cannot be maintained any longer. Rather, it has been shown that the triggering event was often an episode of ischemia, secondary to thrombocytic aggregation with or without spasm, which leads to ventricular fibrillation (Fig. 1). This is often manifested by angina, although it now also has become clear from many studies that "silent ischemia" is much more frequent than previously recognized and may cause death without "warning signs." Even when ischemia manifests itself by threatening symptoms such as in the unstable angina syndrome, it has been shown (1,2) that the clinical distinction between a reversible ischemic state and an already infarcted myocardium cannot clinically be distinguished in many instances.

Accordingly, an entirely new approach to the prevention of sudden cardiac death would be to strive for early and complete revascularization in all those patients who have been shown, in prior contacts with the medical profession, to have obstructive coronary artery disease and who are at risk for complete occlusion. Such revascularization may be carried out by coronary artery bypass surgery, percutaneous transluminal coronary angioplasty (PTCA), or by thrombolysis, for which now a variety of agents have come on the market, such as urokinase, streptokinase, and, most recently, tissue plasminogen activators made by the recombinant technique (rt-PA). It is the purpose of this review to point toward some recent clinical results which will, in part, substantiate this strategy for reducing unnecessary cardiac death.

BYPASS SURGERY

Although no randomized trial has been undertaken in patients known to have ischemia with the express purpose of studying the efficacy of bypass grafting on

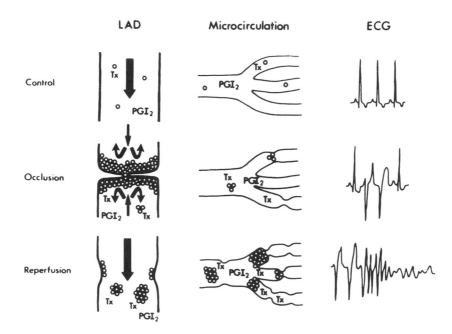

FIG. 1. Schematic of data obtained by Parratt et al. (1) in experimental sudden death, caused by sudden interruption of the microcirculation with reperfusion and release of various substances which can induce ventricular fibrillation.

subsequent death rates, the results of numerous large-scale studies in stable angina have shown an extremely low death rate of approximately 1% per year, which extends to 10 years after the original surgery. From our own experience at the Thoraxcenter, with 1,041 patients followed up for an average of 8 years, it could be shown that the initially low surgical mortality of 1.2% was matched by a similar percentage over the subsequent years (Table 1). Thus, at the end of 10 years as many people were alive after bypass surgery as were alive in a comparable group of healthy Dutch citizens. Of these 1,041 patients, only 123 (12%) required, in the course of 7.5 years on average, another operation, which was a PTCA or CABG for recurrent severe angina. In the 89 CABG patients, operative mortality rose to 6.5%. While part of the low mortality can be explained by the careful preoperative evaluation of each patient, which excluded those with other severe illnesses, the low mortality figures by themselves indicate that death from cardiac causes has been markedly reduced (3). It is only reasonable to assume that this is secondary to the effective revascularization of obstructive lesions. Even in the series recently published by Berg (4), it was shown that when bypass surgery is carried out within hours after the onset of symptoms, in patients known to have an acute infarction, a very low surgical mortality can be achieved in selected cases, which in turn is matched by a very low subsequent mortality.

TABLE 1. *Survival curve after bypass surgery in 1,041 patients*

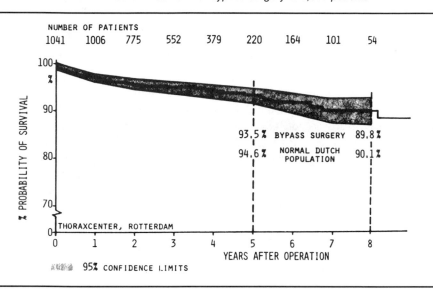

Data obtained during a long-term following of 1,041 patients operated on for angina pectoris at the Thoraxcenter (3).

PERCUTANEOUS TRANSLUMINAL CORONARY ANGIOPLASTY

Now that follow-up studies after PTCA are becoming available, it is again evident that despite a reocclusion rate of between 15% and 20% at the end of 5 years, mortality in those treated has remained equally as low as mortality after successful bypass surgery. Although the procedure heavily favors patients with one-vessel disease, in whom the mortality is low at any rate, increasing numbers of patients with multivessel disease are being treated and similar results are being observed. Again, the only explanation for the low death rate is the timely revascularization, this time by dilatation of the vessel rather than by bypass. In acute unstable angina it also has recently been shown (5,6) that when medical therapy with beta blockers, calcium antagonists, and nitrates is unsuccessful and patients are deemed refractory, that when early PTCA (i.e., within hours after the pharmacological therapy was considered ineffective) has been carried out, 1-year survival rates are remarkable (95–98%). This is in contrast with data reported in the earlier literature, which show the syndrome of unstable angina, when refractory to initial pharmacological treatment, to be associated with death rates of up to 20% (7). Also, when angina returns early after an acute myocardial infarction, recent evidence from our laboratory has shown that the previously reported high death rate (±15%) at the end of the first year can be reduced to a few percent. Again, the most likely explanation is adequate revascularization of a region of the myocardium that was at risk of ischemic episodes and intermittent reperfusion.

THROMBOLYSIS

The most striking circumstantial evidence in favor of the need for early reperfusion comes from recently reported data with streptokinase in acute myocardial infarction. While it is generally accepted that myocardial infarction, when treated with conventional methods, has a 1-year mortality rate ranging from 5% to 15%, depending on the region of the infarction and its size, the age of the patient, and the adequacy of treatment (e.g., availability of CCU), early administration of intravenous streptokinase followed by intracoronary streptokinase within 4 hr after the onset of symptoms has led to a remarkable reduction in death rates (Table 2). From a recent study (8) it has become evident that when an optimal strategy of early revascularization by means of thrombolysis is followed by balloon dilatation of the residual atheromatous lesion, death rates can be brought down to a few percent in the first year of follow-up. In a randomized study involving 533 patients with acute myocardial infarction seen at the hospital within the first few hours after symptoms (reported recently in the Netherlands) (8), it was also reported that the group assigned to a strategy of early reperfusion, regardless of the route of administration of streptokinase, had a death rate that was still half that of the control patients (8.5% vs 16.5%). In the subset that was given intravenous streptokinase within the first 2 hr after the onset of symptoms as they entered the hospital, and who were subsequently treated in an optimal fashion by intracoronary streptokinase and/or PTCA, it could be demonstrated that the 1-year mortality rate had declined to

TABLE 2. *Study of 533 consecutive patients: onset of symptoms to treatment (maximum 4 hr)*

	Conventional	Reperfusion	p-value
Number of patients	264	269	—
Cardiogenic shock	24	13	—
Ventricular fibrillation	61	38	0.01
Pericarditis	46	19	0.0004
Bleeding	8	53	0.0001
Ejection fraction, %	46	53	0.001
Mortality (14 days)	25	14	0.03
Mortality (8 months)	41	23	0.01
	(15.5%)	(8.5%)	

Netherlands Interuniversity Cardiology Institute, 1985.
Data reported from a large randomized multicenter study (8) of 533 patients with acute myocardial infarction. It is evident that early thrombolytic therapy achieves a halving of the major complications and of the death rate after myocardial infarction.

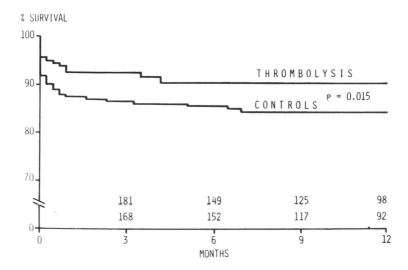

FIG. 2. Persistent improvement in survival when thrombolysis was started early after onset of infarction (8).

just above 1%. Similar data had been reported from the Western Washington Trial conducted by Kennedy, which also revealed a halving of the death rate (8a).

Large-scale trials with intravenous streptokinase are currently under way, as are trials with the much more promising agent, rt-PA. Since the latter affects the thrombus directly, without depressing the general fibrinogen level, the possibility now becomes quite high that such therapy can be given by the general practitioner, as he sees the patient within hours after the onset of symptoms. A general policy of early resolution of the obstructing thrombus, accompanied by a systematic evaluation of the status of the coronary artery system in those individuals who remain symptomatic and have signs of persisting ischemia, should enable us to reduce the risk of subsequent infarction and death in patients sustaining their first infarction to a considerable extent. With further development of strategies to render the postinfarction patient safe from reobstruction, it can be anticipated that the incidence of unnecessary cardiac death can be reduced by this means as well.

OTHER AGENTS

Although many agents have been uncovered that interfere with the clotting process, only the recent large-scale trial reported by Lewis et al. (9) has shown convincingly that the death rate after unstable angina could be reduced by aspirin. In 1,266 men, the death rate and acute infarction rate combined were reduced by 51% (31 patients vs 65 patients in the placebo group, $p < 0.005$). Recently, Cairns (10) reported even more impressive proof of the efficacy of aspirin.

DISCUSSION

It is clearly too early to advocate a general strategy. The purpose of this review is to redirect the reader toward a rather old-time physiological principle, namely, to reestablish blood flow shortly after its interruption to avoid unnecessary loss of myocardial tissue. Since it has now been generally accepted that the degree to which myocardial tissue has been damaged after myocardial infarction is the sole predictor of subsequent sudden cardiac death, it is only logical to attack this problem by reducing the cardiac damage from the outset, i.e., immediately upon the presentation of symptoms. As shown in Fig. 3, there is a curvilinear relationship between the function of the left ventricle at the time of discharge after recovery of the acute myocardial infarction event and the 1-year survival rate. As is evident from that figure, a marked increase in death rates occurs when the ventricular function expressed by the ejection fraction declines below 40%. If, as indicated in that figure, a moderate increase in ejection fraction could be achieved by early reperfusion (it was shown in the Netherlands trial to be a mean of 8%), the improvement in left ventricular function, by itself, could be held responsible for the improvement in the long-term outcome (again, an argument to reestablish blood flow at an early stage).

Whether one talks about stable angina pectoris, unstable angina pectoris, acute myocardial infarction, or angina reoccurring after myocardial infarction, all these clinical states provide clear evidence that the blood supply to the region of the myocardium at risk is impaired. Any strategy aimed at reducing this impairment

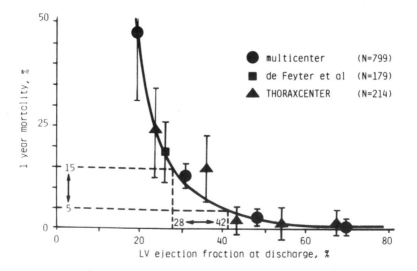

FIG. 3. Composite of data reported on three studies relating ejection fraction at discharge after acute myocardial infarction with subsequent 1-year survival. It is clear that an improvement in ejection fraction from 28% to 40% would entail a reduction in 1-year mortality from 15% to 5%.

in coronary blood flow must, therefore, be judged beneficial, and the remaining question becomes now whether or not the cost benefit ratio of these procedures can justify their general application.

In this context, the large-scale trials with beta blockers and, more recently, with calcium antagonists must be mentioned. Although secondary prevention is, undoubtedly, beneficial in reducing the death rate, the impact of this strategy is much less evident. Large numbers of patients who are not at risk must be treated for the demonstration of benefit in just a few. In the most recent and largest trial with the beta blocker metoprolol (11) it was shown that acute treatment (i.e., within the first 12 hr) with intravenous metoprolol could barely influence the mortality figures in the first 14 days. Even the still larger trial carried out with atenolol, involving over 14,000 patients, could only show a reduction of 14% in the overall death rate in the first 24 hr and, in order to achieve this effect, 150 patients had to be treated to save one life. No long-term follow-up data are available on either the metoprolol or the atenolol trials so that the efficacy of this approach over the first year after the infarction still remains in doubt. When these results and those with the calcium antagonists trials, which are even less convincing (12–15), are contrasted with the data above for early thrombolysis, the benefits of the latter approach are several orders of magnitude higher.

Admittedly, the reperfusion strategy requires a greater initial effort by the medical community than the simple intravenous injection of a beta blocker, with or without a calcium antagonist, but such therapy can only be given to a subset of those patients offered to the coronary care unit. Most beta blocker trials had to be restricted by inclusion or exclusion criteria in 40% to 50% of the patients, and usually involved only those at low risk. The streptokinase reperfusion approach, with or without subsequent aspirin, can be and has been offered to all patients except those showing a hemorrhagic diathesis. Thus, with the promised arrival of more effacious thrombolytic agents with even less complications, the road appears clear toward major trials that should aim at early reperfusion of the vessel leading to the area of the myocardium at risk.

SUMMARY AND CONCLUSION

From this brief overview, the arguments have become clear as to why further studies are needed to verify that the problem of unnecessary sudden cardiac death can best be tackled by a strategy aimed at early and complete revascularization. Whether such a strategy begins with intravenous injection of rt-PA at the home, or requires subsequent intravenous manipulation when obstruction persists (whether by thrombolyisis with other agents, PTCA, or bypass surgery) is, in itself, a moot point. The main aim should be to offer this strategy as the best chance to reduce the unnecessary sudden death rate that currently accounts for between 25% and 50% of all cardiac deaths. It deserves this chance the more, since earlier approaches employing cardioprotective efforts by beta blockade or by antiarrhythmic agents have patently shown that they cannot tackle the problem in a convincing manner.

REFERENCES

1. Parratt, J. R. (1985): Coronary vascular endothelium, spasm and reperfusion arrhythmias; experimental approaches. In: *Unstable Angina,* edited by P. G. Hugenholtz and B. S. Goldman, pp. 19–28. Schattauer, Stuttgart, New York.
2. Report of the Holland Interuniversity Nifedipine/Metoprolol Trial (HINT-Research Group) (1986): Early treatment of unstable angina at the coronary care unit: a randomized double-blind placebo controlled comparison of recurrent ischemia in patients treated with nifedipine and/or metoprolol. *Brit. Heart J.,* 56:400–413.
3. Laird-Meeter, K., Penn, O. C. K. M., Haalebos, M. M. P., van Domburg, R., Lubsen, J., Bos, E., and Hugenholtz, P. G. (1984): Survival in 1041 patients with consecutive aortocoronary bypass operations. *Eur. Heart J.,* 5:35–42.
4. Berg, R., Jr. (1979): Acute myocardial infarction treated as a surgical disease. Florence International Meeting on Myocardial Infarction, pp. 151–158. Excerpta Medica, Amsterdam.
5. De Feyter, P. J., Serruys, P. W., van den Brand, M., Soward, A. L., and Hugenholtz, P. G. (1985): Percutaneous transluminal coronary angioplasty in unstable angina pectoris, The Rotterdam Experience. In: *Unstable Angina,* edited by P. G. Hugenholtz and B. S. Goldman, pp. 229–237. Schattauer, Stuttgart, New York.
6. Meyer, J., Erbel, R., Schmitz, H. J., Pop, T., v. Olshausen, K., Henkel, B., Rupprecht, H. J., Kopp, H., and Effert, S. (1985): PTCA as an emergency treatment in unstable angina: Technical procedure, immediate and follow-up results. In: *Unstable Angina,* edited by P. G. Hugenholtz and B. S. Goldman, pp. 319–329. Schattauer, Stuttgart, New York.
7. Julian, D. G. (1985): The natural history of unstable angina. In: *Unstable Angina,* edited by P. G. Hugenholtz and B. S. Goldman, pp. 65–70. Schattauer, Stuttgart, New York.
8. Simoons, M. L., van den Brand, M., de Zwaan, C., Verheugt, F. W. A., Remme, W., Serruys, P. W., Bar, F., Res, J., Krauss, X. H., and Vermeer, F. (1985): Improved survival after early thrombolysis in acute myocardial infarction. *Lancet,* 2:578–582.
8a. Kennedy, J. W., Ritchie, J. L., Davis, K. B. (1985): The Western Washington randomized trial of intracoronary streptokinase in acute myocardial infarction. *N. Engl. J. Med.,* 312:1973–1978.
9. Lewis, H. D., Davis, J. W., Archibald, D. G., et al. (1983): Preventive effects of aspirin against acute myocardial infarction and death in men with unstable angina: results of a Veterans Administration Cooperative Study. *N. Engl. J. Med.,* X:396–403.
10. Cairns, J. R. (1985): Aspirin and sulfinpyrazone in unstable angina. In: *Unstable Angina,* edited by P. G. Hugenholtz and B. S. Goldman, pp. 219–227. Schattauer, Stuttgart, New York.
11. The Miami Trial Research Group (1985): Metoprolol in acute myocardial infarction (MIAMI). *Eur. Heart J.,* 6:199–226.
12. The Danish Study Group on Verapamil in Myocardial Infarction (1984): Verapamil in acute myocardial infarction. *Eur. Heart J.,* 5:516–528.
13. Muller, J. E., Morrison, J., Stone, P. H., Rude, R. E., Rosner, B., Roberts, R., Pearle, D. L., Turi, Z. G., Schneider, J. F., Serfas, D. H., Tate, C., Schneider, E., Sobel, B. E., Hennekens, C. H., and Braunwald, E. (1984): Nifedipine therapy for patients with threatened and acute myocardial infarction: a randomized double-blind, placebo-controlled comparison. *Circulation,* 69:740–747.
14. Muller, J. E., and the NAMIS Study Group (1985): Nifedipine therapy for unstable angina and myocardial infarction: randomized, double-blind evaluations. In: *Unstable Angina,* edited by P. G. Hugenholtz and B. S. Goldman, pp. 199–210. Schattauer, Stuttgart, New York.
15. Sirnes, P. A., Overskeid, K., Pedersen, T. R., Bathen, J., Drivenes, A., Froland, G. S., Kjekshus, J. K., Landmark, K., Rokseth, R., Sirnes, K. E., Sundoy, A., Torjussen, B. R., Westlund, K. M., and Wik, B. A. (1984): Evolution of infarct size during the early use of nifedipine in patients with acute myocardial infarction: The Norwegian Nifedipine Multicenter Trial. *Circulation,* 70:638–644.

Hammersmith Cardiology Workshop Series, Vol. 3,
edited by A. Maseri, B. E. Sobel, and S. Chierchia.
Raven Press, New York © 1987.

The Treatment of Acute Myocardial Infarction

D. A. Chamberlain

Department of Cardiology, Royal Sussex County Hospital, Brighton BN2 5BE, England

Many of the fundamental principles governing the management of myocardial infarction remain matters of debate for two reasons. The first, understandably, relates to the continuing development of new therapeutic agents, for evaluation and consensus takes time. The second reason, however, is an indictment of those who manage cardiac care units: Very infrequently in the past 25 years has clinical research been undertaken with trial designs capable of providing definitive answers to questions relating to treatment and prognosis. In particular, significant results may require large numbers of patients, but only recently have cooperative studies become common; consequently, type II errors abound and practice is influenced by evidence that is inadequate or misleading.

ANALGESIA

Management for most patients with acute infarction begins with analgesia, and for this at least broad principles are agreed. Sadly, however, the use of intravenous opiates, with dose titrated against need, is common only in hospital practice. Primary care physicians do not always appreciate that prompt relief of pain is likely to reduce the risk of arrhythmias, and that use of the intramuscular route and opiate substitutes are, therefore, inappropriate. Even in hospitals, opiates are given without antiemetics, yet vomiting can be very persistent in patients subjected to sudden movements during transfer from an emergency department. In the United Kingdom, diamorphine is the drug of choice; cyclizine can be used as the diluent for the freeze-dried pellet, but other antiemetics should be given by separate injection. Naloxone should always be available in case undue respiratory depression occurs. The responsibility for poor standards in pain relief lies principally with cardiologists who do not always give high priority to education in matters that seem mundane.

THROMBOLYSIS

Thrombolysis is believed by many to be the most important advance in the treatment of infarction since the introduction of defibrillation, yet results so far hardly warrant such optimism. No consensus exists on the best agent, on optimal doses, or on the most appropriate route of administration. Most experience has been gained with streptokinase; though the first clinical report appeared in 1959 (1), interest was restricted largely to European and Australian centers until its "rediscovery," using the intracoronary route, in the United States (2,3). Recent research on intracoronary streptokinase has been of academic value, though clinical benefit has been modest. The investigation of thrombolysis by sequential angiography during the acute phase of infarction has demonstrated beyond a doubt that most infarcts are associated with fresh thrombus formation and that reperfusion can be obtained relatively quickly. But intracoronary administration is too invasive for routine use, it cannot be administered without some delay, and facilities and skills are not widely available. The intravenous route is more practical for ease and speed of administration, though larger doses must be used and the high systemic concentration may be undesirable. Most interest is now centered on fibrin-specific agents, including tissue plasminogen activator (t-PA) (4), anisolyl plasminogen streptokinase activator complex (APSAC) (5), and pro-urokinase (6). These can be given intravenously yet attain relatively high concentrations at the site of a recent clot, thereby combining the advantages of the other methods of administration.

Yusuf et al. (7) recently reviewed the results of the trials with intracoronary and intravenous streptokinase using bar diagrams showing average mortality results and confidence limits. On this uncontrolled evidence, the intravenous route does not seem inferior overall to intracoronary administration. Few data are available yet on fibrin-specific agents, but early results with t-Pa and APSAC are promising (8,9). In our own randomized study of 149 patients with suspected infarction comparing APSAC with conventional treatment, confirmed infarction was significantly less common in those who had received the active agent; other results were consistent with benefit from early reperfusion (10). Several years will pass before the best modality of treatment is clearly established, but good results will be achieved only in patients admitted to the hospital promptly after the onset of symptoms. Early diagnosis and referral will become increasingly important though, doubtless, depressingly difficult to achieve.

ANTIARRHYTHMIC TREATMENT

When coronary care units were introduced in the 1960s, defibrillation and antiarrhythmic therapy were conceived as the twin strategies to save lives. The former has fulfilled its promise but the latter has not. No one doubts that antiarrhythmic drugs have a role in the treatment of established tachyarrhythmias, but they have proved disappointing in the prophylaxis of those that are life threatening. One well-known randomized placebo-controlled study (11) of 212 patients did show a significant reduction in the incidence of ventricular fibrillation as a result of intravenous lignocaine. But the clinical relevance of the study must be assessed in light of two additional facts: First, an unusually high proportion of control patients developed the arrhythmia and, second, none died because of it. Other studies have failed to show a significant protective effect, yet, this drug and other class I agents continue to be used somewhat uncritically despite theoretical risks from depression of automaticity, conductivity, and contractility—as well as possible proarrhythmic effects. Early administration of metoprolol (12) and propranolol (13) have also been claimed to protect against ventricular fibrillation during the acute phase of infarction though, again, this early effect has not been associated with a concurrent reduction in mortality.

That mortality in the acute phase can be reduced to a small degree by beta blockade is, however, suggested by the large Isis I study of over 16,000 patients (14); after early intravenous administration of atenolol, a 15% decrease in mortality occurred in the first week, and this benefit persisted (without increasing) into late convalescence. No trials of prophylactic antiarrhythmic agents without beta-blocking properties have demonstrated convincingly any reduction in mortality during acute myocardial infarction, if studies of intramuscular lignocaine (15) and oral disopyramide (16) are discounted because they are now considered to have been seriously flawed (17). The conclusion is clear. Although antiarrhythmic therapy may be effective for established rhythm disorders during acute infarction, prophylactic use of agents without beta-blocking activity has not been associated with any reduction in mortality. Atenolol may have a small protective effect, though patient selection in the multicenter trial may (as is inevitably the case) introduce a bias that cannot easily be defined or reliably reproduced.

BETA BLOCKADE

Much has been written on the use of beta blockers in myocardial infarction and the topic has been extensively reviewed (18). Reference has been made already to the important Isis trial of intravenous atenolol. One other agent has been shown to achieve a decrease in mortality when administered early in the acute phase; patients given metoprolol intravenously then orally in the Göteberg trial (19) had, at three months, a mortality rate 36% lower than the placebo group. But when a similar study was conducted on a wider scale, no statistically significant result was obtained (20). Chest pain and indices of infarct size were reduced in the Göteborg study as in others, and in these carefully supervised patients heart failure was not more common in the treated group than in those on placebo. Though the benefits of beta blockade in acute infarction are not striking, the information now available attests to the relative safety of the drugs for this indication, and does suggest that some, at least, may have a small role in improving comfort and decreasing risk. I believe that previous maintenance treatment with beta blockers should be continued after infarction has supervened, provided that neither failure nor bradycardia are prominent. Consideration should be given to starting treatment in the acute phase for patients with sinus tachycardia in the absence of failure, for those with persistent pain who are free of important contraindications, and for those in whom recurrent tachyarrhythmias signify heightened risk. The important issue of secondary prevention in the convalescent phase is outside the scope of this review.

ANTICOAGULATION

Anticoagulation is an older method of secondary prevention, and perhaps one too readily discarded over 20 years ago. This followed disillusionment from expectations set too high and the publication of trials beset (as with antiarrhythmic therapy) by type II errors. In 1948 (21), a trial conducted for the American Heart Association demonstrated a reduction in mortality as a result of anticoagulation, and recommended its use in patients with infarction. But the trial was not properly randomized, and the main advantage of therapy may have been to counter the 4% death rate from thromboemboli (mainly pulmonary) in patients immobilized in hospital after coronary attacks (22). Subsequently, many trials, including that published by the Medical Research Council in 1969 (23), failed to show significant improvement in mortality. Large-scale analyses of death rates have, however, suggested that these might be reduced by anticoagulation (24). Pooling of randomized studies has also indicated that mortality can be lowered by approximately 20% (25). The design of most trials would not have been capable of demonstrating a change of this magnitude, yet, it is as large as that claimed for secondary prevention by beta blockade. Moreover, the results were achieved in an era before anticoagulation was standardized: Dosage in many centers was likely to have been below that now regarded as adequate to achieve prothrombin times within the therapeutic range. Evidence of a favorable effect of anticoagulation on the prognosis of chronic coronary disease came from a Dutch study (26) showing that continuation of treatment in elderly postinfarction patients was significantly safer than withdrawal. Though this does not prove the value of introducing anticoagulation in the acute stage, it does confirm that at least some of the pathological processes in ischemic heart disease can be influenced favorably by anticoagulation. New trials of anticoagulation involving adequate numbers of patients with acute (and chronic) ischemic heart disease are urgently needed yet may never be done.

The value of anticoagulation to prevent pulmonary and cerebral emboli is less contentious and is supported by objective evidence from trials. The Veterans Administration trial (27), for example, showed that clinical cerebrovascular accidents were reduced from 3.8% to 0.8% by heparin and warfarin, with striking reduction also in the incidence of pulmonary emboli. In the same study, markers of risk were identified within the control group, including enzyme rise, age, white count, and heart failure. We ourselves follow the suggestion of Fulton (28) and use fibrinogen concentrations in the acute phase to define a population at special risk, so that anticoagulation beyond a few days can, with reasonable safety and maximum benefit ratio, be restricted to 25% of the infarct population. Comparison of complication rates in the two years before and after our anticoagulation policy was adopted

(50 vs 17 "thrombotic events"; unpublished observations) underlines the need for further randomized trials in this important area. At present, neither heparin nor warfarin are standard treatments for patients with acute infarction.

ANTIPLATELET THERAPY

Interest in antiplatelet agents centers, at present, principally around aspirin. This class of drugs has attracted less passion than anticoagulants, despite the criticism leveled at the much publicized study of sulfinpyrazone (29). The role of antiplatelet agents has been explored mostly in patients with threatened infarction (30) or for secondary prevention after infarction (31). No satisfactory trials have been reported relating to their effects in the course of acute infarction.

ANTIFAILURE THERAPY

The treatment of heart failure in the early phase of myocardial infarction does not differ in any fundamental respect from that of acute left ventricular failure of other etiologies. Some points, however, are worthy of comment. First, special care should be taken not to lower coronary perfusion pressure unduly when intravenous nitrates are used. Optimal doses are difficult to determine clinically at the bedside, but fortunately modest falls in blood pressure with this agent may be associated with improvement in ischemia as judged by ST segment shift (32). Second, the use of inotropes in infarction poses special problems relating to provocation of arrhythmias, increased oxygen requirement aggravating myocardial ischemia, and (with some agents) rises in systemic vascular resistance, which lower cardiac output and increase left atrial pressure (33). Third, digitalis should also be used with special caution. Four studies have identified digitalis as an independent risk factor (34–37) due to its proarrhythmic effect. Another study— the Coronary Artery Surgery Study (38)—also found digoxin to be associated with excess mortality, but analysis failed to show this was independent of other variables. The data should, however, prompt caution. Glycosides should be used for rapid atrial fibrillation and for acute heart failure, but a persuasive case can be made for discontinuing the drug as soon as possible in the convalescent phase.

CONCLUSION

The emphasis in the management of acute myocardial infarction in the second half of this decade should be on prompt admission so that ventricular fibrillation can be treated and, if promise holds good, so that intracoronary clot can be lysed: These will be regarded as first measures in treatment before other steps are taken to reduce the risk of recurrences. A fair summary of appropriate emergency treatment can be offered in brief: "Relieve the pain, dissolve the clot." Bearing in mind the undoubted hazards of antiarrhythmic and other drugs, this may suitably be followed by the aphorism: ". . . electricity's safe, but drugs are not."

REFERENCES

1. Fletcher, A. P., Sherry, S., Alkjaersig, N., Smyrniotis, F. E., and Jick, S. (1959): The maintenance of a sustained thrombolytic state in man. II. Clinical observations on patients with myocardial infarction and other thromboembolic disorders. *J. Clin. Invest.*, 38:1111–1119.
2. Rentrop, P., Blanke, H., Karsch, K. R., Kaiser, H., Kostering, H., and Leitz, K. (1981): Selective intracoronary thrombolysis in acute myocardial infarction and unstable angina pectoris. *Circulation*, 63:307–316.
3. Ganz, W., Buchbinder, N., Marcus, H., Mondkar, A., Maddahi, J., Charuzi, Y., O'Connor, L., Shell, W., Fishbein, M., Kass, R., Miyamoto, A., and Swan, H. J. C. (1981): Intracoronary thrombolysis in evolving myocardial infarction. *Am. Heart J.*, 101:4–13.
4. Matsuo, O., Rijken, D. C., and Collen, D. (1981): Thrombolysis by human tissue plasminogen activator and urokinase in rabbits with experimental pulmonary embolus. *Nature*, 291:590–591.
5. Smith, R. A. G., Dupe, R. J., English, P. D., and Green, J. (1981): Fibrinolysis with acyl-enzymes: a new approach to thrombolytic therapy. *Nature*, 290:505–508.
6. Gurewich, V., Pannell, R., Louie, S., Kelley, P., Suddith, R. L., and Greenlee, R. (1984): Effective and fibrin-specific clot lysis by a zymogen precursor form of urokinase (pro-urokinase). *J. Clin. Invest.*, 73:1731–1739.
7. Yusuf, S., Collins, R., Peto, R., Furberg, C., Stampfer, M. J., Goldhaber, S. Z., and Hennekens, C. H. (1985): Intravenous and intracoronary fibrinolytic therapy in acute myocardial infarction: overview of results on mortality, reinfarction and side-effects from 33 randomized controlled trials. *Eur. Heart J.*, 6:556–585.
8. The TIMI Study Group (1985): The thrombolysis in myocardial infarction (TIMI) trial. Phase I findings. *N. Engl. J. Med.*, 312:932–936.
9. Hillis, W. S., Horning, R. S., and Dunn, F. G. (1984): Coronary reperfusion following single dose intravenous BRL 26921. *Circulation, (Suppl. II)* 70:11–28.
10. Ikram, S., Lewis, S., Bucknall, C., Scram, I., Thomas, N., Vincent, R., and Chamberlain, D. (1986): Treatment of acute myocardial infarction with anisoylated plasminogen streptokinase activator complex. *Br. Med. J.*, 293:786–789.
11. Lie, K. I., Wellens, H. J., Van Capelle, F. J., and Durrer, D. (1974): Lidocaine in the preventation of primary ventricular fibrillation. A double-blind, randomized study of 212 consecutive patients. *N. Engl. J. Med.*, 291:1324–1326.
12. Ryden, L., Ariniego, R., Arnman, K., Herlitz, J., Hjalmarson, A., Holberg, S., Reyes, C., Smedgard, P., Scedberg, K., Vedin, A., Waagstein, F., Waldenstrom, A., Wilhelmsson, C., Wedel, H., and Yamamoto, M. (1983): A double-blind trial of metroprolol in acute myocardial infarction. Effects on ventricular tachyarrhythmias. *N. Engl. J. Med.*, 308:614–618.
13. Norris, R. M., Barnaby, P. F., Brown, M. A., Geary, G. G., Clarke, E. D., Logan, R. L., and Sharpe, D. N. (1984): Prevention of ventricular fibrillation during acute myocardial infarction by intravenous propranolol. *Lancet*, 2:883–887.
14. Isis-I (First International Study of Infarct Survival) Collaborative Group (1986): Randomized trial of intravenous atenolol among 16,027 cases of suspected acuted myocardial infarction: ISIS-I. *Lancet*, 2:57–66.
15. Valentine, P. A., Frew, J. L., Mashford, M. L., and Sloman, J. G. (1974): Lidocaine in the prevention of sudden death in the pre-hospital phase of acute infarction. *N. Engl. J. Med.*, 291:1327–1331.
16. Zainal, N., Carmichael, D. J. S., Kidner, P. H., Gilham, A. D., and Summers, G. D. (1977): Oral disopyramide for the prevention of arrhythmias in patients with acute myocardial infarction admitted to open wards. *Lancet*, 2:887–889.
17. Campbell, R. W. F. (1984): Prophylactic antiarrhythmic therapy in acute myocardial infarction. *Am. J. Cardiol.*, 54 (Suppl.): 8E–10E.

18. Chamberlain, D. A. (1983): Beta adrenoceptor antagonists after myocardial infarction—where are we now? *Br. Heart J.*, 49:105–110.
19. Hjalmarson, A., Elmfeldt, D., Herlitz, J., Holmberg, S., Malek, I., Nyberg, G., Ryden, L., Swedberg, K., Vedin, A., Waagstein, F., Waldenstrom, A., Waldenstrom, J., Wedel, H., Wilhelmsen, L., and Wilhelmsson, C. (1981): Effect on mortality of metoprolol in acute myocardial infarction. *Lancet*, 2:823–827.
20. The Miami Trial Research Group (1985): Metoprolol in acute myocardial infarction (MIAMI). A randomised placebo-controlled international trial. *Eur. Heart J.*, 6:199–226.
21. Wright, I. S., Marple, C. D., and Beck, D. F. (1948): Report of the committee for the evaluation of anticoagulants in the treatment of coronary thrombosis with myocardial infarction. *Am. Heart J.*, 36:801–815.
22. Hilden, T., Raaschou, F., Iverson, K., and Schwartz, M. (1961): Anticoagulants in acute myocardial infarction. *Lancet*, 2:327–331.
23. Report of the Working Party on Anticoagulant Therapy in Coronary Thrombosis to the Medical Research Council (1969): Assessment of short-term anticoagulant administration after cardiac infarction. *Br. Med. J.*, 1:335–342.
24. Modan, B., Shani, M., Schor, S., and Modan, M. (1975): Reduction of hospital mortality from acute myocardial infarction by anticoagulant therapy. *N. Engl. J. Med.*, 292:1359–1362.
25. International Anticoagulant Review Group (1970): Collaborative analysis of long-term anticoagulant administration after acute myocardial infarction. *Lancet*, 1:203–209.
26. Report of the Sixty Plus Reinfarction Research Group (1980): A double-blind trial to assess long-term anticoagulant therapy in elderly patients after myocardial infarction. *Lancet*, 2:989–994.
27. Veterans Administration Hospital Investigators (1973): Anticoagulants in acute myocardial infarction. Results of a cooperative clinical trial. *J.A.M.A.*, 225:724–729.
28. Fulton, R. M., and Duckett, K. (1976): Plasma-fibrinogen and thromboemboli after myocardial infarction. *Lancet*, 2:1161–1164.
29. Anturane Reinfarction Trial Research Group (1980): Sulfinpyrazone in the prevention of sudden death after myocardial infarction. *N. Engl. J. Med.*, 302:250–256.
30. Lewis, H. D., Jr., Davis, J. W., Archibald, D. G., Steinke, W. E., Smitherman, T. C., Doherty, J. E., Schnaper, H. W., LeWinter, M. M., Linares, E., Pouget, J. M., Sabharwal, S. C., Chesler, E., and DeMots, H. (1983): Protective effects of aspirin against acute myocardial infarction and death in men with unstable angina. Results of a Veterans Administration Cooperative Study. *N. Engl. J. Med.*, 309:396–403.
31. May, G. S., Eberlein, K. A., Furberg, C. D., Passamani, E. R., and DeMets, D. L. (1982): Secondary prevention after myocardial infarction: a review of long-term trials. *Prog. Cardiovasc. Dis.*, 24:331–352.
32. Come, P. C., Flaherty, J. T., Baird, M. G., Rouleau, J. R., Weisfeldt, M. L., Greene, H. L., Becker, L., and Pitt, B. (1975): Reversal by phenylephrine of the beneficial effects of intravenous nitroglycerin in patients with acute myocardial infarction. *N. Engl. J. Med.*, 293:1003–1007.
33. Timmis, A. D., Fowler, M. B., and Chamberlain, D. A. (1981): Comparison of hemodynamic responses to dopamine and salbutamol in severe cardiogenic shock complicating acute myocardial infarction. *Br. Med. J.*, 282:7–9.
34. Moss, A. J., Davis, H. T., Conard, D. L., DeCamilla, J. J., and Oderoff, C. L. (1981): Digitalis-associated cardiac mortality after myocardial infarction. *Circulation*, 64:1150–1156.
35. Bigger, J. T., Weld, F. M., Rolnitzky, L. M., and Ferrick, K. J. (1981): Is digitalis treatment harmful in the year after acute myocardial infarction? *Circulation (Suppl. IV)*, 64:83.
36. Muller, J., Turi, Z., Stone, P., Rude, R., Raabe, D., Jaffe, A., Gold, H., Gustafson, N., Pool, K., Smith, T., Braunwald, E., and the MILIS Group (1983): Does digoxin therapy increase mortality following myocardial infarction? *Circulation (Suppl. III)* 68:368.
37. Moss, A. J., Davis, H. T., Odoroff, C. L., and Bigger, J. T. (1983): The Multicenter Postinfarction Research Group. Digitalis-associated mortality in postinfaraction patients. *Circulation*, 67:735–742.
38. Ryan, T. J., Bailey, K. R., McCabe, C. H., Luk, S., Fisher, L. D., and Mock, M. B. (1983): The effects of digitalis on survival in high-risk patients with coronary disease (CASS). *Circulation*, 67:735–742.

Hammersmith Cardiology Workshop Series, Vol. 3,
edited by A. Maseri, B. E. Sobel, and S. Chierchia.
Raven Press, New York © 1987.

Précis of the Discussion: Section IX

UPDATE: ORGANIZATION AND POLICIES IN CCU

Attilio Maseri

Desmond Julian insisted that a most crucial point was early referral or self-referral because whatever forms of treatment we believe in, early institution of therapy is absolutely vital. Douglas Chamberlain described his experience with early referral in a British environment: "In the last six months of 1970, the median time for admission to our CCU after the onset of major symptoms was six hours and 20 minutes. We then had a resuscitation ambulance and that created a new awareness of the need to get into hospital quickly. Then, over a period of two or three years, that time went down to somewhere between two and two-and-a-half hours median. It varies from year to year, but we have found it incredibly difficult to get below that."

Desmond Julian commented that it may be easy to make some bogus figures on this admission time. "At the beginning of CCUs, the admission criteria included everybody within 48 hr. Later policies were instituted whereby patient admission later than six hours was discouraged. In this way, the median time can be improved without necessarily getting patients in really early. We must be very careful in interpreting figures of this kind."

Nina Rehnqvist commented on the Swedish experience: "In Sweden we have the system of self-referral so the patient can phone the ambulance himself and get to the hospital, but that does not mean that the time is better than in Brighton or anywhere else. Rather to the contrary, I think the 'hoo-haa' that goes with a mobile CCU might have put the figures a little down. In Stockholm with the short transportation time, the delay is still over four hours."

Paul Lichtlen reported his experience: "In Northern Germany we also have a self-referral system and ambulances with a doctor usually can be there quite quickly, but also our referral time is approximately three hours. It came down from about four hours in the early 1970s when I started in Hanover. It is difficult to get lower because the decision time of the patient is still so long; I think that is the major factor."

Douglas Chamberlain commented that their data indicate that people don't do any better the second time around, even though they have been instructed.

Attilio Maseri said that we have to try to improve the perception of the community and not only to infarction. It would be desirable to get patients into the hospital during an unstable phase of angina, as chest pain often precedes the onset of myocardial infarction; in this way, we would be in a position to try and prevent infarction, rather than cure it or reduce it. This is not an alternative to alerting the patient who has the full-blown picture of infarction to come in, but rather to extend this to other patients. The problem then would be moved to the need for sophisticated or invasive procedures which would require a stratified system of centers so that when patients require procedures not available locally (such as angioplasty), they can be transferred.

Paul Hugenholtz reported on his experience: "One of the things we have tried is what we call 'free call,' that is, a patient once seen by a physician or a specialist, and having been recognized as being at increased risk of a subsequent event, is given a telephone number which he can call. It really has broken the barrier; all of a sudden they now feel they can decide on their fate. We have now broken this barrier because the patient can, without feeling that he is bothering his doctor, contact the hospital directly. By this method we also get the patients with unstable angina."

Editorial comment: A. Maseri

In the past two decades, the outlook for patients with acute coronary syndromes has greatly improved. This result has been achieved by early recognition and better management of arrhythmias, of the consequences of myocardial ischemia, and, more recently, by prevention and reduction of ischemia.

Along the same lines I can see room for further refinements: on the one hand, by development of better drugs and techniques, on the other by defining more precisely which subsets of patients, and in which phase of their disease, benefit most by the various forms of treatment. Indeed, patients with infarction, and with acute coronary syndromes in general, represent a wide spectrum in terms of severity of coronary obstruction, ventricular function, impairment, and prevailing pathogenetic mechanisms of ischemia. Therefore, the current tendency to think in terms of management of "unstable angina" or of "acute infarction," as if they were homogeneous entities, although quite convenient for drug companies and for lazy physicians, should be corrected. Both for the optimal medical treatment of the individual patient and for limiting the costs it is necessary to identify (a) which type of patient benefits most from nitrates, calcium antagonists, beta blockers, antithrombotic therapy, thrombolitic therapy, angioplasty, or surgery, and (b) in which phase of their disease should each form or combination of treatments be used. This goal cannot be achieved by large-sized clinical trials which, by definition, examine the average benefit for the average patient following an average treatment (for example, the same dose of beta blockers used in a trial is not necessarily the best for all eligible patients, nor will all eligible patients have the same beneficial or unwanted effects from this treatment). Until we learn more about the mechanisms of the disease and their clinical correlates, this goal is more likely to be achieved by careful consideration of each individual patient, beginning with what appears the most reasonable first line of treatment of that particular case, and stepping up or modifying the treatment as indicated by unwanted effects, by the persistence of symptoms and signs of ischemia, or by the anticipated short-term prognosis.

Along different lines, further improvement of the outlook for patients with acute coronary syndromes can be achieved by (a) gaining a better understanding of why they occur in a given patient at that time of his or her life, (b) trying to identify the elements that make patients different from one another rather than on those that make them similar, and (c) increasing the awareness of society or, at least, of the patients at risk so that an efficient system of self-referral can shorten the time for intervention possibly in the unstable phase, or in the early onset of infarction.

Hammersmith Cardiology Workshop Series, Vol. 3,
edited by A. Maseri, B. E. Sobel, and S. Chierchia.
Raven Press, New York © 1987.

Early Thrombolysis in Acute Myocardial Infarction

Burton E. Sobel

*Cardiovascular Division, Washington University School of Medicine,
St. Louis, Missouri 63110*

The effects of reperfusion on myocardium are complex (1–7). They depend markedly upon the interval of antecedent ischemia. Delayed reperfusion may not only fail to restore myocardial intermediary metabolism and function, but also exacerbate injury in jeopardized cells because of accumulation of calcium, potentiating irreversible injury. Thus, despite numerous reports attesting to coronary recanalization after intravenous or intracoronary administration of activators of the fibrinolytic system, many issues remain unresolved. Obviously, although very early reperfusion can preclude cell death, late reperfusion cannot possibly restore viability to already dead cells even in the face of angiographically documented recanalization.

CLINICAL CRITERIA OF THE EFFICACY OF CORONARY THROMBOLYSIS

As stated by Hugenholtz and Rentrop (8), there is "no doubt that intracoronary lysis of the thrombus . . . will reestablish blood flow through the acutely occluded coronary artery in approximately 80% of cases." The question is, however, whether or not the recanalization is accompanied by salutary effects on the heart. Accelerated resolution of ST segment elevation and rapid evolution of Q waves are typical, but their interpretation may be ambiguous. Effects of coronary thrombolysis on ventricular function may be obscured by temporal disparities between the return of function and the restoration of nutritional blood flow. Furthermore, apparent improvements in global function may be attributable to changes in the physical properties of the reperfused zone, such as increased stiffness despite lack of restoration of its contractile function. Alterations of blood viscosity associated with fibrinogenolysis accompanying the use of conventional activators, compensatory changes in previously hyperfunctioning well-perfused tissue that dissipate as the previously jeopardized myocardium resumes contraction, and difficulties in delineating identical regions of the ventricle for sequential wall motion analysis in serial studies, make interpretation of changes in indexes of global and regional ventricular function far from certain after coronary thrombolysis. Scintigraphy with single-photon emitters, such as thallium-201, may be misleading because of delayed clearance of tracer from hypoperfused zones obscuring ischemia initially, possible effects of streaming of tracer, or unavoidable physical limitations of imaging modalities impairing quantification of the distribution of tracer in reperfused zones.

In view of these considerations, we have utilized positron emission tomography in experimental animals and patients to define the effects of coronary thrombolysis on the heart. When reperfusion was initiated early after the onset of ischemia in dogs, improvement of regional metabolism in jeopardized tissue was evident. Ischemia for intervals greater than 3 hr, however, was associated with persistence rather than resolution of metabolic impairments detectable tomographically. In patients in whom coronary thrombolysis was initiated within approximately 6 hr after the onset of symptoms or less, accumulation of carbon-11 labeled palmitate, diminished in jeopardized tissue prior to reperfusion, was augmented in the reperfused zone. More than 75% of such patients exhibited improvement of 20% or more in regional myocardial metabolism defined tomographically. Thus, in experimental animals and patients, recovery of myocardial intermediary metabolism is inducible in at least some instances by well-timed, early reperfusion.

FACTORS INFLUENCING THE EFFICACY OF CORONARY THROMBOLYSIS

Ultimately, the clinical impact of coronary thrombolysis is likely to depend on several characteristics of the activator of the fibrinolytic system utilized. Because of the need for rapid implementation, activators devoid of risks otherwise requiring extensive pretreatment monitoring or low dose intracoronary administration are likely to be particularly useful. Activators with short biological half-lives are attractive because of the frequent need for restoration of hemostasis promptly when patients require invasive diagnostic procedures or surgery soon after successful coronary thrombolysis. Clot-selective thrombolysis is particularly attractive because it provides a wide therapeutic-to-toxic ratio for the activator employed, and because it permits administration of activator intravenously in generous but still safe doses. Perhaps the most promising agent undergoing evaluation currently is tissue-type plasminogen activator (t-PA). This moiety has a high binding affinity for fibrin but a low affinity for circulating plasminogen. Thus, it elicits lysis of fibrin in the clot without flooding the circulating blood with plasmin and without inducing marked fibrinogenolysis that could compromise hemostasis.

INDUCTION OF CORONARY THROMBOLYSIS WITH t-PA

After experimentally induced thrombosis in dogs, intravenously administered human t-PA harvested from melanoma cell tissue culture supernatant fractions consistently elicited coronary thrombolysis within 15 to 30 min. When regional myocardial metabolism was evaluated tomographically with intravenously administered carbon-11 labeled palmitate and regional perfusion was quantified with intravenously administered oxygen-15 labeled water, it became clear that restoration of both myocardial perfusion and metabolism could be accomplished. In marked contrast to the case with urokinase, neither intravenous nor intracoronary t-PA induced a systemic lytic state. Thus, circulating concentrations of alpha$_2$-antiplasmin did not decline, marked fibrinogenolysis did not occur, and circulating plasminogen was not depleted. In subsequent studies, similar results were achieved with human t-PA synthesized by recombinant DNA technology. Coronary thrombolysis was induced in each of 9 dogs studied after an average of only 13.7 ± 1.9 min, with doses that did not induce marked depletion of circulating fibrinogen. Improvement of regional myocardial perfusion and intermediary metabolism assessed tomographically was evident.

In the initial clinical study of coronary thrombolysis with t-PA, we administered material harvested from human melanoma cell tissue culture fluid to 7 patients in doses of 20,000 to 40,000 IU per minute for 30 to 60 min. Recanalization occurred in 6 to 7 patients. A systemic lytic state was not induced. Subsequently, we administered human t-PA produced by recombinant DNA technology to 45 randomized patients in a multicenter cooperative trial. Successful lysis was achieved in 75% of patients given 0.5 mg/kg of the agent and in 87% of those given 0.75 mg/kg (approximately 60,000 and 83,000 IU/min, respectively, for 60 min). Fibrinogen declined by an average of only 8% in posttreatment compared with pretreatment samples. Initial results of the National Heart, Lung, and Blood Institute-supported double-blind, random assignment trial, Thrombolysis in Myocardial Infarction (TIMI), in which we are participating have confirmed those observations in more than 140 treated patients.

FUTURE DIRECTIONS

Tissue-type plasminogen activator exhibits several attributes likely to make it a particularly useful pharmaceutical. Because it is a naturally occurring human protein, the likelihood of allergic reactions is low. Its short half-life in the circulation is potentially advantageous in avoiding risks that would preclude or impair the safety of invasive diagnostic procedures or cardiac surgery early after successful coronary thrombolysis to prevent reocclusion. Its lack of induction of a systemic lytic state in doses capable of inducing coronary thrombolysis facilitates its use in generous doses intravenously, with predictable therapeutic responses without toxocity, and reduces the need for extensive monitoring of the status of the coagulation and fibrinolytic systems prior to and during treatment. Successful synthesis of human tissue-type plasminogen activator with recombinant DNA technology increases the likelihood of widespread availability of the agent in the near future.

REFERENCES

1. Sobel, B. E., and Bergmann, S. R. (1982): Coronary thrombolysis: Some unresolved issues. *Am. J. Med.*, 72:1.
2. Bergmann, S. R., Lerch, R. A., Fox, K. A. A., Ludbrook, P. A., Welch, M. J., Ter-Pogossian, M. M., and Sobel, B. E. (1982): Temporal dependence of beneficial effects of coronary thrombolysis characterized by positron tomography. *Am. J. Med.*, 73:573.
3. Bergmann, S. R., Fox, K. A. A., Ter-Pogossian, M. M., Sobel, B. E. (Washington University), and Collen, D. (University of Leuven) (1983): Clot-selective coronary thrombolysis with tissue-type plasminogen activator. *Science,* 220:1181.
4. Van de Werf, F., Bergmann, S. R., Fox, K. A. A., de Geest, H., Hoyng, C. F., Sobel, B. E., and Collen D. (1984): Coronary thrombolysis with intravenously adminstered human tissue-type plasminogen activator produced by recombinant DNA technology. *Circulation,* 69:605.
5. Sobel, B. E., and Bergmann, S. R. (1985): The impact of coronary thrombolysis and tissue-type plasminogen activator (t-PA) on acute myocardial infarction. In: *Thrombolysis,* edited by D. Collen and M. Verstraete. Churchill Livingstone, Edinburgh.
6. Van de Werf, F., Ludbrook, P. A., Bergmann, S. R., Tiefenbrunn, A. J., Fox, K. A. A., de Geest, H., Verstraete, M., Collen, D., and Sobel, B. E. (1984): Coronary thrombolysis with tissue-type plasminogen activator in patients with evolving myocardial infarction. *N. Engl. J. Med.,* 310:609.
7. Sobel, B. E., Geltman, E. M., Tiefenbrunn, A. J., Jaffe, A. S., Spadaro, J. J., Jr., Ter-Pogossian, M. M., Collen, D., and Ludbrook, P. A. (1984): Improvement of regional myocardial metabolism after coronary thrombolysis induced with tissue-type plasminogen activator or streptokinase. *Circulation,* 69:983.
8. Hugenholtz, P. G., and Rentrop, P. (1982): Thrombolytic therapy for acute myocardial infarction: quo vadis? *Eur. Heart J.,* 3:395–403.

Hammersmith Cardiology Workshop Series, Vol. 3,
edited by A. Maseri, B. E. Sobel, and S. Chierchia.
Raven Press, New York © 1987.

Précis of the Discussion: Section X

EARLY THROMBOLYSIS IN ACUTE MYOCARDIAL INFARCTION

Attilio Maseri

Burton Sobel addressed considerations pertinent to coronary thrombolysis in general, such as the time of onset of the intervention with respect to the time of onset of ischemia on the one hand, and considerations pertinent to the selection of a specific activator of the fibrinolytic system, such as tissue-type plasminogen activator (t-PA), on the other. Although the temporal window during which thrombolysis can be expected to restore myocardial metabolic activity, as well as recanalize vessels, has not been defined unequivocally in man, the bulk of evidence from studies in experimental animals and from clinical research suggests that its boundary is only a few hours. Thus, although angiographic evidence of successful recanalization can be acquired readily after intravenous administration of streptokinase or urokinase in patients with occlusive coronary thrombi, the intervention offers little benefit to the myocardium or to the patient if it cannot be implemented promptly after the onset of ischemia.

In practical terms, universal implementation of fibrinolysis on suspicion of myocardial ischemia may not be justified because of the attendant risks of systemic bleeding that are invariably encountered with the use of conventional activators of fibrinolysis. However, the advent of clot-specific activators that do not induce substantial fibrinogenolysis or elevation of circulating fibrinogen degradation products, themselves potent and persistent anticoagulants, has led to consideration of the strategy of rapid implementation of agents such as t-PA in an effort to abort myocardial infarcts in progress and to salvage as much myocardium as possible prior to definitive coronary arteriography or mechanical revascularization when indicated.

Residual coronary stenosis is common after coronary thrombolysis, whether implemented with conventional activators or t-PA. Conventional wisdom dictates that heparin should be used to prevent reocclusion, despite the absence of definitive information justifying its use or providing confidence regarding its efficacy. One factor that has been identified as pivotal with respect to the potential for early reocclusion is the magnitude of the residual stenosis. Patients with very high grade residual stenosis have a high probability of early reocclusion. Those with widely patent recanalized vessels are likely to exhibit persistent patency. Tissue-type plasminogen activator is effective in recanalizing coronary arteries in approximately 75% of patients studied prospectively with preinterventional and postinterventional coronary angiograms. In selected subjects, metabolic improvements of myocardium in the jeopardized zone has been evident tomographically. In general, however, marked functional improvement after coronary thrombolysis with any agent has been difficult to document. One factor responsible may be the relatively late implementation of coronary thrombolysis, particularly when preinterventional angiography is required when thrombolysis is evaluated in the context of a research protocol governing its use.

Paul Hugenholtz agreed that between 20% and 40% of patients with successful coronary thrombolysis may require additional interventions because of high grade residual stenosis. Several contributors concurred with the view that we must focus on the overall long-term objective, namely, protracted protection of myocardium in the originally jeopardized zone rather than simply the short-term objective of initial recanalization. Douglas Chamberlain indicated that logistics often precludes the stepwise implementation of coronary arteriography and PTCA soon after thrombolysis is achieved with intravenous administration of activators of the fibrinolytic system, underscoring the social and economic implications of the profound change in management of acute myocardial infarction that may evolve as a result of the availability of safe activators of the fibrinolytic system and changes in practice increasingly entailing interventional angiography and early surgery. Wolfgang Kübler felt that we must seek to stratify patients selected for aggressive management such that a genuinely beneficial response can be anticipated in the individual patient. Although no specific time limit will apply to all patients, the contributors concurred in recognizing the crucial need for implementing revascularization promptly after the onset of ischemia, generally within 3 hr or less.

The potential benefit and potential complexities encountered in attempting to induce coronary thrombolysis in critically ill patients were underscored by Graham Davies, who illustrated sequential angiographic responses to intracoronary streptokinase. As indicated by the work of many investigators, coronary patency appears to be a dynamic process, particularly when high grade stenosis is present. Graham Davies showed graphic illustration of the possibility that cyclic reflow, so well documented in experimental animals, may occur in patients as well.

Differences between the biological half-life of specific activators in the circulation, biological half-lives of activators at the loci of thrombi, and biological half-lives of products of some activators, such as fibrinogen degradation products elaborated with streptokinase, were considered and differentiated. The potential value of activators that compromise hemostatic mechanisms with respect to prevention of reperfusion was addressed, but alternative strategies were considered as well, such as the continuing infusion of subthrombolytic doses of an agent such as t-PA. The consensus was that thrombolysis should not be viewed in a vacuum but, rather, as a component of a set of potential, therapeutic options designed to achieve revascularization during an interval in which the myocardium can still respond favorably to reperfusion. It was agreed that the ultimate impact of thrombolysis per se, or thrombolysis in concert with other interventions designed to induce or sustain recanalization on mortality and quality of life, remains to be defined.

Hammersmith Cardiology Workshop Series, Vol. 3,
edited by A. Maseri, B. E. Sobel, and S. Chierchia.
Raven Press, New York © 1987.

Endothelial Damage: Could It Be Prevented or Treated?

John L. Gordon

Department of Vascular Biology, MRC Clinical Research Centre, Harrow HA1 3UJ, England

THE NATURE OF ENDOTHELIAL DAMAGE

In its crudest form, endothelial damage manifests as the death (and subsequent removal) of the endothelium. There are, however, more subtle forms of damage: The concept of the "biochemical lesion" applies to the endothelium as it does to other cell types. The damage need not be lethal: Cellular function may be compromised but physical integrity can be retained intact. Within the extremes of cell death and minimal biochemical change, there is a spectrum of effects; for example, peroxide-induced damage to endothelial cells can induce loss of cell viability at high concentrations, while cellular functions are variously impaired by concentrations up to 1,000-fold lower, with no morphological effects (1).

Thus, "damage" is an imprecise term: It can be defined in different ways; it need not be irreversible; it can encompass everything from a modest change in a single cellular function to physical alterations and cell death. Gordon and Pearson (2) discuss this concept in more detail, with specific reference to endothelial cells.

CAUSES OF ENDOTHELIAL DAMAGE

Physical damage to endothelium can be induced by invasive procedures, for example, indwelling catheters. Moore and colleagues (3) showed that a free-floating catheter tip in a rabbit artery led to platelet-dependent thrombosis, followed by atherosclerotic lesions, and Baumgartner and Spaet (4) demonstrated that the passage of an inflated Fogarty balloon catheter along an artery resulted in denudation of the endothelium and subsequent platelet deposition. In time, the endothelium regenerated, with the formation of a proliferative lesion resembling an atherosclerotic plaque. Studies of milder physical injury to the endothelium (5,6) have provided more information on the nature and kinetics of endothelial responses (and the responses of the vessel wall as a whole) to focal injury.

Endothelium can be damaged by the administration of chemical agents, or by the generation *in vivo* of biochemical mediators. Examples of chemicals administered intravascularly that damage endothelium include radiographic contrast media. Early investigations of the effects of these agents on isolated endothelial cells (7) used long incubation times (e.g., 24 hr), but even short exposures to contrast media can affect endothelial functions *in vitro* and *in situ,* especially if hyperosmolar formulations are used (8,9). Examples of endogenous mediators that can damage endothelial cells include homocysteine (10), oxygen radicals generated during granu-locyte activation (1,11,12), and proteases from leukocytes or platelets (13,14). Immunological damage to endothelium has also been observed. This need not be complement-dependent: Fab fragments of antibodies directed against endothelial surface proteins (for example, angiotensin-converting enzyme) can induce damage (15). Complement components such as C5a can, however, affect endothelial cells (16). Mediators generated by activated macrophages, such as interleukin I, can alter the composition of the endothelial surface and affect the secretion of biologically active constituents from the endothelium (17,18). Lymphokines (e.g., γ interferon) have a variety of effects on endothelial cells, including the induction of Ia antigen expression (19). Injury to endothelial cells (e.g., by viral infection) can cause changes in morphology and function that include the expression of Fc and C3b receptors (20,21).

CONSEQUENCES OF ENDOTHELIAL DAMAGE

If endothelial cells are physically removed, this can result in platelet deposition (i.e., thrombosis), increased vascular permeability, and an alteration in various biochemical functions of the vessel wall; longer-term consequences include the formation of local, proliferative intimal lesions (3,4).

Sublethal damage can result in changes to the endothelial surface and/or to intracellular functions. Examples of the former include the expression of procoagu-lant activity (thus, reducing the thromboresistant properties of the endothelium), and the appearance of new surface antigens and receptors that affect the local regulation of immune function (17,19–21). Endothelial injury can change the pattern of biochemical mediators secreted in response to stimuli: for example, decreased production of prostacyclin and/or endothelium-derived relaxing factor (22), which can affect platelet function and the regulation of vascular tone. This can be induced by environmental factors such as the oxygen tension.

PREVENTION AND TREATMENT OF ENDOTHELIAL DAMAGE

Because our knowledge of endothelial biology and the responses of endothelium to injury is still in its infancy, attempts at preventing endothelial damage are directed mainly at the damaging stimuli themselves rather than the endothelium.

It is desirable to minimize endothelial exposure to intravascular catheters, hypertonic solutions, hypoxia, and hyperoxia. Treatment of bacterial and/or viral infections should reduce damage to endothelium as well to other affected tissues. In some circumstances, it may be appropriate to consider therapeutic intervention aimed at reducing the generation of endogenous stimuli that could damage endothelium: for example, counteracting homocysteinemia or reducing the secretion of constituents from activated leukocytes and platelets. Agents may also be administered that are designed to substitute for the lack of constituents secreted by the endothelium: for example, vasodilators to compensate for a reduced production of endothelium-derived relaxing factor or prostacyclin.

Above all, an awareness of possible initiators and consequences of endothelial damage is necessary; "endotheliology" is a new science, and our understanding of how endothelium contributes actively to many biological regulatory systems has mainly been gained in the last decade or so. It is safe to predict that our knowledge of endothelial biology and pathology will increase rapidly in the foreseeable future, and this will have implications for the prevention and treatment of endothelial damage.

REFERENCES

1. Ager, A., and Gordon, J. L. (1984): Differential effects of hydrogen peroxide on indices of endothelial cell function. *J. Exp. Med.*, 159:592–603.
2. Gordon, J. L., and Pearson, J. D. (1982): Responses of endothelial cells to injury. In: *Pathobiology of the Endothelial Cell*, edited by H. L. Nossel and H. J. Vogel, pp. 433–454. Academic, New York.
3. Moore, S., Friedman, R., Signal, D. P., Gauldie, J., Blajchman, M. A., and Roberts, R. S. (1976): Inhibition of injury-induced thromboatherosclerotic lesions by anti-platelet serum in rabbits. *Thromb. Haemost.*, 35:70–81.
4. Baumgartner, H. R., and Spaet, T. H. (1970): Endothelial replacement in rabbit arteries. *Fed. Proc.*, 29:710–719.
5. Reidy, M. A., and Schwartz, S. M. (1981): Endothelial regeneration III. Time course of intimal changes after small, defined injury to rat aortic endothelium. *Lab. Invest.*, 44:301–308.
6. Walker, L. N., and Bowyer, D. E. (1984): Endothelial healing in the rabbit aorta and the effect of risk factors for atherosclerosis. *Arteriosclerosis*, 4:479–488.
7. Laerum, F., Borsum, T., and Reisvaag, A. (1983): Human endothelial cell culture as an evaluation system for the toxicity of intravascular contrast media. *Invest. Radiol.*, 18:199–206.
8. Bettmann, M. A. (1985): Effects of contrast agents on endothelial cell function. *Radiology*, 157:55211.
9. Morgan, D., and Bettmann, M. A. (1986). In vitro effects of radiographic contrast media and radiation of human endothelial cells. *Invest. Radiol.*, 21:551.
10. Harker, L. A., Ross, R., Slichter, S. J., and Scott, C. R. (1976): Homocystine-induced arteriosclerosis. The role of endothelial cell injury and platelet response in its genesis. *J. Clin. Invest.*, 58:731–741.
11. Sacks, T., Moldow, C. F., Craddock, P. R. Bowers, T. K., and Jacob, H. S. (1978): Oxygen radicals mediate endothelial cell damage by complement-stimulated granulocytes. *J. Clin. Invest.*, 61:1161.
12. Weiss, S. J., Young, J., LoBuglio, A. F., Slivka, A., and Nimeh, N. F. (1981): Role of hydrogen peroxide in neutrophil mediated destruction of cultured endothelial cells. *J. Clin. Invest.*, 68:714.
13. Harlan, J. M., Killen, P. D., Harker, L. A., Striker, G. E., and Wright, D. G. (1981): Neutrophil-mediated endothelial injury *in vitro*. *J. Clin. Invest.*, 68:1394–1403.

14. LeRoy, E. C., Ager, A., and Gordon, J. L. (1984): Effects of neutrophil elastase and other proteases on porcine aortic endothelial prostaglandin I_2 production, adenine nucleotide release and responses to vasocative agents. *J. Clin. Invest.,* 74:1003–1010.
15. Caldwell, P. R. B., Wigger, H. J., Butler, V. P., and Gigli, I. (1982): Pulmonary endothelial cell injury induced by antibody fragments to angiotensin converting enzyme. In: *Pathobiology of the Endothelial Cell,* edited by H. L. Nossel and H. J. Vogel, pp. 425–430. Academic, New York.
16. Rampart, M., Bult, H., and Herman, A. G. (1983): Activated complement and anaphylatoxins increase the *in vitro* production of prostacyclin by rabbit aorta endothelium. *N-S Arch. Pharmacol.,* 322:158–165.
17. Bevilacqua, M. P., Pober, J. S., Majeau, G. R., Cotran, R. S., and Gimbrone, M. A. (1984): Interleukin I induces biosynthesis and cell surface expression of procoagulant activity in human vascular endothelial cells. *J. Exp. Med.,* 160:618–623.
18. Dejana, E., Breviario, F., Balconi, G., Remuzzi, G., de Gaetano, G., and Mantovani, A. (1984): Stimulation of PGI_2 synthesis in vascular cells by mononuclear cell products. *Blood,* 64:1280–1283.
19. Pober, J. S., Collins, T., Gimbrone, M. A., et al. (1983): Lymphocytes recognize human vascular endothelial and dermal fibroblast Ia antigens induced by recombinant immune interferon. *Nature,* 305:726–729.
20. Ryan, U. S., Schultz, D. R., and Ryan, J. W. (1981): Fc and C3b receptors on pulmonary endothelial cells: induction by injury. *Science,* 214:557–558.
21. Cines, D. B., Lyss, A. P., Bina, M., Corkey, M., Kefalides, N. A., and Friedman, H. M. (1982): Fc and C_3 receptors induced by herpes simplex virus on cultured human endothelial cells. *J. Clin. Invest.,* 69:123–128.
22. Furchgott, R. F., Cherry, P. D., Zawadzki, J. V., and Jothianandan, D. (1984): Endothelial cells as mediators of vasodilation of arteries. *J. Cardiovasc. Pharmacol. (Suppl. 2),* 6:336–344.

Hammersmith Cardiology Workshop Series, Vol. 3,
edited by A. Maseri, B. E. Sobel, and S. Chierchia.
Raven Press, New York © 1987.

Antiplatelet and Anticoagulant Drugs: Which, When?

J. A. Davies

University Department of Medicine, The General Infirmary, Leeds LS1 3EX, England

TREATMENT OF ACUTE MYOCARDIAL INFARCTION

Anticoagulants can prevent formation and extension of thrombi but do not affect formed fibrin. Anticoagulation for patients admitted with acute infarction is, therefore, not likely to alter the basic disease process, though occasionally infarct size might be limited by inhibition of clot extension in the coronary arteries. Early enthusiasts for anticoagulant treatment thought that "it appears physiologically sound to use it whenever there is a definite tendency for a thrombus to propagate or multiple thrombi or embolic phenomena to occur" (1). Unfortunately, the clarity of this aim has been clouded subsequently by largely irrelevant consideration of the part played by coagulation mechanisms in coronary artery occlusion.

At the time of the early trials of anticoagulants, thromboembolic complications accounted for about 20% of hospital deaths (2). The rate is now about 1%, probably because the period of bed rest has been reduced from two or three weeks to a few days (3). About 30% of patients develop small, isotopically detectable calf-vein thrombi, and intracardiac mural thrombi will occur in 12% to 15%; however, deaths and serious sequelae are uncommon. Not only has our aim been clouded but the target has become smaller.

There have been six randomized, controlled trials of anticoagulants in the treatment of myocardial infarction. Only one showed a statistically significant reduction in deaths, but when the results were pooled, the mean case fatality rate fell from 19.6% to 15.4% in treated patients (4). Whether statistical pooling techniques are legitimate is disputed (5), but if these results are accepted, what should physicians be doing today? The issue is complicated because mortality in hospital has dropped in the last 20 years, sufficiently enough to be detectable in the mortality figures in the United States (6). Fatalities now occur from pump failure and dysrhythmias, and these are not likely to be prevented by using anticoagulants. Nonetheless, occasional serious thromboemboli occur which anticoagulants can largely prevent (7). The residual argument, therefore, is not when but which?

Full anticoagulation with heparin and a coumarin is the best way to prevent thrombosis, but it carries risk. Eight percent of patients in the combined studies suffered significant hemorrhage (4). Prophylaxis must, therefore, be chosen on the basis of inadequate information: an unknown level of effectiveness against a complication with a low incidence, and an imponderable reduction in thrombotic deaths, set against an unquantified increase in fatal hemorrhage. The dilemma is unlikely to be resolved by new data because the problems of mounting further trials are probably insuperable. I think many clinicians in the United Kingdom share my compromise and treat patients with low-dose subcutaneous heparin until they are walking. This is less effective than full anticoagulation but it does not cause bleeding. Whether it prevents major thromboembolism and death is unknown, but the information is not available for any form of antithrombotic treatment under today's conditions.

PROPHYLAXIS FOLLOWING MYOCARDIAL INFARCTION

Whether to give prophylaxis against reinfarction in the patient who leaves the hospital is a related but distinct issue. There is a logical basis for the use of antithrombotic medication. Although mortality is related to the extent of myocardial damage, the risk of reinfarction is higher in these patients than in the general population, and thrombotic occlusion of coronary arteries is the precipitating event in most cases.

A straightforward approach is to anticoagulate the patient on admission and continue anticoagulants for life. The case for reevaluating anticoagulants has been persuasively argued (7), but the available evidence in favor of long-term anticoagulant prophylaxis is not impressive. With one exception, published trials have been small and inconclusive. The results have been pooled, and suggest that anticoagulation might reduce the fatal reinfarction rate by about 20% in younger men with previous symptoms of ischemic heart disease (8). The single large study was of unusual design (9): In the Netherlands, long-term anticoagulation has been accepted practice and so the intervention arm consisted of discontinuing treatment. Total mortality over two years rose from 7.6% in patients continuing on coumarins to 13.4% in the 439 patients randomly allocated to stop. The study was carefully executed and anticoagulant control was exemplary, but a surprisingly large number of patients in the intervention group died. And can the possible risks of stopping anticoagulants, on average six years after an infarct, necessarily be equated with benefit from starting them?

Greater attention has been given to evaluating antiplatelet agents. Most of the clinical trials have been carried out with aspirin (Table 1). None has shown unequivocal benefit and the largest single study had more deaths in the treated group (10–14). These trials have also been pooled (15,16), and the data are consistent with an effect of aspirin in reducing deaths by 5% to 10% and the rate of reinfarction by about 20%. At the dosage used in these trials, aspirin is unpleasant for many people to take and the use of low doses, which might be an advantage in theory,

TABLE 1. *Total mortality and coronary event rate (coronary deaths and nonfatal reinfarction) in five controlled trials: Treatment of patients following myocardial infarction*

	Reference	Total mortality (%)		Coronary events (%)	
		Placebo	ASA	Placebo	ASA
MRC 1 (1974)	10	10.9	8.3	na	na
CDP (1976)	11	8.3	5.8	10.2	8.0
MRC 2 (1979)	12	14.8	12.3	22.2	16.0
AMIS (1980)	13	9.7	10.8	14.8	14.1
PARIS (1980)	14	12.8	10.5	18.5	14.0

na, not available.

has not been tested. Nor has aspirin administration been evaluated in combination with beta blockers, for which there is more convincing proof of efficacy.

The problem of whether or not to use antiplatelet drugs in secondary prevention is unlikely to be easily resolved. Most trials were too small, patients were not recruited soon enough after the initial infarct, and randomization was not stratified for risk factors. Circumstantial supportive evidence of benefit from aspirin administration has come from the Boston Collaborative Drug Surveillance Program, which found that regular aspirin users were less likely than nonusers to be admitted to hospital with myocardial infarction (17). And recently, treatment of patients with unstable angina has been shown significantly to reduce the risk of death and infarction (18).

Sulfinpyrazone has been evaluated in two studies, but the results are not consistent (19,20). Dipyridamole has only been tested in combination with aspirin (14). Encouraging, though statistically insignificant, results were obtained, particularly in patients recruited without six weeks of infarction. A second trial has been completed with patients entered within six weeks, and preliminary reports suggest that mortality has not been significantly affected.

The case for anticoagulant or antiplatelet prophylaxis following myocardial infarction has not been established. There are probably significant reductions to be made in mortality for large populations of patients, but the evidence for this is not conclusive. Against the arguable individual benefit must be set the risks, discomforts, and inconveniences of treatment. I do not think the balance favors treatment.

REFERENCES

1. Wright, I. S. (1946): Experiences with dicumarol in the treatment of coronary thrombosis with myocardial infarction. *Am. Heart J.*, 32:20–31.
2. Selzer, A. (1978): Use of anticoagulant agents in acute myocardial infarction: Statistics or clinical judgement? *Am. J. Cardiol.*, 41:1315–1317.
3. Miller, R. R., Lies, J. E., Carretta, R. F., Wampold, D. B., DeNardo, G. L., Kraus, J. F.,

Amsterdam, E. A., and Mason, D. T. (1976): Prevention of lower extremity venous thrombosis by early mobilization. *Ann. Int. Med.*, 84:700–703.

4. Chalmers, T. C., Matta, R. J., Smith, H., and Kunzler, A-M. (1977): Evidence favoring the use of anticoagulants in the hospital phase of acute myocardial infarction. *N. Engl. J. Med.*, 297:1091–1096.

5. Goldman, L., and Feinstein A. R. (1979): Anticoagulants and myocardial infarction. The problems of pooling, drowning and floating. *Ann. Int. Med.*, 90:92–94.

6. Pell, S., and Fayerweather, W. E. (1985): Trends in the incidence of myocardial infarction and in associated mortality and morbidity in a large employed population, 1957–1983. *N. Engl. J. Med.*, 312:1005–1011.

7. Mitchell, J. R. A. (1981): Anticoagulants in coronary heart disease—retrospect and prospect. *Lancet*, 1:257–262.

8. International Anticoagulant Review Group (1970): Collaborative analysis of long-term anticoagulant administration after acute myocardial infarction. *Lancet*, 1:203–209.

9. Report of the Sixty-Plus Reinfarction Study Research Group (1980): A double-blind trial to assess long-term oral anticoagulant therapy in elderly patients after myocardial infarction. *Lancet*, 2:989–994.

10. Elwood, P. C., Cochrane, A. L., Burr, M. L., Sweetnam, P. M., Williams, G., Welsby, E., Hughes, S. J., and Renton, R. (1974): A randomized control trial of acetylsalicylic acid in the secondary prevention of mortality from myocardial infarction. *Br. Med. J.*, 1:436–440.

11. The Coronary Drug Project Research Group (1976): Aspirin in coronary heart disease. *J. Chronic Dis.*, 29:625–642.

12. Elwood, P. C., and Sweetnam, P. M. (1979): Aspirin and secondary mortality after myocardial infarction. *Lancet*, 2:1313–1315.

13. Aspirin Myocardial Infarction Study Research Group (1980): A randomized, controlled trial of aspirin in persons recovered from myocardial infarction. *J.A.M.A.*, 243:661–669.

14. The Persantine-Aspirin Reinfarction Study Research Group (1980): Persantine and aspirin in coronary heart disease. *Circulation*, 62:449–461.

15. Editorial (1980): Aspirin after myocardial infarction. *Lancet*, 1:1172–1173.

16. Canner, P. L. (1983): Aspirin in coronary heart disease. Comparison of six clinical trials. *Isr. J. Med., Sci.*, 19:413–423.

17. Boston Collaborative Drug Surveillance Group (1974): Regular aspirin intake and acute myocardial infarction. *Br. Med. J.*, 1:440–443.

18. Lewis, H. D., Davis, J. W., Archibald, D. G., Steinke, W. E., Smitherton, T. C., Doherty, J. E., Schnaper, H. W., Le Winter, M. M., Linares, E., Pouget, J. M., Sabharwal, S. C., Chesler, E., and De Motts, H. (1983): Protective effects of aspirin against acute myocardial infarction and death in men with unstable angina. *N. Engl. J. Med.*, 309:396–403.

19. The Anturane Reinfarction Trial Research Group (1980): Sulfinpyrazone in the prevention of sudden death after myocardial infarction. *N. Engl. J. Med.*, 302:250–256.

20. The Auturan Reinfarction Italian Study (1982): Sulphinpyrazone in post-myocardial infarction. *Lancet*, 1:237–242.

Hammersmith Cardiology Workshop Series, Vol. 3,
edited by A. Maseri, B. E. Sobel, and S. Chierchia.
Raven Press, New York © 1987.

Précis of the Discussion: Section XI

ANTIPLATELET AND ANTICOAGULANT THERAPY

Burton E. Sobel

This section addressed the potential contributions of endothelial damage as well as atherosclerosis to thrombosis and their implications regarding the potential benefit of antiplatelet and anticoagulant drugs for clinical syndromes associated with vascular occlusive disease. John Gordon pointed out that endothelial damage as seen in experiment of nature, such as homocystinuria or simulated conditions induced in experimental animals, contributes to vascular occlusive phenomena and to platelet aggregation. The severity of the vascular disease can be blunted in some settings by reduction of platelet counts and/or platelet aggregation, but endothelial damage also may account for the precipitation of occlusive disease under analogous, but less severe, conditions, such as physiological stress associated with strenuous activity or damage to the vasculature after intravascular catheterization. To the extent that endothelial damage is a complex phenomenon and that it contributes in complex ways to platelet aggregation and vascular occlusion, agents such as aspirin may not be effective prophylactically when endothelial damage is present. An alternative, such as prostacyclin, may exert salutary effects, but its use may be limited by systemic hypotension unless it is administered directly into the coronary circulation.

Endothelium may mediate not only obstruction but also alterations in coronary vasomotor tone by altering the relative contributions of eicosanoids of different classes, or by virtue of the impairment of elaboration of relaxing factor or other mediators.

Andrew Davies considered different types of therapy that may be useful in the context of the role of endothelium as a contributor to vasospasm and as a nidus for thrombus and atherogenesis. He pointed out that the nonspecific acetylation of proteins by aspirin was a disadvantage, potentially offsetting its value as an inhibitor of platelet cyclo-oxygenase and, hence, elaboration of thromboxane. He also pointed out that stimulation of platelet aggregation by thrombin, and perhaps by other mechanisms, is not amenable to inhibition by aspirin. Results of several clinical trials indicate that antiplatelet agents are useful in reducing occlusion after bypass grafting of the coronary vascular tree and possibly after endarterectomy. Ken Taylor addressed the relative value of antiplatelet and anticoagulant drugs in these settings, but emphasized that results of coronary endarterectomy are inconclusive regardless of the form of medication used after the intervention.

Consideration of aspirin for the treatment of patients with unstable angina elicited lively exchanges. Dose considerations are likely to be crucial. Andrew Davies noted that 24 mg of aspirin can totally suppress prostacyclin synthesis in vascular endothelium, clearly an undesirable concomitant of the inhibition of thromboxane synthesis in platelets. He pointed out as well that such a dose is not sufficient to inhibit thrombin-induced platelet aggregation *in vitro*. The possibility was considered that thrombin antagonists, under development by the pharmaceutical industry, may be particularly useful because of the exquisite sensitivity of platelet aggregation to thrombin *in vivo*. Despite theoretical limitations, David Kelly gave an analysis of pooled data from postmyocardial infarction trials and interpreted them to imply a beneficial effect with respect to reinfarction and mortality.

Editorial comment: B. E. Sobel

Despite the intensity and the enthusiasm of advocates of diverse points of view, the beneficial effects of treatment with aspirin after myocardial infarction are neither consistent nor conclusive. Although benefit may be conferred, the clinical impact of the approach is apparently only modest. The possibility that an ideal dose has not been defined is appealing to advocates of aspirin regimens, but theoretical arguments favoring reduction of dosage are not necessarily unequivocally convincing because of a subtle interplay between endothelial mediators and platelet mediators of vasospasm and thrombosis. A growing consensus supports the view that the solution to the vexing issues raised lies not in yet additional randomized prospective double-blind and exorbitantly expensive trials, but rather in efforts designed to expand the base of knowledge needed to develop targeted prophylactic and therapeutic regimens with more definitive efficacy.

Hammersmith Cardiology Workshop Series, Vol. 3,
edited by A. Maseri, B. E. Sobel, and S. Chierchia.
Raven Press, New York © 1987.

Nitrates: Are Cellular Mechanisms of Action Related to Prostaglandins?

Babette B. Weksler

Department of Medicine, SCOR Center in Thrombosis, The New York Hospital-Cornell Medical Center, New York, New York 10021

The relaxation of vascular smooth muscle involves many different mechanisms. The precise mechanism by which nitrates induce vasodilatation has not been fully elucidated (1), although nitrates are among the oldest drugs used for this purpose. Since the discovery of prostacyclin, the endogenous vasodilatory prostaglandin produced by vascular cells (2), much interest has centered on the possible role of prostacyclin as an intermediate in nitrate-induced vasodilatation. Vascular prostacyclin synthesis is markedly depressed by doses of aspirin prescribed to control platelet function in patients with cardiovascular and cerebrovascular disease (3,4). Therefore, the concern has arisen that such aspirin usage in patients who are taking nitrates might abrogate the vasodilatory effect of the nitrates.

This chapter will focus on two questions: First, are prostaglandins, prostacyclin in particular, involved in vascular responses to nitrates? Second, do drugs that inhibit prostaglandin formation in vascular tissue prevent the beneficial clinical effects of nitrates?

RESEARCH

The hypothesis that nitrates might cause vasodilation by inducing prostacyclin synthesis in vascular endothelium was examined first by Levin et al. (5) in our group, in a tissue culture system. Using cultured human umbilical vein endothelial cells, we showed that low concentrations of nitroglycerin, comparable to those achieved in plasma during administration *in vivo,* stimulated the production of prostacyclin measured in the medium overlying the cells as the stable hydrolytic product, 6-keto $PGF_{1\alpha}$. Supernatant medium from cultures of endothelial cells stimulated with nitroglycerin inhibited the aggregation of human platelets in plasma, whereas medium from unstimulated endothelial cell cultures did not. Nitroglycerin alone at concentrations similar to those present in the medium failed to inhibit platelet aggregation, although higher concentrations of nitroglycerin directly prevented platelet aggregation. We interpreted these experimental results to indicate that clinically achievable (nanomolar) concentrations of nitroglycerin induced a modest (70%), dose-related increase in endothelial cell prostacyclin production. Similar results were reported for human saphenous vein or umbilical vein rings by Mehta et al. (6), and for bovine coronary artery by Schror et al. (7). In each case, the stimulation of prostacyclin was modest, about two times basal release, but platelets exposed to the nitroglycerin-treated tissue or the medium derived therefrom showed depression of aggregation or thromboxane production.

We recently restudied the effect of nitrates on endothelial prostacyclin production in greater detail, testing in addition to nitroglycerin the drug isosorbide dinitrate and its active metabolite, isosorbide-5-mononitrate (8). A wide range of drug concentrations were studied with each drug. Endothelial cells in several passages and differing growth states were examined. The results were different from those of the earlier study. Neither nitroglycerin nor the dinitrates induced significant production of prostacyclin from cultured endothelial cells, as indicated by the lack of increased 6-keto $PGF_{1\alpha}$ in the medium following either brief or prolonged incubation with each drug. Growth conditions, state of confluency, or passage number did not affect these results. While variation in baseline production of prostacyclin in different control preparations of endothelial cells might have obscured a change in production of as much as 50% the basal level of PGI_2, it was clear that such an amount of prostacyclin would be unlikely to have a significant biologic effect on platelets or on vasodilatation.

In separate experiments we also examined the effects of nitrates on prostacyclin production by cultured human vascular smooth muscle cells. No increase in prostacyclin was observed in these cells after exposure to nitrates (unpublished observations).

In order to extend these studies from tissue culture models to a more physiologic setting, we next examined the effect of nitrates on prostacyclin production by freshly excised human saphenous vein, mesenteric artery, or atrial appendage (8). These tissues, obtained during cardiac surgery, were chosen to represent venous, arterial, and microvascular settings. No increase in prostacyclin production by any of these tissues was detected after exposure to nitroglycerin, isosorbide dinitrate, or isosorbide-5-mononitrate. No dose-related induction of prostacyclin synthesis was observed for any of these preparations, although inherent variability in baseline prostacyclin formation in these tissues might have concealed small changes. Therefore, it must be concluded that nitrates do not elicit significant prostacyclin production from cultured human endothelial cells or from human vascular fragments *in vitro*.

Experimental and clinical evidence that prostaglandins might be involved in the vasodilatory effects of nitrates has been based mainly on studies in which the cyclo-oxygenase inhibitor, indomethacin, was administered prior to measurement of blood flow or vessel diameter (9,10). Other studies have not shown a lessening of nitrate vasodilatory effect after indomethacin (11,12). Indomethacin has now been recognized to have vasoconstrictor activity, which may have confounded the interpretation of studies in which nitrate effects were diminished. In animal studies in which indomethacin was used, alteration in autoregulatory mechanisms, specifically the reflex response to hypotension, could be an alternative mechansim for apparent attenuation of nitrate effect (12). Clinical studies in which aspirin was used as the cyclo-oxygenase blocker instead of indomethacin have had clearer results, suggesting that prostaglandins were not involved. Hirsch directly infused nitroglycerin into the coronary arteries of human subjects who had been given aspirin or placebo treatment (13). The increases in coronary artery diameter induced by nitrate infusion were the same in both groups of subjects, suggesting that the coronary vasodilation induced by nitroglycerin was just as effective in patients taking aspirin as in those who did not. Also, when the level of prostacyclin in coronary sinus blood was measured, a low level of prostacyclin after aspirin (50% of the pre-aspirin level) was not associated with any impairment of coronary vasodilatation. Thus, coronary vasodilatation in response to nitroglycerin also appeared independent of circulating prostacyclin level.

Simonetti et al. (14) similarly observed that vasodilatation induced by intracoronary infusion of isosorbide dinitrate during coronary angiography was equivalent before and after intravenous aspirin administration to the subjects. Both coronary artery diameter and coronary flow were measured and supported the concept that inhibition of prostaglandin synthesis did not alter the vasodilatory responses to nitrates.

Coronary vascular responses to nitroglycerin were correlated with coronary sinus blood flow, vascular resistance, and thromboxane level in plasma by Rehr et al. (15), designed to examine the effects of aspirin therapy. Aggregation of platelets in the coronary circulation, accompanied by release of thromboxane, has been considered a possible cause of coronary vasoconstriction. These authors found that coronary blood flow was the same at baseline in aspirin-treated and aspirin-free subjects and increased to the same or greater extent (about 60%) after nitroglycerin. Coronary sinus vascular resistance fell similarly in both groups after aspirin (35% vs 33%). The plasma thromboxane B_2 level in coronary sinus blood was not significantly increased after nitroglycerin in the aspirin-free group. Plasma thromboxane B_2 was markedly inhibited in the aspirin-treated subjects. There was no correlation between the plasma thromboxane level and changes in the coronary sinus blood flow or vascular resistance, suggesting that aspirin treatment did not impair the vascular response to nitrates, and that thromboxane in flowing blood appeared to play no part in nitroglycerin-related vasodilatation.

The excretion of prostacyclin metabolites into the urine in relationship to nitrate infusion was studied by Fitzgerald et al. (16), who could not demonstrate an increase in metabolites of vascular prostacyclin by the sensitive technique of gas chromatography-mass spectroscopy. Since previous work by this group showed that amounts of prostacyclin in the circulation that exerted a hemodynamic effect were easily detectable by measuring urinary metabolites of PGI_2 with this technique, they concluded that nitroglycerin did not induce clinically significant amounts of prostacyclin formation by vascular tissues.

The known actions of prostacyclin and the proposed action of organic nitrates represent two different, indeed opposite, mechanisms (Fig. 1). Prostacyclin stimu-

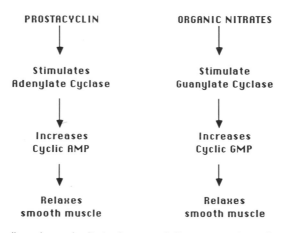

FIG. 1. Prostacyclin and organic nitrates have parallel but separately mediated effects resulting in the relaxation of vascular smooth muscle, hence producing vasodilatation.

lates the enzyme adenylate cyclase (17), leading to increased intracellular levels of cyclic AMP in vascular smooth muscle cells, platelets, and many other cell types. The raised cyclic AMP level, in turn, induces relaxation of vascular smooth muscle. Other substances beside prostacyclin cause vasodilation by this mechanism, for example, PGE_1 and isoproterenol (18). In contrast, organic nitrates stimulate guanylate cyclase, leading to increased intracellular levels of cyclic GMP (18,19). The raised cyclic GMP induces relaxation of vascular smooth muscle by a mechanism still not fully understood. Thus, the net effects of prostacyclin and of nitrates on vascular smooth muscle are similar: vasodilation, but the mechanism by which vasodilation takes place is markedly different. In fact, the vasodilatory effect of these two classes of compounds might be expected to summate.

Organic nitrates, amyl nitrite, or nitroprusside appear to enter vascular smooth muscle cells and release nitrite or nitrate intracellularly to contribute, by a sulfhydryl-dependent mechanism (20), to the formation of nitrosothiols (21). The nitrosothiol derivatives are now considered to be the key intermediates that stimulate guanylate cyclase and induce smooth muscle relaxation responses to nitrates. Application of nitrosothiol compounds directly to vascular smooth muscle produces a more rapid increase of cyclic GMP and more rapid induction of vascular relaxation than does application of an organic nitrate (22). Cysteine is needed for the action of nitroglycerin, although other thiols can combine more actively with other organic nitrates. Semipurified, isolated guanylate cyclase reponds only to high doses of nitroglycerin and yields only a modest elevation of cyclic GMP (23). Cysteine alone as a thiol source has no effect on guanylate cyclase in such a preparation, but the combination of nitroglycerin and cysteine strongly activates guanylate cyclase (23). This activation is blocked by the inhibitor, methylene blue. The different responses of arterial and venous vessels to nitrates may also be related to quantitative differences in the levels of cyclic GMP achieved in response to guanylate cyclase stimulation in different vascular beds. For example, nitrates appear to stimulate venous guanylate cyclase more than arterial guanylate cyclase (24). The differential effect of nitrates on arterial and venous vessels contrasts with the vasodilating effect of prostacyclin, which affects both arterial and venous tissue similarly.

The potentiating effect of thiols on nitrate-induced vasodilation can be demonstrated in a clinical context. Intravenous acetylcysteine potentiates the cardiovascular effects of nitroglycerin (25). Conversely, tolerance develops to nitrates when tissue thiols are exhausted (20,26). The tolerance is associated with a reduced cyclic GMP response (26). Replenishment of thiol levels might serve as a useful adjunct in prolonged nitrate therapy.

To complete the discussion of nitrate actions, one should contrast the organic nitrates with nitroprusside, itself a potent vasodilator. Both types of agents directly affect platelets in a dose-dependent manner. Nitroglycerin (5,27) and dinitrates (28) inhibit platelet aggregation and thromboxane release by platelets at doses achievable clinically. Nitroglycerin can increase the bleeding time transiently (29). Nitroprusside given intravenously at high levels directly inhibits platelet function and can induce a bleeding tendency (30). Low concentrations of nitroprusside alone do not inhibit platelet aggregation. Prostacyclin and nitroprusside act synergistically to inhibit platelet aggregation (31). Nitroprusside does not stimulate prostacyclin formation by vascular endothclial cells, even though it potentiates the platelet inhibitory effect of prostacyclin (32,33).

CONCLUSION

The studies reviewed above clearly demonstrate that nitrate-induced vasodilation is not mediated by prostacyclin. Neither the organic nitrates nor nitroprusside stimulates endothelial cells to produce prostacyclin to any significant extent. It is interesting that agents which induce prostacyclin synthesis in endothelium also raise the cyclic GMP level, but raising endothelial cyclic GMP does not induce prostacyclin synthesis (33). Conversely, cyclo-oxygenase inhibition of vascular endothelium or smooth muscle does not interfere with the vasorelaxant effects of organic nitrates. Indomethacin, which appeared in some earlier studies to interfere with nitrate-induced vasodilation, probably has a direct vasoconstrictor effect on vascular smooth muscle that is quite independent of prostaglandin synthesis. High dose nitrates, clinically achievable by intravenous infusion, can inhibit platelet activation and, in the presence of other vasoactive drugs such as beta blockers and calcium channel blockers, can inhibit platelet function. This antiplatelet effect of nitrate therapy may offer ancillary benefit.

In conclusion, prostacyclin and nitrates have separate mechanisms of inducing vasodilation of human blood vessels. Inhibition of prostacyclin production does not affect the vasodilatory action of short- or long-acting nitrates.

REFERENCES

1. Kreye, V. A. W. (1984): Direct vasodilators with unknown modes of action: the nitro-compounds and hydralazine. *J. Cardiovasc. Pharmacol. (Suppl. 4)*, 6:S646–655.
2. Moncada, S., Gryglewski, R., Bunting, S., and Vane, J. R. (1976): An enzyme isolated from arteries transforms prostaglandin endoperoxides to an unstable substance that inhibits platelet aggregation. *Nature*, 263:663–665.
3. Weksler, B. B., Pett, S. B., Alonso, D., Richter, R. C., Stelzer, P., Subramanian, V., Tack-Goldman, K., and Gay, W. A., Jr. (1983): Differential inhibition by aspirin of vascular and platelet prostaglandin synthesis in atherosclerotic patients. *N. Engl. J. Med.*, 308:800–805.
4. FitzGerald, G. A., Oates, J. A., Hawiger, J., Maas, R. L., Roberts, L. J., and Brash, A. R. (1983): Endogenous synthesis of prostacyclin and thromboxane and platelet function during chronic aspirin inhibition in man. *J. Clin. Invest.*, 71:676–688.
5. Levin, R. I., Jaffe, E. A., Weksler, B. B., and Tack-Goldman, K. (1980): Nitroglycerin stimulates synthesis of prostacyclin by cultured human endothelial cells. *J. Clin. Invest.*, 67:762–769.
6. Mehta, J., Mehta, P., and Ostrowski, N. (1983): Effects of nitroglycerin on human vascular prostacyclin and thromboxane A2 generation. *J. Lab. Clin. Med.*, 102:116–125.
7. Schror, K., Grodzinska, L., and Darius, H. (1981): Stimulation of coronary vascular prostacyclin and inhibition of human platelet thromboxane A2 after low-dose nitroglycerin. *Thromb. Res.*, 23:59–67.
8. De Caterina, R., Dorso, C. R., Tack-Goldman, K., and Weksler, B. B. (1985): Nitrates and endothelial prostacyclin production: studies *in vitro. Circulation*, 71:176–182.
9. Morcillo, E., Reid, P. R., Dubin, N., Ghodgaonkar, R., and Pitt, B. (1980): Myocardial prostaglandin E release by nitroglycerin and modification by indomethacin. *Am. J. Cardiol.*, 45:53–57.
10. Friedman. P. L., Brown, E. J., Jr., Gunther, S., et al. (1981): Coronary vasoconstrictor effect of indomethacin in patients with coronary artery disease. *N. Engl. J. Med.*, 305:1171–1175.
11. Winniford, M. D., Jackson, J., Malloy, C. R., Rehr, R. B., Campbell, W. B., and Hillis, D. (1984): Does indomethacin attenuate the coronary vasodilatory effect of nitroglycerin? *J. Am. Coll. Cardiol.*, 4:1114–1117.
12. Panzenbeck, M., Baez, A., and Kaley, G. (1984): Nitroglycerin and nitroprusside increase coronary blood flow in dogs by a mechanism independent of prostaglandin release. *Am. J. Cardiol.*, 53:936–940.
13. Hirsh, P. D. (1984): Nitroglycerin-induced coronary artery dilation in humans is not mediated by prostacyclin and is not blocked by aspirin. *Clin. Res.*, 43:175A.
14. Simonetti, I., De Caterina, R., Michelassi, C., Marzilli, M., De Nes, M., and L'Abbate, A. (1985): Coronary vasodilation by nitrates: any role for prostaglandins? *Adv. Prostaglandin Thromboxane Leukotriene Res.*, 13:327–332.
15. Rehr, R. B., Jackson, J. A., Winniford, M. D., Campbell, W. B., and Hillis, L. D. (1984): Mechanism of nitroglycerin-induced coronary dilatation: Lack of relation to intracoronary thromboxane concentrations. *Am. J. Cardiol.*, 54:971–974.
16. Fitzgerald, D. J., Roy, L., Robertson, R. M., and FitzGerald, G. A. (1984): The effect of organic nitrates on prostacyclin biosynthesis and platelet function in humans. *Circulation*, 70:297–302.
17. Best, L. C., Martin, T. J., Russel, R. G., and Preston, F. E. (1977): Prostacyclin increases cyclic AMP levels and adenylate cyclase activity in platelets. *Nature*, 267:850–852.
18. Hardman, J. G. (1984): Cyclic nucleotides and regulation of vascular smooth muscle. *J. Cardiovasc. Pharmacol. (Suppl. 4)*, 6:S639–645.
19. Galvas, K. E., and DiSalvo, J. (1983): Concentration and time-dependent relationships between isosorbide dinitrate-induced relaxation and formation of cyclic GMP in coronary arterial smooth muscle. *J. Pharmacol. Exp. Ther.*, 224:373–377.
20. Needleman, P., Jakschick, B., and Johnson, E. M. (1973): Sulfhydryl requirement for relaxation of vascular smooth muscle. *J. Pharmacol. Exp. Ther.*, 187:324–331.
21. Ignarro, L. J., Lippton, H., Edwards, J. C., Baricos, W. H., Hyman, A. L., Kadowitz, P. H., and Gruetter, C. A. (1981): Mechanism of vascular smooth muscle relaxation by organic nitrates, nitrites, nitroprusside and nitric oxide: evidence for the involvement of s-nitrosothiols as active intermediates. *J. Pharmacol. Exp. Ther.*, 218:739–749.
22. Edwards, J. C., Ignarro, L. J., Hyman, A. L., and Kadowitz, P. J. (1984): Relaxation of intrapulmo-

nary artery and vein by nitrogen oxide-containing vasodilators and cyclic GMP. *J. Pharmacol. Exp. Ther.*, 228:33–42.

23. Laustiola, K., Vuorinen, P., Vapaatalo, H., and Metsa-Ketela, T. (1983): Effects of cysteine and nitroglycerin on bovine heart guanylate cyclase and on tissue cyclic GMP and lactate of rat atria. *Eur. J. Pharmacol.*, 91:301–304.

24. Mackenzie, J. E., and Parratt, J. R. (1978): Comparative effects of glyceryl trinitrate on venous and arterial smooth muscle *in vitro;* relevance to antianginal activity. *Br. J. Pharmacol.*, 60:155–160.

25. Horowitz, J. D., Antman, E. M., Lorell, B. H., Barry, W. H., and Smith, T. W. (1983): Potentiation of the cardiovascular effects of nitroglycerin by N-acetylcysteine. *Circulation,* 68:1247–1253.

26. Axelsson, K. L., and Andersson, R. G. (1983): Tolerance towards nitroglycerin, induced *in vivo,* is correlated to a reduced cGMP response and an alteration in cGMP turnover. *Eur. J. Pharmacol.*, 88:71–79.

27. Schafer, A. I., Alexander, R. W., and Handin, R. I. (1980): Inhibition of platelet function by organic nitrate vasodilators. *Blood,* 55:649–652.

28. De Caterina, R., Giannessi, D., Crea, F., Chierchia, S., Bernini, W., Gazetti, P., and L'Abbate, A. (1984): Inhibition of platelet function by injectable isosorbide dinitrate. *Am. J. Cardiol.*, 53:103–107.

29. Ring, T., Knudsen, F., Kristensen, S. D., and Larsen, C. E. (1983): Nitroglycerin prolongs the bleeding time in healthy males. *Thromb. Res.*, 29:553–559.

30. Saxon, A., and Kattlove, H. E. (1976): Platelet inhibition by sodium nitroprusside, a smooth muscle inhibitor. *Blood,* 47:957–962.

31. Levin, R. I., Weksler, B. B., and Jaffe, E. A. (1982): The interaction of sodium nitroprusside with human endothelial cells and platelets: nitroprusside and prostacyclin synergistically inhibit platelet function. *Circulation,* 66:1299–1307.

32. Mehta, J., Mehta, P., Roberts, A., Faro, R., Ostrowski, N., and Brigmon, L. (1983): Comparative effects of nitroglycerin and nitroprusside on prostacyclin generation in adult human vessel wall. *J. Am. Coll. Cardiol.*, 2:625–630.

33. Brotherton, A. F. A. (1986): Induction of prostacyclin biosynthesis is closely associated with increased guanosine 3',5'-cyclic monophosphate accumulation in cultured human endothelium. *J. Clin. Invest.*, 78:1253–1260.

Hammersmith Cardiology Workshop Series, Vol. 3,
edited by A. Maseri, B. E. Sobel, and S. Chierchia.
Raven Press, New York © 1987.

Nitrates, Pharmacology, and Tolerance

K. M. Fox

National Heart Hospital, London W1M 8BA, England

Nitrates, particularly in the sublingual form, have been used for over 100 years in the acute treatment of angina pectoris. Much more controversy surrounds their use for chronic therapy of angina pectoris.

PHARMACODYNAMICS

Nitrates act in three ways. First of all, and most importantly, they are venodilators, causing a fall in cardiac preload. They also, particularly when used acutely, cause a fall in cardiac afterload. Finally, they cause coronary vasodilation. The importance of coronary vasodilatation in exertional angina is probably small, but it is much greater in patients with variant angina.

Thus, nitrates will cause a fall in mean arterial pressure and a rise in heart rate. An initial increase in cardiac output due to arterial dilation will be followed by a fall in output as the venodilatation occurs and, likewise, the fall in total peripheral resistance that occurs initially will be followed by a rise in peripheral resistance. The net effect is a marked reduction in cardiac work. Blood flow to the major organs and the kidneys and gut will, therefore, initially be increased, followed by a fall in flow as venodilatation occurs.

PHARMACOKINETICS (1)

The most commonly used nitrates are Glyceryl Trinitrate (nitroglycerin) and isosorbide dinitrate. For acute administration, either Glyceryl Trinitrate or isosorbide dinitrate may be given. This is usually given sublingually or by aerosol. Alternatively, in patients with frequent recurrent episodes, both Glyceryl Trinitrate and isosorbide dinitrate may be given intravenously.

For chronic administration, Glyceryl Trinitrate or isosorbide dinitrate may be given via the skin, in which case first pass metabolism is avoided. For oral administration, isosorbide dinitrate is given and is metabolized on first pass through the liver to the isosorbide-2-mononitrate and the isosorbide-5-mononitrate. Recently, to avoid the variabilities of first pass metabolism, the mononitrate has been produced.

ACUTE EFFECTS OF ORAL THERAPY

There is now ample evidence that following the oral administration of isosorbide dinitrate, there will be a fall in systolic blood pressure together with some increase in heart rate, which will last up to 4 hr following the oral dose. This will be accompanied by an improvement in exercise walking time and ST segment depression in angina subjects (2).

LONG-TERM THERAPY: TOLERANCE

Much more controversy exists regarding the use of nitrates in long-term therapy. It has been shown that a fall in pulmonary wedge pressure may be present after three months' therapy (3). Early studies of the response in angina after one month's therapy showed that the effects of nitroglycerin upon exercise walking time were maintained after one month's therapy with isosorbide dinitrate (4). However, more recent studies have shown that the heart rate and blood pressure effect was markedly attenuated within a period of five oral doses (5). This attenuated effect was also seen in the walking time to angina. The cause of this tolerance must be related to end-organ effect, since the blood levels on sustained therapy were equal to the blood levels on acute therapy.

CONCLUSIONS

Nitrates have a firm, established place in the treatment of acute anginal episodes where they are given sublingually or intravenously. For chronic prophylaxis, whether skin preparations, dinitrate, or mononitrate is used, at least partial tolerance is likely to occur. However, since tolerance not only develops rapidly, but also regresses equally quickly, it is likely that, provided the blood levels are not sustained over the full 24 hr period, tolerance may not occur (6). New formulations of nitrates such as the mononitrates will not prevent the development of tolerance, but will be advantageous in providing predictable levels in patients since first pass metabolism does not occur. New preparations of nitrates are being developed that allow for peak effects during the day, with a fall in blood levels at night to prevent tolerance from occurring.

REFERENCES

1. Chasseaud, L. F. (1984): Pharmacokinetics and bioavailability of different nitrate preparations. *Vascular Medicine*, 2:176–186.
2. Glang, D. L., Ritcher, M. A., Ellis, E. V., and Johnson, W. (1977): Effect of swallowed isosorbide dinitrate on blood pressure, heart rate and exercise capacity in patients with coronary artery disease. *Am. J. Med.*, 62:39–47.

3. Franciosa, J. A., and Cohn, J. N. (1980): Sustained hemodynamic effects without tolerance during long-term isosorbide dinitrate treatment of chronic left ventricular failure. *Am. J. Cardiol.,* 45:648–654.
4. Lee, G., Mason, D. T., and De Maria, A. N. (1978): Effects of long-term oral administration of isosorbide dinitrate on the anti-anginal response to nitroglycerin. Absence of nitrate cross tolerance and self tolerance shown by exercise testing. *Am. J. Cardiol.,* 41:82–87.
5. Thadani, U., Fung, H. L., Darke, A. C., and Parker, J. (1982): Oral isosorbide dinitrate in angina pectoris: comparison of duration of action and dose response relationship during acute and sustained therapy. *Am. J. Cardiol.,* 219:411–417.
6. Parker, J. O., Fung, H. L., Ruggirello, D., and Stone, J. A. (1983): Tolerance to isosorbide dinitrate: rate of development and reversal. *Circulation,* 68:1074–1080.

Hammersmith Cardiology Workshop Series, Vol. 3,
edited by A. Maseri, B. E. Sobel, and S. Chierchia.
Raven Press, New York © 1987.

Précis of the Discussion: Section XII

NITRATE THERAPY

Colin T. Dollery

Colin Dollery wondered if Kim Fox really meant that no one had ever done a proper randomized controlled trial of the long-term efficacy of oral nitrates in angina. Dr. Fox replied that the hope was that low plasma concentrations at night, when anginal attacks are less frequent, would minimize the development of tolerance. He went on that up to now, there had been very few well-designed studies of once daily dosing, although some were in progress and should be reporting very soon.

Dr. Silber said that his institution, in Munich, had done a study that was randomized and double-blind, but not placebo controlled. The problem of tolerance to the antianginal effects of prolonged treatment with nitrates did not seem to arise with a high dose given once a day. Unfortunately, some patients needed twice daily dosing to obtain relief from symptoms. Patients on regimens that gave low plasma concentrations during the night did not seem to develop tolerance. He went on to say that he was concerned that these patients might suffer episodes of painless ischemia during the night, but that Sergio Chierchia's data suggested that these occur mainly during the day.

Colin Dollery commented that if tolerance was a problem, sustained release formulations would be more likely to induce it. Kim Fox agreed, but added that a long-acting preparation that was effective for 12 hr and given once a day in the morning might prove to be the best solution.

Attilio Maseri then commented on the mechanism by which nitrates relieve chronic stable exertional angina. He said that there is good evidence to show that dilatation of stenoses in the coronary arteries does make a contribution. Kim Fox didn't deny that, but he was not sure how important it was in someone exercising.

David Kelly asked Babette Weksler if a receptor for nitrates had been identified, and she replied that although a specific receptor has been sought for many years, none had so far been found. Wolfgang Kübler also asked her if there was any pharmacological means whereby tolerance could be prevented or reversed. Dr. Weksler replied that a number of studies in animals have suggested that tolerance can be reversed by increasing the thiol pool. The only clinical study she know of used N-acetyl cysteine, which was very unpleasant for the patient. The thiol mechanism seemed most likely to be important with nitroglycerin, but it didn't seem to apply to other substances such as amyl nitrate.

Attilio Maseri commented that it was difficult enough to show that one drug was effective in angina, then to compare two drugs, which differ only slightly in efficacy, would be an enormous task. Colin Dollery added that if the number of anginal attacks in a given time was predictable and an estimate could be made of the expected reduction with two different treatments, it would be perfectly possible to calculate the number of patients required to reach a given level of statistical significance and power (that a negative result is true). Conclusions that two drugs are of similar efficacy are often, wrongly, based on small trials that would not have been able to detect a difference unless it were very large. He went on that on a practical level, it may be that there isn't enough difference to make it worthwhile finding out exactly what it is, but that was a different issue.

Attilio Maseri said that one of the major problems in studying tolerance is the highly variable course of the disease in individual patients. However, preliminary studies with long-term infusions of Glycerol Trinitrate (nitroglycerin) suggest that substantial tolerance develops within two days, but it can be reversed by stopping the infusion overnight. Richard Conti said that he doubted whether tolerance was a major clinical problem. In the United States, it would be rare for a patient with severe angina to be treated with a single type of drug. Lionel Opie added that by using beta blockers and calcium antagonists as the basic therapy, supplemented where necessary with short-acting nitrates, the problem could be avoided.

Editorial comment: S. Chierchia

Nitrates have been used, clinically, since the last century and yet, their efficacy and mode of action in the various clinical manifestations of ischemic heart disease are a matter of controversy. Although their ability to relieve episodes of angina is well recognized, there is less consensus on whether or not they can also prevent myocardial ischemia and, hopefully, improve prognosis. Available evidence indicates that intravenous and long-acting oral nitrates can, respectively, reduce the number of ischemic attacks in patients with vasospastic angina and in those with chronic stable effort angina. They can improve hemodynamics and, possibly, reduce ischemia in acute myocardial infarction.

The mechanism of action of nitrates is dual; they improve myocardial perfusion by relieving or preventing coronary vasoconstriction and they also decrease myocardial oxygen demand, primarily by reducing the venous return to the heart.

In the individual patient, the prevalence of each of these effects in preventing and/or relieving ischemia is dependent upon the prevailing pathophysiological mechanism operating in that specific individual. Coronary vasodilatation is obviously more relevant when symptoms mainly result from transient impairment in regional myocardial perfusion. Conversely, a reduction in cardiac work has to be considered in patients presenting with effort-related angina and exhibiting a fixed, limited coronary flow reserve. Recent data obtained in our institution in patients with effort-related angina and severe coronary artery disease indicate that, although nitrates are more effective in preventing exercise-induced ischemia when given systemically, a definite coronary vasodilator effect is present, even when coronary flow reserve is extremely impaired. The effect is both related to dilatation of epicardial coronary arteries, with decrease in severity of pliable stenoses, and to dilatation of smaller vessels and improvement of collateral flow.

Although a large variety of nitrate preparations exist, with buccal, nasal, respiratory, gastrointestinal, and topical routes of administration, only a few are suitable for effective long-term treatment. Also, the clinical use of nitrates for the prophylactic treatment of angina has so far been complicated by the relatively poor bioavailability of some of these compounds, related to the variable degree of first pass liver metabolism and by the development of tolerance.

The first problem has been, at least partially, circumvented by shunting the hepatic circulation with alternative routes of administration (buccal, transdermal) and by the use of mononitrates. The second can be obviated with appropriate preparations and/or administration schedules that allow for peak effects during the day and a fall in blood levels during the night. Obviously, such a solution can only be applied to patients whose attacks are predominantly and consistently concentrated in one part of the day. Conversely, for those patients whose symptoms occur unpredictably, "continuous protection" may be needed for a discreet period or indefinitely.

The most appropriate formulation and dosing should be established to maximize the effect while minimizing tolerance and side effects. The efficacy of treatment should be established in the individual patient on the basis of the prevailing pathophysiological mechanism that one is attempting to counteract and prevent.

Hammersmith Cardiology Workshop Series, Vol. 3,
edited by A. Maseri, B. E. Sobel, and S. Chierchia.
Raven Press, New York © 1987.

Morbidity in Coronary Artery Surgery: The Importance of Myocardial and Cerebral Protection

Kenneth M. Taylor

*Department of Cardiac Surgery, Royal Postgraduate Medical School,
Hammersmith Hospital, London W12 0HS, England*

Coronary artery surgery has progressed to the point where, at least with elective procedures, mortality is no longer a real issue. Most large centers are carrying out elective coronary revascularization with an operative mortality of around 1%. The focus of attention is, therefore, increasingly on morbidity. This is surely a sign of progress since the success of the operation is no longer able to be defined simply in terms of the patient's survival. Attention is being focused on quality of life following surgery and on the avoidance of vital organ damage sustained during the cardiac surgical procedure. It is increasingly appreciated that there is a significant morbidity associated with coronary artery surgery and that much further work requiries to be done in order to address this problem and, hence, provide even safer coronary artery surgical therapy.

MYOCARDIAL PROTECTION

One principal area in which progress has already been made is in the field of myocardial protection. The myocardium is rendered ischemic during the coronary artery surgical procedure when the aorta is cross-clamped. In the early days, this additional period of myocardial cellular insult often resulted in further infarction of ventricular muscle. There is no doubt that this apparently unavoidable ischemic insult contributed to the poor results in coronary surgery for patients with already impaired left ventricular function (1). It was also associated with a high level of perioperative myocardial infarction. The concept of myocardial protection has passed through various phases since the early work of Shumway's group, who introduced the technique of topical hypothermia (2). Considerable volumes of 4°C electrolyte solution were continuously instilled into the pericardial cavity and discarded by suction, thus providing external cooling of the heart during the ischemic period when the aorta was cross-clamped. This technique was combined with core hypothermia to around 28°C and with reduced bypass flow to reduce collateral re-warming of the myocardium. Studies clearly demonstrated a reduction in perioperative myocardial infarction and in operative mortality figures when topical hypothermia was employed.

Myocardial protection advanced more significantly when crystalloid cardioplegia preservation of the myocardium was introduced. This technique employs the infusion of 4°C cardioplegia solution into the aortic root after the aorta has been cross-clamped. The coronary circulation is thus perfused with cardioplegic solution and arrest of the heart occurs. The principles of cardioplegic techniques have been well described (3,4) and, in addition to providing excellent myocardial cellular protection, also provide the surgeon with excellent operating conditions with a relaxed flaccid heart facilitating coronary arterial anastomosis. Crystalloid cardioplegia is now employed by the vast majority of cardiac surgeons around the world. Though few challenge the principles, debate continues as to the exact chemical composition of the ideal cardioplegic solution. Opinion has been divided between proponents of an extracellular-based electrolyte composition (5) and those who favor an intracellular-based solution (6). Recent work has suggested that there may be other additive agents, for example, calcium blockers, which may provide additional myocardial cellular protection, though their use has not been accepted universally. Buckberg and colleagues have advocated the use of cold blood cardioplegia (7). Though experimental and clinical evidence suggest a degree of superiority over crystalloid techniques, cold blood cardioplegia entails additional complexity in delivery systems, which some have found a significant negative feature.

CEREBRAL PROTECTION

It is striking that as most aspects of coronary artery surgery practice have improved over the past years, one area of morbidity that has not changed significantly is that of brain damage associated with cardiac surgery. Brain damage may be defined in terms of definitive stroke where the incidence is around 2% in most published series. Where more sensitive techniques, for example, neurological or psychometric testing, are employed, the incidence is accepted as around 15% to 20%. If biochemical marker techniques are used, measuring the level of suitable markers of brain cell injury (for example, creatinine kinase BB-isoenzyme), there is evidence of brain cell damage in more than 60% to 70% of patients. As a result of an increased awareness of the problem, considerable effort is currently directed toward identification of the principal etiological factors involved and toward therapy that will reduce this unacceptably high morbidity.

There is little doubt that the two most likely etiological mechanisms are the following:

1. The altered perfusion of cardiopulmonary bypass (especially nonpulsatile flow).
2. The occurrence of microembolism as a result of microbubbles or microaggregates generated in the extracorporeal circuit.

Classical teaching that the brain is particularly susceptible to the reduced perfusion of cardiopulmonary bypass is now increasingly called into question. The measurement of cerebral blood flow during cardiopulmonary bypass has shown that though the levels are reduced by nonpulsatile flow, they are not reduced to a level consistent with the occurrence of cerebral cell death (8). Further studies have shown that the classical areas of watershed ischemia and infarction in the boundary zones susceptible to global reduction in cerebral perfusion are not a histological feature of the cerebral injury associated with open-heart surgery. The only group of patients who are particularly at risk from perfusion-related cerebral injury are those who have flow-limiting carotid stenosis. In these patients the flow distal to the stenosis becomes pressure passive, and only in these patients is it worth recommending that the mean arterial perfusion pressure during cardiac surgery be maintained at above 50–60 mm Hg.

It must be said, however, that it is still possible to produce optimal cerebral perfusion by modifying cardiopulmonary bypass techniques. There is clear and extensive evidence that there is functional disturbance in the brain as a result of conventional nonpulsatile perfusion and that the response of the hypothalamus, the anterior pituitary, and stress responses in general may be returned to normal by using pulsatile flow (9,10). More recent evidence has shown that pulsatile perfusion at the same levels of mean flow and pressure produces a significantly higher level both of cerebral blood flow and also of cerebral metabolism. Since modified roller pump systems that produce safe and acceptable pulsatile flow are now clinically available, the use of these systems is recommended as routine.

The role of microembolism in the production of brain damage in cardiac surgery patients is more significant and less easy to modify. Despite improvements in equipment and in materials used, it is still impossible to prevent two events:

1. Microbubble generation by artificial oxygenation and the cardiotomy suction return in the extracorporeal circuit.
2. Cellular activation (particularly of platelets and white blood cells), with the production of potentially pathological microaggregates.

The traditional view of microaggregates and microembolism has been rather too simplistic. It is now evident that microaggregates are not inert particles that exercise pathological effects simply by blocking small blood vessels. They are, in fact, biologically active. They release vasoactive substances, including thromboxane, histamine, and serotonin, and may be associated with free radical liberation and consequent cellular injury. These aspects have important ramifications in relation to therapy.

The current approach to the therapy of cerebral damage during cardiopulmonary bypass includes

1. *Filtration of the blood passing through the extracorporeal circuit.* This technique is directed toward providing mechanical retention of both microbubbles and particulate aggregates, preventing their passing into the patient's ascending aorta and, hence, cerebral circulation. The optimal pore size for the arterial line

is around 30–40 μm. This pore size provides optimal filtration with minimal blood trauma.

2. *Inhibition of platelet aggregation.* This is a newer approach in which the prostaglandin substance, prostacyclin (PGI2) has been used most extensively. The naturally occurring prostacyclin or its synthetic carbacyclin derivatives have been shown to preserve platelet numbers and function during cardiopulmonary bypass and to prevent platelet aggregation (11).

3. *Protection of the brain by cerebral protective drugs.* This form of therapy has not yet shown itself to have significant value. Various studies are in progress using pharmacological agents varying from corticosteroids through short-term intravenous anesthetic agents such as Pentothal Sodium (thiopental sodium) to the use of calcium antagonists as cerebral protectives.

REFERENCES

1. Taylor, K. M. (1985): Surgical possibilities and results in coronary patients with poor left ventricular function. In: *Hammersmith Cardiology Workshop Series, Vol. 1,* edited by A. Maseri and J. F. Goodwin, pp. 195–201. Raven Press, New York.
2. Griepp, R. B., Stinson, E. B., and Shumway, N. E. (1973): Profound local hypothermia for myocardial protection during open-heart surgery. *J. Thorac. Cardiovasc. Surg.,* 66:731–746.
3. Hearse, D. J., Braimbridge, M. V., and Jynge, P. (1981): *Protection of the ischemic myocardium: Cardioplegia.* Raven Press, New York.
4. Kirklin, J. W., Conti, V. R., and Blackstone, E. H. (1979): Prevention of myocardial damage during cardiac operations. *N. Engl. J. Med.,* 301:135–141.
5. Braimbridge, M. V., Chayen, J., Bitensky, L., Hearse, D. J., Jynge, P., and Cankovic-Darracott, S. (1977): Cold cardioplegia or continuous coronary perfusion? *J. Thorac. Cardiovasc. Surg.,* 74:900–906.
6. Bretschneider, H. J. (1980): Myocardial protection. *Thorac. Cardiovasc. Surg.,* 28:295–302.
7. Follette, D. M., Mulder, D. G., Maloney, J. V., and Buckberg, G. D. (1978): Advantages of blood cardioplegia over continuous coronary perfusion or intermittent ischemia. *J. Thorac. Cardiovasc. Surg.,* 76:604–619.
8. Taylor, K. M. (1982): Brain damage during open-heart surgery. Editorial. *Thorax,* 37:873–876.
9. Taylor, K. M., Jones, J. V., Walker, M. S., Rao, L. G. S., and Bain, W. H. (1976): The cortisol response during heart-lung bypass. *Circulation,* 54(1):20–26.
10. Taylor, K. M., Wright, G. S., Bain, W. H., Caves, P. K., and Beastall, G. S. (1978): Comparative studies of pulsatile and non-pulsatile flow during cardiopulmonary bypass. III. Anterior pituitary response to thyrotrophin-releasing hormone. *J. Thorac. Cardiovasc. Surg.,* 75(4):579–584.
11. Walker, I. D., Davidson, J. F., Faichney, A., Wheatley, D. J., and Davidson, K. G. (1981): A double-blind study of prostacyclin in cardiopulmonary bypass surgery. *Br. J. Haematol.,* 49:415–423.

Hammersmith Cardiology Workshop Series, Vol. 3,
edited by A. Maseri, B. E. Sobel, and S. Chierchia.
Raven Press, New York © 1987.

Veins, Internal Mammary Artery, or Artificial Grafts?

Floyd D. Loop

*Department of Thoracic and Cardiovascular Surgery, The Cleveland Clinic Foundation,
Cleveland, Ohio 44106*

Three operative descriptors affect long-term survival after myocardial revascularization: (a) mortality and morbidity, (b) performance of internal mammary artery (IMA) grafting, and (c) complete revascularization.

The gradual rise in death rates, beginning 3 to 5 years after saphenous vein bypass grafting, may relate more to graft closure than to progression of coronary atherosclerosis. Approximately half the saphenous vein grafts show atherosclerotic change or closure by the tenth postoperative year. Since atherosclerosis is observed rarely in the internal mammary artery, use of this conduit has escalated.

Given the wide separation in late graft patency in favor of the IMA graft (Fig. 1), we reviewed the records of patients who had undergone coronary artery surgery from 1971 through 1978 (1). Only patients with bypass grafts to the anterior descending artery were included; the study included 2,306 patients who had an IMA graft alone or combined with one or more saphenous vein grafts, and 3,625 patients who had saphenous vein bypass grafting only. Exclusive of hospital deaths, actuarial survival of IMA groups compared with that of the vein grafts group showed these differences: one-vessel, 93.4% versus 88.0% ($p = 0.05$); two-vessel, 90.0% versus 79.5% ($p < 0.0001$); and three-vessel, 82.6% versus 71.0% ($p < 0.0001$).

The demographic and clinical differences were adjusted by Cox multivariate analysis with the finding that patients who had vein grafts only had 1.61 times greater risk of death throughout 10 years, 1.41 times the risk of late myocardial infarction ($p < 0.0001$), 1.25 times the risk of hospitalization for cardiac causes ($p < 0.0001$), 2.00 times the risk of cardiac reoperation ($p < 0.0001$), and 1.27 times the risk of all late cardiac events ($p < 0.0001$) compared with patients who had received an IMA graft to the anterior descending artery.

This effect of the IMA graft on 10-year survival and the reduction in cardiac events among those who had received an IMA graft to the anterior descending artery strongly suggest that wider use of the IMA graft is beneficial.

In previous studies, we determined that extension of IMA graft usage through bilateral IMA grafting has resulted in excellent long-term survival for selected

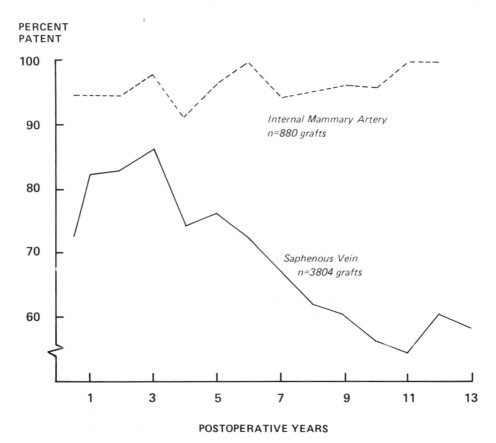

FIG. 1. Patency for internal mammary artery and saphenous vein grafts is shown at one-year intervals. The advantage of the internal mammary artery graft is evident at each interval.

patients (2). Most surgeons who use the internal mammary artery have already extended its use to sequential grafting (3). In our experience, no additional hospital mortality has occurred with IMA grafting (4).

In view of the consistent deterioration of the vein graft in the aortocoronary position and the results of long-term survival in patients who have received one IMA graft to the anterior descending artery, the therapeutic implications are that patients who have severe stenosis of the anterior descending artery should receive an IMA graft to that vessel, along with other grafts as indicated. The saphenous vein graft is no longer the preferred conduit for coronary artery surgery.

Synthetic grafts in the 4–5 mm size have not shown a consistently reasonable patency rate. No new materials hold promise as acceptable aortocoronary bypass conduits.

REFERENCES

1. Loop, F. D., Lytle, B. W., Cosgrove, D. M., Stewart, R. W., Goormastic, M., Williams, G. W., Golding, L. A. R., Gill, C. C., Taylor, P. C., Sheldon, W. C., and Proudfit, W. L. (1986): Influence of the internal–mammary–artery graft on 10-year survival and other cardiac events, 314:1–6.
2. Lytle, B. W., Cosgrove, D. M., Saltus, G. L., Taylor, P. C., and Loop, F. D. (1983): Multivessel coronary revascularization without saphenous vein: long-term results of bilateral internal mammary artery grafting. *Ann. Thorac. Surg.,* 36:540–547.
3. Tector, A. J., Schmahl, T. M., Canino, V. R., Kallies, J. R., and Sanfilippo, D. (1984): The role of the sequential internal mammary artery graft in coronary surgery. *Circulation (Suppl. I),* 70:222–225.
4. Cosgrove, D. M., Loop, F. D., Lytle, B. W., Goormastic, M., Stewart, R. W., Gill, C. C., and Golding, L. R. (1985): Does mammary artery grafting increase surgical risk? *Circulation (Suppl. II),* 72:170–174.

Hammersmith Cardiology Workshop Series, Vol. 3,
edited by A. Maseri, B. E. Sobel, and S. Chierchia.
Raven Press, New York © 1987.

Précis of the Discussion: Section XIII

ADVANCES IN CORONARY SURGERY

Kenneth M. Taylor

Regarding the reversibility of brain damage in coronary surgery patients, Ken Taylor indicated that available evidence suggests that if psychometric testing is still abnormal two to three months postoperatively, the change tends to be persistent. In addition, studies have also shown that patients who have persistent abnormality on psychometric testing have poorer prognosis following coronary surgery than patients whose psychometric tests do not change. Gerry Klassen raised the possibility of detecting a subset of patients with a higher potential for cerebral damage during coronary surgery. In Ken Taylor's opinion, patients with flow-limiting carotid stenotic lesions were at risk from impaired cerebral perfusion during cardiopulmonary bypass. He recommended maintenance of perfusion pressures in excess of 50–60 mm Hg mean in such patients. In reply to a question regarding the possible beneficial effect of calcium antagonists, Ken Taylor felt that their use in cardioplegic solutions was still an open question, though interesting work from Richard Clark in Bethesda, Maryland, reported improved myocardial protection when calcium antagonists were added to crystalloid cardioplegia. The use of calcium antagonist cerebral protective agents is currently being studied at the Hammersmith Hospital.

Celia Oakley raised the important point of the degree to which carotid or vertebral artery disease should be sought in patients requiring coronary surgery. She had not been impressed with the results of preoperative carotid endarterectomy carried out prior to coronary bypass surgery. Ken Taylor felt that asymptomatic patients who have no carotid bruits should not be investigated further, but that patients with a clear history suggestive of transient ischemic attacks, or who have carotid bruits, should have their carotid artery anatomy characterized before undertaking coronary arterial surgery. Finally, in a brief discussion of the role of antiplatelet therapy in reducing microembolic brain damage, the point was made by Celia Oakley that when aspirin is given preoperatively, bleeding problems encountered during and after coronary surgery can be significantly increased.

Floyd Loop's review on the use of the internal mammary artery provoked considerable discussion. Henry Neufeld voiced his belief in internal mammary artery grafts and raised the question of atherosclerosis in the internal mammary artery and the progression of atherosclerosis following grafting. Dr. Loop reported that at the Cleveland Clinic, they had seen very few cases of recognizable atherosclerosis in mammary artery grafts. There was also some evidence to indicate that the progression of proximal lesion atherosclerosis was less following mammary grafting as opposed to simple vein grafting. Dr. Loop indicated that inadvertent transection of the mammary artery graft in reoperations had occurred in 8% of patients in their early experience, but that with additional expertise, the incidence of this complication was much lower. He recommended the initial use of single left mammary to anterior descending anastomosis for surgical teams beginning to use the internal mammary artery graft. Once confidence had been built up, he said, the team could progress to bilateral mammary grafts and perhaps also to sequential grafting. Dr. Loop said that there was little information yet available regarding the patency of sequential internal mammary grafts. It was true that the average flow in an internal mammary graft was less than that in an average saphenous vein graft, though measurement of internal mammary graft flow had satisfied the Cleveland Group that the flow was certainly adequate and was probably capable of significant increase following implantation. William Grossman related Boston's experience in saying that preoperative angiography, to define the health of the internal mammary artery in suitable patients, was not worth doing since they had failed to demonstrate significant atherosclerosis, even in patients whose other arteries were significantly affected by atheroma.

Regarding artificial graft materials, Ken Taylor related the experience of his colleague, Ralph Sapsford, at the Hammersmith who, using Goretex grafts in a sizable number of patients, had demonstrated that patency was significantly poorer than saphenous vein. It was true that many of the major manufacturing companies were hard at work trying to develop biocompatible graft materials, but as yet synthetic grafts should be considered bottom of the list for coronary revascularization.

John Goodwin said that he was convinced that there was room for improvement in coronary surgery. He identified the main problem as graft occlusion and also the possible understanding of the 10% of patients who failed to obtain a good symptomatic result after apparently successful coronary surgery. Hugh Bentall agreed wholeheartedly with the concept of internal mammary usage, particularly in view of the data indicating significantly better survival in patients receiving internal mammary artery grafts compared with patients, matched in other respects, receiving only vein grafts. Celia Oakley felt that it was most important to continue to treat aspects of coronary disease in patients following surgery, for example, encouraging them to stop smoking, adjusting lipid levels, and controlling blood pressure. She encouraged the view that surgery should be considered as part of the overall treatment of coronary disease. Spencer King asked Floyd Loop if competitive flow between the mammary graft and the native artery could not be a problem in relation to long-term patency. Dr. Loop stressed that a view often expressed regarding the inadequacy of mammary arteries as a conduit in small blood vessels and in female patients was nonsense. His group had found internal mammaries an excellent conduit in women aged 50–70. He stressed the importance of thinking in the long term if using bilateral mammary artery implants. Gerry

Klassen put forward the suggestion that the gastroepiploic artery might be a conduit suitable for revascularization of arteries on the inferior surface of the heart.

In reply to Desmond Julian's question, Floyd Loop said that patients receiving only internal mammary artery grafts did not receive any antiplatelet drugs. Patients receiving saphenous vein grafts with or without mammary artery grafts had aspirin and persantine (dipyridamole) therapy according to the Mayo Clinic regimen. Attilio Maseri voiced the concept that flow dynamics, including pulsatility, might be important in determining graft patency. He also wondered if preservation of the vasa vasorum accounted for the superiority of mammary artery over radial artery grafts. Floyd Loop suggested that more careful preparation of the radial artery might produce results similar to that with a mammary. Sergio Chierchia asked if Dr. Loop would recommend total abandoning of saphenous vein grafts. Dr. Loop felt that would be too radical since there were, anatomically, only two mammary arteries and the versatility was significantly inferior to that of the vein graft. The question was the best use of vein grafts and internal mammary grafts in dealing with individual patients. In reply to John Goodwin, Floyd Loop concluded by saying that the Cleveland Clinic experience was one in which the use of the internal mammary graft had evolved and increased markedly over the past few years. Internal mammary artery grafts were now employed in over 90% of the coronary surgery patients. Improved results in coronary surgery were, in part, related to the use of better conduits, but the preoperative cardiological management and improved cardiothoracic anesthesia had also made great contributions. Finally, the introduction of better organ protection during cardiopulmonary bypass, including the use of cardioplegic myocardial preservation, had been a step forward.

Editorial comment: A. Maseri

Improvement of the results of cardiac revascularization concerns not only increased survival and higher and longer graft patency rates, but also reduction of complications. The achievement of these goals depends on improvement of surgical techniques, anesthesia, and myocardial and cerebral protection. I can see two aspects of this improvement, which are eventually related to a variable extent: on the one hand, innovations as a fruit of research and on the other, elevation of the standard of results in average hospitals.

When considering surgery one is often emotionally influenced by the appearance of the angiogram, by the possible unpredictable progression of the disease, and by the results of surgery published or presented by leading authorities from major centers. However, it may be unwise to extrapolate these results to all centers. In the majority of institutions, graft patency is only occasionally checked because of the cost and inconvenience of repeat angiography; the occurrence of complications is not systematically reported, but surgical mortality varies considerably among centers participating in multicenter trials, and it may be even higher in centers not participating in trials. In the United Kingdom, average mortality for bypass surgery in 1982 was 3.2%, which contrasts with the much lower figures reported by some centers. A greater severity of the disease is unlikely to be the only explanation of the higher mortality; it is also likely that the complication rate may be greater and graft patency lower in centers with a higher mortality. Therefore, when making individual decisions, it is essential to consider the results of the institution where the patient should be operated on rather than those published by the best centers.

Hammersmith Cardiology Workshop Series, Vol. 3,
edited by A. Maseri, B. E. Sobel, and S. Chierchia.
Raven Press, New York © 1987.

Percutaneous Transluminal Coronary Angioplasty in Multivessel Coronary Artery Disease

Spencer B. King III

Cardiovascular Laboratory, Emory University, Atlanta, Georgia 30322

Therapy for ischemic heart disease is aimed at restoring the altered supply-demand relationships of coronary blood flow. Medical therapy is largely directed at the demand side of the formula, while revascularization procedures address the supply side. There are two goals of revascularization procedures. One is to relieve the symptoms of ischemic heart disease; the other is to prevent the complications of the disease and, thereby, prolong the useful productive life of the patient.

CORONARY BYPASS SURGERY AND PTCA

How effective has coronary bypass surgery been in this regard? Symptomatic relief has been demonstrated by coronary bypass surgery in many studies, and its superiority to medical therapy alone has been well demonstrated in the American Veteran's Administration study (1), the Coronary Artery Surgery Study (CASS) (2), and in the European multicenter trial (3). Prolongation of life, however, has been limited to those patients with more severe coronary obstructive disease. In establishing the cost-benefit relationships for coronary bypass surgery, the rules of the game are relatively straightforward. Few would argue with the proposition that an open artery is superior to a closed one; however, the cost of the procedure both from a monetary point of view and in terms of morbidity tempers the enthusiasm except in subsets where clear symptomatic or life-extending benefits can be well demonstrated. Few would offer coronary artery bypass surgery to an asymptomatic patient unless severe forms of life-threatening coronary disease are present. Such constraints do not always prevail in considering coronary angioplasty. First, the cost may be one-half to one-third that of coronary bypass surgery (4), and the morbidity is preceived to be significantly less.

How effective has percutaneous transluminal coronary angioplasty (PTCA) been in alleviating symptoms in patients with single vessel disease? Improved flow has been documented angiographically, hemodynamically, and by various forms of exercise stress testing to be equally effective in PTCA as compared to coronary bypass surgery. In our center approximately 4,500 cases have been performed so far, with a primary success rate of 90%, an emergency surgery rate of 3%, and a mortality risk of just over 0.01% (5). The long-term patency of the dilated segment has improved from 67% of successfully dilated patients in 1980–1981 to 74% of patients undergoing angiograms in 1983. Follow-up of Gruentzig's original patients, now greater than seven years, has taught that once a patient passes 4–6 months without recurrence of a lesion, then late recurrence is indeed a rarity (6). When restenosis occurs, repeat angioplasty is almost always successful with an acceptable second restenosis rate (7).

Given this good track record there is understandable interest in expanding the technique to multivessel disease. The initial selection of patients with single-vessel disease for the technique was not because of the impossibility of performing multivessel angioplasty or entirely because of safety considerations, but rather because single-vessel angioplasty lent itself best to a clear-cut objective assessment of the result over time. With the development of the steerable guidewire system and low profile catheters, it is now possible to dilate most segments of the arterial tree.

Although the results of the National Heart, Lung, and Blood Institute Registry of Angioplasty showed the highest complication rate and mortality in patients with multivessel disease (8), those results should not be used as a standard to be expected. Much of those data were accumulated during the early learning phase of angioplasty both in terms of the individual operator and in terms of collective experience regarding the technique. Our selection criteria for multivessel angioplasty at Emory have been relatively conservative. The majority have been performed in patients with discreet stenoses, but not total occlusion, located in accessible portions of the coronary arteries. Patients with stenoses and also total occlusion of large contralateral arteries with or without extensive myocardial infarction are not generally accepted.

Using these criteria we have now performed angioplasty on approximately 500 patients with multivessel coronary artery disease. In these carefully selected patients results have been gratifying both in terms of the initial success and complication rate and in terms of long-term patency of the artery measured angiographically. Primary success has been achieved in 88% of the patients with multivessel disease. Coronary bypass surgery has been required in 5%, Q-wave myocardial infarctions in 2%, and mortality in 0.4%. Three-fourths of the patients, despite having multivessel disease, have undergone angioplasty on only one artery by design and, despite the fact that only one artery was attempted, this group of patients had a higher complication rate than the patients with single-vessel disease. Emergency bypass surgery was required in 5.2%, myocardial infarction occurred in 2.3%, and death in 0.5%. The 25% of patients who underwent a dilatation of two separate arterial beds had an emergency bypass graft surgery rate of 3%, myocardial infarction rate of 1%, and no deaths. There was an increased risk of closure of a vessel in this group with multiple dilatations so that 9% of the patients suffered closure of some vessel, usually the second, less important vessel. This fact was the reason that despite the high closure rate, only 3% went for coronary bypass graft surgery as an emergency. Utilizing the experience we've gained we have developed a strategy for PTCA in multivessel disease.

The overriding consideration is the safety of the patient. If the judgment is made that sudden closure of an arterial segment will result in such massive overall left ventricular ischemia as to likely produce cardiogenic shock, then these patients are not selected for multivessel angioplasty. An example would be a patient with a totally occluded large right coronary artery served by collaterals from a left anterior descending (LAD) artery which has high grade proximal disease. If sudden closure occurs during attempts at angioplasty of the LAD, then the amount of myocardium affected will be extensive, placing the patient in jeopardy for movement to emergency bypass surgery.

The preferred strategy in multivessel disease is to dilate the most severe lesion first, especially if this artery has the potential for supplying collateral vessels to another diseased vessel. This is true even in totally occluded arteries. If the most severe lesion is suitable for angioplasty then it is approached first, and only after satisfactory completion of that angioplasty will subsequent vessels be attempted. Throughout the process the rule of thumb is kept in mind that if sudden closure occurs in one vessel, which would result in massive left ventricular ischemia, then angioplasty should not be chosen. If the first vessel dilated has an extensive dissection or other indices that would lead us to worry about the possibility of an early reclosure, then the second vessel is not attempted. The patient would then be brought back to the laboratory in one to two days for a reexamination of the dilated segment. If the segment stood the test of time and remained open or improved its appearance, then the second vessel can safely be attempted. This staged-type approach to multivessel angioplasty has been used in only 15% of our multivessel dilatation procedures.

Symptomatic relief and objective exercise evaluation of patients who have had multivessel angioplasty is comparable to those with single vessel angioplasty. Even the patients who were selected for dilatation of only one vessel have had very excellent symptomatic improvement and reversion of objective signs of ischemia. In many cases we find it unnecessary to dilate moderately stenosed vessels or totally occluded vessels when the area of myocardium served is relatively small.

Major unanswered questions in multivessel angioplasty relate to the percentage of patients who can be approached with this technique with a high degree of safety. Clearly, that percentage is higher than the 15% to 20% of multivessel patients that we are currently treating in our center. Others have attempted multivessel angioplasty in upwards of 50% of patients who would otherwise have gone for coronary bypass surgery. Such extension of the technique has resulted in significantly higher complication rates (9). Another problem facing multivessel PTCA is that of recurrence of the stenosis. Since there is not a direct one-to-one correlation between recurrent symptoms and recurrent stenosis, we have chosen to evaluate recurrence by angiography. Most symptomatic patients agree to angiography, and many of those patients who are asymptomatic also agree. We have been encouraged by the improving recurrence rate which showed that in 1983, 26% of the patients undergoing angiography had a recurrence. When multiple dilatation patients are analyzed, the recurrence rate is approximately 17% per lesion, with an overall multidilatation recurrence rate per patient of 33%. We have been somewhat more successful in obtaining restudies in asymptomatic, multivessel patients and this may account for the slightly lower recurrence rate per lesion. One lesson we have learned is that the recurrence seems to be lesion-specific rather than patient-specific. That is, many patients have had recurrence of one lesion while other dilated areas remain fully patent. Finally, the objective assessment of the efficacy of multivessel angioplasty in a broad range of patients awaits a randomized trial comparing that form of therapy to coronary bypass surgery and medical therapy. Although such trials have been encouraged, our attempt to institute such a trial has not yet been supported with adequate funding. We plan a scaled down version of our randomized trial in the near future.

REFERENCES

1. Read, R. C., Murphy, M. L., Hultgren, H. N., et al. (1978): Survival of men treated for chronic stable angina pectoris: A cooperative randomized study. *J. Thorac. Cardiovasc. Surg.,* 75:1.
2. Coronary Artery Surgery Study (CASS) (1983): A randomized trial of coronary artery bypass surgery, survival data. *Circulation,* 68(5):939–950.
3. European Coronary Surgery Study Group (1982): Long-term results of prospective randomized study of coronary artery bypass surgery in stable angina pectoris. *Lancet,* 2:1173–1180.
4. Jong, G. C., Block, P. C., Cowley, M. J., et al. (1984): Relative cost of coronary angioplasty and bypass surgery in a one-vessel disease model. *Am. J. Cardiol.,* 53:C52–C55.
5. Bredlau, C. E., Leimgruber, P. P., Douglas, J. S., King, S. B., and Gruentzig, A. R. (1985): In-hospital morbidity and mortality in elective coronary angioplasty. *Circulation,* X:XXX–XXX (submitted for publication).
6. Gruentzig, A. R., Schlumpf, M., and Siegnthaler, W. (1984): Long-term results after coronary angioplasty. *Circulation,* 70:II–323 (abstract).
7. Meier, B., King, S. B., Gruentzig, A. R., Douglas, J. S., Hollman, J., Ischinger, T., Galen, K., and Tankersley, R. (1984): Repeat coronary angioplasty. *J. Am. Coll. Cardiol.,* 4:463–466.
8. Cowley, M. J., Dorros, G., Kelsey, S. F., VonRaden, M., and Detre, K. M. (1984): Acute coronary events associated with percutaneous transluminal coronary angioplasty. *Am. J. Cardiol.,* 53C:12–21.
9. Dorros, G., Singh, S., and Janke, L. M. (1984): Coronary angioplasty in multivessel coronary disease. *Circulation,* 70:II–107 (abstract).

Hammersmith Cardiology Workshop Series, Vol. 3,
edited by A. Maseri, B. E. Sobel, and S. Chierchia.
Raven Press, New York © 1987.

Technical Advances and Future Perspectives Concerning Coronary Angioplasty

William Grossman

*Cardiovascular Division, Harvard-Thorndike Laboratory, Beth Israel Hospital,
Boston, Massachusetts 02215*

Coronary angioplasty has evolved with extreme rapidity since its clinical introduction (1) by Dr. Andreas Gruentzig in September 1977. The first patients treated by Gruentzig in Zurich underwent coronary angioplasty with a system that utilized a fixed balloon and catheter, without a leading guidewire. Over the next 3 to 4 years, major technological advances occurred, including the introduction of steerable balloon angioplasty systems. In the currently utilized steerable systems, a separately moveable guidewire leads the balloon angioplasty catheter (2). The guidewire is manipulated around bends and beyond obstructions, and subsequently serves as a "monorail track" upon which the balloon angioplasty catheter can be advanced into the coronary segment requiring dilatation. A second major technological advance has been the development of low-profile angioplasty catheters, whose shaft diameter is 3.2 French (0.042 in.). Standard angioplasty catheters today have a shaft diameter of 4.3 French (0.057 in.), and are led by guidewires which are 0.014–0.018 in. in diameter. An additional advance in the technology of angioplasty catheter design has involved the materials used in construction of the dilatation balloon itself. Initially, dilatation balloons would not withstand an inflation pressure of greater than 4–5 atm (60–75 pounds per square inch). However, substantial improvement in materials and design has enabled current balloons to withstand up to 10 atm inflation pressure without rupture.

These technological advances in balloon catheter and guidewire design have resulted in a substantial improvement in the success of coronary angioplasty. Primary success (ability to reach a lesion, cross it with guidewire and balloon, and achieve substantial luminal enlargement following balloon inflation) currently exceeds 90% in most large centers.

The use of very fine guidewires has also permitted cardiologists performing balloon angioplasty to approach lesions that previously were not considered appropriate for coronary angioplasty. In particular, total coronary occlusions can be crossed safely with a fine guidewire in many cases, particularly when dealing with coronary occlusions of relatively recent onset. The success rate in dilatations of patients with total coronary occlusion is currently 60% to 70% in most centers (3,4). In the last 120 cases of chronic total coronary occlusion where angioplasty was attempted at the Beth Israel Hospital in Boston, dilatation was successful in 83 patients (69%). These lesions are considered safe for coronary dilatation since the territory distal to a chronic coronary occlusion is usually subserved by well-developed collaterals. Successful dilatation of coronary occlusion has enabled collaterals to be used in reverse, to provide support for vessels that had previously provided collateral flow to the myocardium subserved by the occluded coronary artery. The reversal of coronary flow has increased the safety of coronary angioplasty of the second coronary stenosis, and has permitted development of a technique known as "bootstrap" angioplasty. This technique is applicable to the patient with a total coronary occlusion *and* a severe stenosis in a second coronary artery whose distal branches give rise to collaterals that perfuse the area of total occlusion. In such a case, the total occlusion is attacked first; if successful opening of the total occlusion is achieved, the reversed collaterals now provide protection for angioplasty of the second stenosis.

CORONARY ANGIOPLASTY AND LASER TECHNIQUES

An important potential advance with regard to invasive therapy for coronary artery disease is the marriage of coronary angioplasty and laser techniques. In particular, Dr. J. Richard Spears in Boston is developing a method for laser fusion of dissected coronary segments (5). In this technique, a tiny laser filament is inserted down the central lumen of a balloon angioplasty catheter, so that its diffusion tip is located in the middle of the fluid-filled angioplasty dilatation balloon. Abrupt heating of the fluid within the balloon to 80°C for 5–15 sec has been shown experimentally to produce a weld of dissected and separated tissues. This is currently undergoing experimental testing and, if successful, may prove to be of great benefit in the prevention and/or treatment of abrupt reclosure, one of the persistent problems of coronary angioplasty today.

CORONARY RESTENOSIS

A word should be added concerning coronary restenosis. The two major problems in coronary angioplasty today are abrupt reclosure and coronary restenosis. As discussed earlier, new laser fusion techniques may play an important role in reduction of the incidence of abrupt reclosure, which is commonly associated with a progressive coronary dissection. Insofar as abrupt reclosure is associated with *in situ* thrombosis on the raw, exposed atheromatous plaque, new thrombolytic agents such as tissue plasminogen activator may play an important role. However, the problem of restenosis is a challenging one for which no dramatic solutions are currently on the horizon. Symptomatic restenosis appears to occur in 20% of cases, and restenosis as defined by angiographic criteria probably occurs in 30%

of lesions dilated. Gruentzig has reported that the incidence of restenosis may be inversely related to the degree of success of the initial procedure, with patients in whom significant residual gradients were present across the stenosis following angioplasty having a higher incidence of restenosis. Currently, it is believed that the incidence of restenosis can be reduced by aggressive postangioplasty treatment with aspirin/dipyridamole together with a calcium blocker (6). The potential role of serum lipids, and in particular high density lipoprotein subfractions, needs further definition. Since restenosis resembles accelerated atherosclerosis, it seems likely that antiatherogenic measures may influence its incidence.

PTCA AND MYOCARDIAL INFARCTION

The role of percutaneous transluminal coronary angioplasty in patients with acute myocardial infarction is still unsettled. Several groups, including the group of Dr. Harzler in Kansas City, Dr. Meier in Aachen, West Germany, as well as others, have reported on the use of balloon angioplasty either immediately following thrombolysis in acute myocardial infarction or instead of the use of thrombolysis. It is clear that rapid opening of the occluded artery can be achieved by primary angioplasty in many patients, but the eventual effect (beneficial or harmful) on myocardial salvage using this technique is unknown. The National Institutes of Health-sponsored TIMI (Thrombolysis in Myocardial Infarction) trial currently under way in the United States will examine in a randomized prospective protocol the potential value of coronary angioplasty carried out within the first 48 hr following successful thrombolysis. Until the results of this and other studies are available, there is no firm evidence either in favor or against the use of angioplasty in a setting of acute myocardial infarction.

REFERENCES

1. Gruentzig, A. R., Senning, A., and Siegenthaler, W. E. (1979): Nonoperative dilatation of coronary-artery stenosis. Percutaneous transluminal coronary angioplasty. *N. Engl. J. Med.,* 301:61–68.
2. Simpson, J. B., Baim, D. S., Robert, E. W., and Harrison, D. C. (1982): A new catheter system for coronary angioplasty. *Am. J. Cardiol.,* 49:1216–1222.
3. Dervan, J. P., Baim, D. S., Cherniles, J., and Grossman, W. (1983): Transluminal angioplasty of occluded coronary system. *Circulation,* 68:776–784.
4. Holmes, D. R., Jr., Vlietstra, R. E., Reeder, G. S., Bresnahan, J. F., Smith, H. C., Bove, A. A., and Schaff, H. V. (1984): Angioplasty in total coronary artery occlusion. *J. Am. Coll. Cardiol.,* 3:845–849.
5. Hiehle, J. F., Bourgelais, D. B. C., Shapshay, S., Schoen, F. J., Kim, D., and Spears, J. R. (1985): Nd:YAG laser fusion of human atheromatous plaque-arterial wall separations *in vitro. Am. J. Cardiol.,* 56:953–957.
6. Thornton, M. A., Gruentzig, A. R., Hollman, J., King, S. B., III, and Douglas, J. S. (1984): Coumadin and aspirin in prevention of recurrence after transluminal coronary angioplasty: a randomized study. *Circulation,* 69:721–727.

Hammersmith Cardiology Workshop Series, Vol. 3,
edited by A. Maseri, B. E. Sobel, and S. Chierchia.
Raven Press, New York © 1987.

Determining Factors of Restenosis After Percutaneous Transluminal Coronary Angioplasty

Michel E. Bertrand, Jean M. Lablanche, J. L. Fourrier, and G. Traisnel

Hopital Cardiologique, Lille University, 59037 Lille, France

Many previous reports have clearly established that percutaneous transluminal coronary angioplasty (PTCA) is a very effective method of myocardial revascularization. However, restenosis remains one of the most difficult problems in the follow-up of the patients treated with PTCA. In this chapter, the following questions will be addressed: What is the frequency of restenosis after a successful PTCA? What are the possible mechanisms of restenosis? How does one predict restenosis? And how can we prevent restenosis?

FREQUENCY OF RESTENOSIS AFTER PTCA

Restenosis is difficult to define. Various angiographic criteria have been used. Five definitions of restenosis have been proposed: (a) an increase of at least 30% from the immediate post-PTCA stenosis to the following PTCA stenosis, (b) an immediate post-PTCA stenosis of less than 50% that increased to greater than or equal to 70% at follow-up, (c) an increase in stenosis at follow-up to 10% below predilatation stenosis or higher, (d) a loss of at least 50% of the gain achieved at PTCA, and (e) a follow-up PTCA stenosis higher than 50%. Definition (d) is the most commonly used, and a report of the National Heart, Lung, and Blood Institute showed that this definition identified all patients. However, it must be noticed that this definition is only angiographic, and it could be useful in the future to take into account other markers (functional capacity or exercise test). For example, in our experience 21% of the patients with angiographically defined restenosis were totally asymptomatic.

From various publications (1–7) (Table 1), the incidence of restenosis varied from 18% to 43%, with an average of 31%. Among 550 patients who underwent PTCA in our institution, the first 184 patients with successful PTCA achieved

TABLE 1. *Frequency of restenosis after PTCA*

Author	Year	Number of I success	Restenosis
Scholl (1)	1982	45	24%
Jutzki (2)	1982	30	40%
Gruentzig (3)	1982	116	25%
Holmes (4)	1982	397	18%
Dangoisse (5)	1982	103	30%
Hollman (6)	1983	276	43%
NHLBI (8)	1984	557	33%
Meier (7)	1984	514	33%
Levine	1985	92	40%
Bertrand	1985	184	30%
	Total	2,314	31.6%

complete follow-up with angiography: 56, or 30%, had restenosis defined by criterion (d).

HYPOTHESES CONCERNING THE MECHANISMS OF RESTENOSIS AFTER PTCA

The cause of restenosis is totally unknown. Pre-PTCA clinical variables, details of the procedure, and treatment after PTCA may affect the restenosis rate. Even more, the mechanisms of PTCA itself are still not well understood. Initially, it was thought that a compression and even a remodeling of the atherosclerotic plaque could explain the increase of luminal diameter. Some authors had evoked the release of the fluid components of the plaque. Nowadays it is more likely that the beneficial effects result from a disruption and splitting of the plaque, associated with gradual stretching of the outer layers of the arterial wall.

Moreover, the intima is damaged and denuded; the "healing" of the split atherosclerotic plaque is complex and not well understood. Fibrous retraction of the split plaque and a recoil of the outer layers of the wall can occur. Some authors have suggested a proliferation of collagen. It is more likely that the damaged and denuded endothelium can expose the neo-intima to platelet adhesion. Once adhesion occurs, release of platelet factors such as adenosine diphosphate, thromboxane, or platelet growth factor may promote aggregation, vasospasm, or smooth muscle proliferation (8,9). Therefore, intimal damage from the angioplasty balloon may, in some situations, actually accelerate the atheromatous process and may account for the recurrence of narrowing within 4 to 6 months after a successful procedure. However, all these mechanisms are speculative, and we need further studies to understand the "healing" process after angioplasty and to delineate the mechanisms of restenosis.

HOW TO PREDICT RESTENOSIS?

In the report from the National Heart, Blood, and Lung Institute (N.H.L.B.I.) PTCA registry (8), a univariate and multivariate analysis was performed. Four variables are significantly associated with an increased incidence of restenosis: male sex, Canadian heart class III or IV, angina pectoris, and no history of myocardial infarction. Univariate comparisons revealed other variables associated with increased restenosis: large gradient before and after PTCA, short duration of the symptoms, diabetes, and the degree of narrowing.

A study from the Montreal Heart Institute suggests that the degree of residual stenosis immediately after PTCA is the most important determinant of restenosis. Other variables include variant angina, multivessel disease, coronary calcifications, type of coronary dissection, and balloon catheter size.

In 184 patients who were successfully dilated and with complete angiographic follow-up, we performed a univariate analysis to determine whether clinical and technical factors can be predictive of restenosis. We studied 21 variables: 6 clinical parameters, 8 angiographical variables, and 7 technical parameters. The clinical factors are not predictive of restenosis. Neither age, sex, risk factors, history of previous myocardial infarction, symptoms, nor the duration of symptoms was predictive of restenosis. The number of vessel disease, the location of the narrowing, and left ventricular end-diastolic volume index were not predictive, but ejection fraction was significantly lower in the group of patients with restenosis (n = 56). The type of the lesions, the severity of the narrowing, and the transtenotic gradient were not predictive.

In our institution, it is usual to test the vasomotor reactivity of the narrowing by the combination of two tests, one with vasoconstrictor effect (methylergometrine 0.4 mg single i.v. bolus) followed by a test of vasodilatation with 3 mg isosorbide dinitrate i.v. injected. This procedure was done in 155 patients (110 without restenosis, and 45 in the group of 56 patients with restenosis). The incidence of spasm defined as the total obstruction of the vessel at the site of the dilated narrowing was significantly higher in the group with restenosis. From the technical parameters, it was observed that maximal pressure of inflation and the size of the balloon were predictive of restenosis, while the number, the duration, and the degree of residual stenosis or transtenotic gradient were not predictive. However, the patients with restenosis had a slight but significantly ($p < 0.05$) lower gain than the other group. At the time of the reinvestigation, the two previously mentioned tests (methylergometrine followed by isosorbide dinitrate administration) were performed in all the patients except nine. There was again a significant difference between the two groups, and the incidence of spasm was significantly higher in the group with restenosis. Therefore, we identified four predictive factors of restenosis after PTCA: pressure of inflation, size of the balloon, the initial gain, and dynamic coronary stenosis. It is well known that the results of PTCA are less satisfactory in patients with variant angina than in the other groups (10). Our study supports these results and stresses the role of spasm in the pathogenesis of restenosis. Moreover, if we consider a group of 155 patients who had the two tests before PTCA and at the time of the restudy, we observed that those who were still in active phase at the time of the restudy (6 months), have a significantly higher chance to have restenosis. These results support the hypothesis of Block (9) who suspected the role of platelet factors and spasm.

HOW TO PREVENT RESTENOSIS?

The first question that arises concerns the technical problems: Can we influence the incidence of restenosis by larger balloon size and higher pressure inflation? However, these modifications could increase the risk of dissection and need careful. examination. Second, can medical regimens, post-PTCA, decrease the incidence of restenosis? Thornton et al. (11) showed that Coumadin (sodium warfarin) was not superior to aspirin for prevention of recurrence after PTCA. More recently, Corcos et al. (12) published a randomized trial of diltiazem for prevention of restenosis, but the drug did not prevent the incidence of recurrence after PTCA. However, the patients had no spasm before PTCA. Similar results were obtained by Whitworth (13) in 1985 with nifedipine. In contrast, in patients with spasm treated by calcium antagonists after PTCA the incidence of restenosis was significantly lower than in the other group.

Finally, the restenosis rates are occurring despite the use of various drugs, including antiplatelet regimens. Therefore, we need further studies with properly controlled regimens since the problem of restenosis is really crucial for the future of PTCA.

REFERENCES

1. Scholl, J. M., David, P. R., Chaitman, B. R., Lesperance, J., Crepeau, J., Dyrda, I., and Bourrassa, M. G. (1982): Recurrence of stenosis following percutaneous transluminal coronary angioplasty. *Circulation (Suppl. I)*, 66:331.
2. Jutzki, K. R., Berte, L. E., Alderman, E. L., Rotts, J., and Simpson, J. B. (1982): Coronary restenosis rates in a consecutive patient series one year post successful angioplasty. *Circulation (Suppl. II)*, 66:331.
3. Gruentzig, A. R. (1984): Percutaneous transluminal coronary angioplasty: six years' experience. *Am. Heart J.*, 107:818–819.
4. Holmes, D. R., Jr., Vliestra, R. E., Smith, H. C., Vetrovec, G. W., Cowley, M. J., Kent, K. M., Detre, K. M., and Myler, R. (1982): Restenosis following PTCA: a report from the N.H.L.B.I. PTCA registry. *Am. J. Cardiol.*, 49:905 (abstract).
5. Dangoisse, V., Gruteros, Val P., David, P. R., Lesperance, J., Crepeau, J., Dyrda, I., and Bourrassa, M. G. (1982): Recurrence of stenosis after successful PTCA. *Circulation (Suppl. II)*, 66:331 (abstract).
6. Hollman, J., Gruentzig, A., Meier, B., Bradford, J., and Galan, K. (1983): Factors affecting recurrence after successful coronary angioplasty. *J. Am. Coll. Cardiol.*, 1:644.
7. Meier, B., King, S., III, Gruentzig, A., et al. (1984): Repeat coronary angioplasty. *J. Am. Coll. Cardiol.*, 4:463–466.

8. Holmes, D. R., Vliestra, R. E., Smith, H. C., Vetrovec, G. W., Kent, K. M., Cowley, M. J., Faxon, D. P., Gruentzig, A. R., et al. (1984): Restenosis after percutaneous transluminal coronary angioplasty. A report from the PTCA registry of the National Heart, Lung, and Blood Institute. *Am. J. Cardiol.,* 53:77c–81c.
9. Block, P. C. (1984): Mechanism of transluminal angioplasty. *Am. J. Cardiol.,* 53:69c–71c.
10. David, P. R., Waters, D. D., Scholl, J. M., Crepeau, J., Szlechcic, J., Lesperance, J., Hudon, J., and Bourrassa, M. G. (1982): Percutaneous transluminal coronary angioplasty in patients with variant angina. *Circulation,* 65:695–698.
11. Thornton, M., Gruentzig, A., Hollman, J., Kings, S. B., and Douglas, J. S. (1984): Coumadin is aspirin in prevention of recurrence after PTCA. *Circulation,* 69:721–727.
12. Corcos, Th., David, P. R., Renkin, J., Dangoisse, V., Gruteros, Val P., Ropold, H., and Bourrassa, M. G. (1984): Diltiazem for prevention of restenosis after PTCA. *Circulation,* 70:175.
13. Whitworth, H. B., Gruentzig, A. R., Hollman, J., Galan, K., and Gershon, L. (1985): Effect of nifedipine on recurrence stenosis after percutaneous transluminal angioplasty (PTCA). *J.A.C.C.,* 5:524 (abstract).

Hammersmith Cardiology Workshop Series, Vol. 3,
edited by A. Maseri, B. E. Sobel, and S. Chierchia.
Raven Press, New York © 1987.

Précis of the Discussion: Section XIV

Percutaneous Transluminal Angioplasty

Sergio Chierchia

Spencer King said that the first absolute contraindication to multivessel angioplasty would be represented by the patient's safety being jeopardized. The potential consequences of an acute coronary occlusion due to PTCA should always be kept in mind before the procedure. Another contraindication would be the fact that the immediate predicted result is inferior to that of surgery. For long-term results, it is difficult to compete with surgery. However, angioplasty gives the opportunity to come back again and again, if necessary, and does not need to produce complete revascularization in every patient with multivessel disease.

A contributor asked why the recurrence rate was higher in patients with multivessel disease, even if only one vessel had been dilated: Which drugs were used to prevent recurrence? Spencer King said he had no answer to the first question. As far as the second was concerned, he said that the current treatment they used was either a combination of Persantine (dipyridamole) and high-dose or low-dose aspirin alone. They had compared Coumadin (warfarin sodium) with aspirin and found that Coumadin was not superior. Also, the addition of the calcium blocker nifedipine to the standard aspirin treatment did not improve the recurrence rate.

Sergio Chierchia stressed the point that in patients with multivessel coronary artery disease, only one vessel is often responsible for the patient's symptoms at a given time. One of the major advantages of angioplasty is the fact that it allows us to deal with that particular vessel at a given time, leaving the possibility to go back in, if needed. He emphasized the need for sensitive techniques to identify the ischemia-related vessel.

Spencer King said that the major question that still had to be answered was whether angioplasty represented an effective approach to improve prognosis. In this respect, a randomized trial to compare surgery with PTCA needed to be done urgently.

Richard Conti asked Spencer King to give his definition of surgical complication. In Spencer King's view, a case had to be classified as a surgical complication when the patient had to be taken to theater because of ongoing ischemia resulting from PTCA. If the procedure was a failure and the patient underwent surgery the next day, then it does not qualify as an emergency. He felt that surgical backup was an absolute necessity for every case.

Paul Lichtlen asked Michel Bertrand to report on the experience of early restenosis.

Dr. Bertrand replied that this occurs very often in patients with variant angina, within two months of the dilatation.

Raphael Balcon noted that the incidence of spasm appeared very high in Michel Bertrand's series. Dr. Bertrand answered that the reason for this was probably the fact that ergonovine testing is routinely used in his institution in all patients undergoing coronary arteriography.

Sergio Chierchia commented that on the one hand, Dr. Bertrand's series showed a higher recurrence rate in patients with ergonovine-induced spasm; on the other, previous reports had shown no effect or restenosis rate with calcium blockers. He wondered if spasm was the cause of restenosis or, more likely, the marker of some arterial damage predisposing the wall to both vasoconstriction and recurrence.

Paul Lichtlen asked Michel Bertrand the rationale for giving ergonovine to his patients. Michel Bertrand said he wanted to know if the lesion was "fixed" or "dynamic" because, if this was the case, calcium blockers would be indicated for medical treatment. Obviously, the information is not as relevant from the clinical point of view if PTCA was the treatment of choice.

Richard Conti asked William Grossman if he thought that the rabbit atherosclerotic model was relevant to human atheroma, especially with relation to hematoporphyrin uptake. Dr. Grossman replied that hematoporphyrin may be taken up by any area of abnormal endothelial permeability. The idea of using the pigment in conjunction with photoablation came from an oncologist who observed that it is concentrated in tumors. It now seems that it is also taken up by an atheromatous plaque although, obviously, there are still quite a lot of details to work out. William Grossman's major concern about the vaporization approach was the difficulty, in coronary angioscopy, in identifying what you are looking at and in telling diseased from normal wall.

Attilio Maseri asked Spencer King for his definition of restenosis. Spencer King answered that, at Emory, they elected to take a 50% diameter reduction as a significant obstruction. If the lesion comes back to over 50%, then it is recurrent; otherwise, it is defined a continued success.

Celia Oakley asked why a more physiological assessment, for instance the recurrence of a positive exercise test, was not used instead. Spencer King answered that "significant" lesions greater than 50% were seen in approximately 20% of asymptomatic patients: Many of these also have a negative exercise test.

Celia Oakley asked which patient population would have been considered for the randomized trial comparing angioplasty and coronary bypass surgery. Spencer King said that this would be limited to patients with multivessel disease (50% diameter reduction of two or more major arteries). Accurate clinical characterization and exercise testing would also be included. Attilio Maseri emphasized the problems related to a patient's classification mainly based on the number of vessels critically diseased. Dr. King agreed, but also pointed out that to stratify patients in any different way would probably result in so many different subsets that the numbers required for the possible differences to reach statistical significance would be huge.

The policy of the centers involved for entering patients into the trial was also discussed. It was agreed that randomization was probably going to be ethical for quite some time, since, for the time being, it is impossible to say whether surgery or angioplasty is prognostically better.

The contributors discussed their experiences in dilating venous grafts. Spencer King said that good results could only be obtained if the stricture involved the distal anastomosis or if the graft was occluded and the native vessel had to be dilated. The results of angioplasty of the proximal anastomosis or of the graft itself were usually poor.

The indications for coronary angioplasty were discussed at length. It was agreed that angioplasty had to be advised not just for removing coronary stenosis but had to be considered when coronary stenosis was found in association with symptoms and evidence for myocardial ischemia. It was felt that this was a very important point and that in day-to-day practice, these criteria were not always used for establishing the indications.

Most agreed that, whenever possible with a low risk, angioplasty was probably preferable to coronary bypass surgery.

Editorial comment: S. Chierchia

There are, in medicine, very few discoveries and new techniques that have the power of conditioning our way of thinking and the capability to influence profoundly our way of practicing medicine. Coronary angioplasty is certainly one of these. This is not only because it has represented the first successful attempt of nonsurgical cardiac revascularization, but also because it has contributed to create a completely new and daring attitude to the study and treatment of the human coronary circulation. Techniques and procedures that were difficult even to dream of only a few years ago are today not only possible, but are part of our day-to-day clinical routine. As a result, a number of new ideas for approaching the coronary circulation with a view to nonsurgical revascularization have been produced.

It is somewhat ironical that, while a considerable amount of energy was spent by both basic and clinical scientists in a rather sterile search for better understanding of the coronary circulation in health and disease, a major clinical advance in the treatment of ischemic heart disease came from a relatively crude, unsophisticated idea. However, the fact that angioplasty, at least in good hands, is a rather simple and effective technique has some potential disadvantages. The risk for the technique to be exploited for financial rather than medical purposes has to be carefully controlled, especially when one considers the continuously growing number of procedures performed in the United States and Europe. The temptation to treat coronary rather than ischemic heart disease should be avoided, and rigorous criteria should be applied in establishing indications. Likewise, relief of symptoms and/or ischemia, rather than a purely anatomical success, should be considered for evaluating results.

Finally, although almost a decade has passed since the first angioplasty was performed successfully, we don't know yet the answer to a basic question: Does angioplasty influence prognosis? Does it affect survival and occurrence (or recurrence) of acute myocardial infarction? The appropriate trials to answer these questions are long overdue.

Hammersmith Cardiology Workshop Series, Vol. 3,
edited by A. Maseri, B. E. Sobel, and S. Chierchia.
Raven Press, New York © 1987.

Medical Treatment of Ischemic Heart Disease: Nitrates in Combination with Other Drugs

C. Richard Conti

*Division of Cardiovascular Medicine, University of Florida, College of Medicine,
Gainesville, Florida*

The most common indication for the use of nitrates is to treat and prevent myocardial ischemia in patients with exertional angina or resting angina. Nitrates are available in many preparations; these include parenteral, sublingual, buccal, oral, and transdermal. In the near future, a lingual spray preparation will be available. The most common route of administration is sublingually, yet the intravenous preparation is being used more frequently, especially in the acute situation, that is, patients with unstable angina and acute myocardial infarction.

When used in appropriate patients and in appropriate doses, nitrates can be effective therapy of myocardial ischemia. However, in clinical practice it is naive to think that they will be used alone to manage the complex problems associated with ischemic heart disease. It is highly likely that nitrates, calcium antagonists, and beta blockers will be used in combination rather than separately. Other than hypotension and adverse effects of the drug, there seems to be no contraindication to the combination of nitrates and calcium antagonists or beta blockers.

COMBINATION THERAPY FOR THE TREATMENT OF ANGINA

Each of the antianginal drug classes possesses somewhat different properties. The physiologic effects of nitrates, beta blockers, and calcium blockers on the determinants of myocardial oxygen consumption and coronary blood flow are summarized in Table 1. The combination of one or more of these agents makes physiologic sense because detrimental effects may be counterbalanced by the beneficial effects of another drug. In order to provide individualized therapy for the single patient, physicians should understand the benefits and drawbacks of the various drugs.

Nitrates and Beta Blockers

The benefits of combining a nitrate with a beta-blocking drug are obvious. Nitrates act predominantly on the venous system. As a result of peripheral venous

TABLE 1. *Physiologic effects of nitrates, beta blockers, and calcium blockers on determinants of myocardial oxygen consumption (MVO$_2$) and coronary blood flow*

| | Nitrates | Beta Blockers | Calcium Antagonists | | |
			Diltiazem	Verapamil	Nifedipine
Myocardial Oxygen Consumption					
Contractility	↑	↓↓↓↓	↓	↓	↑
Heart Rate	↑	↓↓↓↓	↓	↓↑	↑
LV Wall Tension					
Volume	↓↓↓↓	↑	?	↑	↓
Systolic Pressure	↓	↓	↓	↓	↓
Diastolic Pressure	↓↓↓↓	↑	NC	↑	NC
Coronary Blood Flow					
Aortic Pressure	↓	↓	↓	↓	↓
Coronary Resistance	↓↓↓↓	↑	↓↓↓	↓↓↓	↓↓↓
Epicardial Artery Size	↑↑↑↑	↓	↑↑	↑↑	↑↑

↑↑↑↑, Significant effect; ↑, minor effect; NC, no change.

dilation, venous return is decreased and consequently pulmonary artery pressure, left ventricular filling pressure, and left ventricular volume are decreased. Nitrates also act by decreasing peripheral vascular resistance and lowering systolic blood pressure. However, a side effect of these physiologic responses is a reflex tachycardia and an increased myocardial contractility. Both of these latter two effects could be detrimental for patients with angina. The beta-blocking agents counter this effect by their negative chronotropic and inotropic activity.

A recent report by Muller and colleagues (1) illustrates the effectiveness of the combination of nitrates and beta blockers. They reported a randomized double-blind trial comparing nifedipine to the combination of propranolol and isosorbide dinitrate in 126 patients with unstable angina. This trial lasted 14 days. Their observations indicated that there was no significant difference in time to relief of angina, decrease in anginal attacks for 24 hr, decrease in number of nitroglycerin tablets consumed, percentage of patients requiring morphine on day one, or percentage of patients who develop infarction (14% in both groups), when nifedipine was compared to the combination of isosorbide dinitrate and propranolol.

Nitrates and Calcium Antagonists

The effects of combining nitrates with calcium antagonists also can provide a complementary and beneficial effect for patients. For example, nifedipine, a potent peripheral arterial dilator, may exert its major clinical effect by decreasing after-load in combination with its coronary dilatory effect, i.e., maintenance of coronary artery size or the prevention of vasoconstriction. In contrast, the nitrates, which clearly dilate epicardial coronary arteries significantly, may be effective because of this action plus a marked effect on decreasing ventricular volume and ventricular end-diastolic pressure. Specific calcium antagonists, such as verapamil and diltiazem, may limit any tachycardia resulting from nitrate administration.

Perhaps one of the best ways to manage patients with ischemic heart disease utilizes a combination of calcium antagonists and nitrates. This will result in (a) dilation of the coronary arteries to maintain coronary blood flow, (b) decrease in systemic arterial pressure and, thus, a decrease in peripheral vascular resistance, and (c) dilation of peripheral veins, and, thus, a decrease in ventricular volume and pressure. When proper doses are used, the combination of nitrates and a calcium antagonist may be more effective than either drug alone.

To illustrate the effectiveness of combining a calcium blocker to nitrate therapy, Hugenholtz and his colleagues (2) reported 73 patients admitted to the coronary care unit for "impending myocardial infarction." All were treated with beta blockers and nitrates in high doses, but 52 remained symptomatic. Subsequently added to the regimen was 60 mg of nifedipine for a 24-hr period. Within 8 hr after administration, 42 of the 52 patients became asymptomatic. Gerstinblith et al. (3) reported similar results in 138 patients with unstable angina pectoris who were treated with either beta-blockade and nitrates or a combination of nitrates, beta blockers, and nifedipine. Over a 3-month period, there was no difference in the mortality or myocardial infarction rate when the two therapies were compared. However, those who received nifedipine in combination with nitrates and beta blockers had less requirements for cardiac surgery than those receiving only nitrates and beta blockers.

Beta Blockers and Calcium Antagonists

The combination of a beta blocker and a calcium antagonist can have both additive and complementary effects (4). In the case of nifedipine, the slight tachycardia that might ensue after nifedipine therapy will be blocked by beta-blocker therapy. Additionally, patients with mild conduction abnormalities may tolerate the combination of nifedipine and beta blocker better than a beta blocker alone. In these patients, verapamil and/or diltiazem might not be appropriate drugs to combine with a beta blocker, since both classes of drugs decrease heart rate and myocardial contractility. Although this latter effect of decreasing myocardial contractility may offer benefit to some patients with angina by further decreasing myocardial oxygen consumption, it can also cause harm by precipitating congestive heart failure. Despite this concern, in the experience of many, heart failure is a rare consequence of treatment with the combination of a beta blocker and a calcium antagonist. However, should the occasion arise, I would recommend the use of the calcium antagonist nifedipine with a beta blocker rather than combining a beta blocker with verapamil or diltiazem in a patient who is in borderline heart failure.

One could make a logical argument that the combination of a calcium antagonist

Hammersmith Cardiology Workshop Series, Vol. 3,
edited by A. Maseri, B. E. Sobel, and S. Chierchia.
Raven Press, New York © 1987.

Medical Treatment of Ischemic Heart Disease: Beta Blockers and Combination

Nina Rehnqvist

Department of Medicine, Danderyd Hospital, S-182 88 Danderyd, Sweden

The aim for treating ischemic heart disease with beta blockers is twofold: (a) to relieve symptoms, and (b) to improve prognosis. Various studies have been performed in the different stages of ischemic heart disease to elucidate both mechanisms.

ACUTE MYOCARDIAL INFARCTION

In acute myocardial infarction, four large major studies have been performed, one with propranolol showing a reduced incidence of ventricular fibrillation (VF) in the acute phase (1), and two with metoprolol, one showing reduced incidence of VF in the acute phase and reduction in enzymatically estimated infarct size (2,3). The other larger metoprolol trial was intended to shed light on effects on mortality but did not confirm the data on VF or reduce mortality significantly (4). The recently performed ISIS study, in which 16,105 patients were given atenolol 5–10 mg i.v. followed by oral doses of 50 and 100 mg for seven days, showed a $p < 0.04$ significant reduction in mortality (ISIS II; personal communication). A smaller multicenter study using timolol showed that infarct size was reduced when estimated enzymatically or vectorcardiographically (5). In all the studies there was also reduced need of morphine, indicating less pain among the treated patients. The beneficial effects, however, were predominantly confined to those patients entered early into the study. In these patients other modes of treatment with the purpose of reducing infarct size, such as thrombolysis or nitroglycerin infusion to relieve spasm, have also been proposed to be beneficial, and the match between these three therapies is not solved. Combination therapies have not been studied systematically, even though some beneficial protection by the beta-blockade may be anticipated while thrombolysis is under way. However, reperfusion arrhythmias reported to be alpha-mediated and, thus, theoretically enhanced by beta-blockade may be observed in a higher frequency. This is also not studied. In our department we are currently using the combination without noticing negative effects.

UNSTABLE ANGINA

Patients with unstable angina are currently the focus of much interest. Depending on resources, different measures are taken and everything from conservative therapy with bed rest and slow mobilization to acute coronary angiography and bypass surgery or PTCA, if feasible, is advocated (6). What are the results with beta-blockade in this setting? In the study by Telford et al. (7), atenolol had no effect on the development of myocardial infarction, death, or readmission due to angina pectoris whereas heparin had such an effect. However, in this study atenolol was abruptly withdrawn, which could count for some of the events in the later phase of the study. In the Dutch HINT study, metoprolol seemed superior to placebo or nifedipine. Nifedipine may, on the other hand, improve symptomatology when added to beta-blocker therapy, as shown by Ouyang et al. (6,7). Thus, patients with unstable angina pectoris should be treated aggressively medically, including the use of beta blockers. Symptom relief is the target of therapy and improvement should be documented when a new therapeutic principle is added. For instance, when nitrates are combined with beta blockers in adequate doses as estimated by decreased pulse and blood pressure, this should be accompanied by objectively measured improvement either in the form of reduced nitroglycerin consumption or increased performance. Negative effects are encountered as often as in 30% when vasodilation is combined with oxygen-sparing agents. Coronary flow must, in the case of unstable angina, be optimized. However, also the patients' previous history must be taken into account. As shown by Muller et al. (8), those patients already on propranolol therapy were improved by adding nifedipine therapy in unstable angina, whereas those patients not on propranolol therapy had a better prognosis when given propranolol than when given nifedipine.

STABLE ANGINA

When first introduced, beta blockers were used to treat patients with stable angina pectoris at effort. The logic of this is obvious. Heart work is reduced when blood pressure and heart rate are reduced, leading to reduced oxygen demand. Various studies have been performed with all the beta blockers claiming effects on exercise tolerance and signs of ischemia on the exercise test. However, angina pectoris patients are difficult to study, especially in temperate climates, due to the important influences of the weather. Therefore, the initial studies claiming increased effects by increased doses may not be relevant. Instead, the maximal effect is achieved on a moderate dose and the dose response curve shows a knee-form for most beta blockers (9). However, also when taking the study difficulties into account, it must be remembered that patients with chronic angina pectoris are down-regulated as regards their physical performance. Although angina is relieved, total performance is not necessarily dramatically improved. Recently,

Kenny et al. published a study where both diltiazem and propranolol increased performance in angina patients, and the combination was shown to be even more effective (10). That also alpha-blockade may be beneficial is shown in a study with labetalol (11). Metoprolol and nifedipine have also been compared in a Scandinavian study where patients responding to metoprolol were weaned off the beta blocker and put on nifedipine or the combination (12). Nifedipine was, in this study, shown to be less effective than metoprolol which, in turn, was less effective than the combination. However, nifedipine was tested when a rebound situation was most often proposed, three weeks after metoprolol withdrawal, and this could account for some of the failures as well as the unwanted side effects. That "optimal therapy," i.e., triple therapy with nitrates, calcium antagonists, and beta blockers, is not always the best has been shown by Tollins et al., where two of 16 patients were unable to perform the exercise tolerance test and, further, seven had poorer tolerance on the three drugs than on double therapy (13). Again, individual titration and careful monitoring should be performed.

POST AMI

This is a thoroughly investigated field and today there is no doubt that at least certain beta blockers reduce sudden deaths and total deaths in the postinfarction period by about 30% (14). The patients with poor prognosis as regards death can now also be identified reasonably well, thereby identifying those in whom the benefit of the blockade is to be expected. The methods used are those identifying a large myocardial damage, left ventricular failure, and premature ventricular complexes. It has also been shown that the reinfarction rate can be reduced by metoprolol, propranolol, sotalol, and timolol. The risk for reinfarction, however, is not as readily identified even though some clues are given. Patients with previous cardiac history and hypertension may especially benefit. This has, however, not been tested prospectively.

What does it cost to treat all patients with documented ischemic heart disease with beta-blockade? In a postinfarction population, we have shown that the proportion of patients who are asymptomatic, both regarding symptoms of ischemia and side effects, increase with time among those treated with beta-blockade compared with placebo-treated patients, where this proportion diminishes. On the other hand, when beta-blockade is gradually withdrawn, 25% perceive a general improvement in fitness, accounting for the negative effects of beta blockers (15). The tolerability of the beta blockers shown to reduce mortality is acceptable but not perfect. Calcium channel blockers are, perhaps, better tolerated; this has not, however, been studied in the same number of patients as has beta blockers. Furthermore, the protective effects of calcium blockers and nitrates have not been shown.

What mechanisms are responsible for the beneficial effects of the beta blockers? An antifibrillatory effect is probable since many of the ischemia-induced ventricular arrhythmias are catecholamine-dependent (16,17). Furthermore, anti-ischemic effects both in the myocardium and other tissues may occur. These effects are cate-cholamine-mediated but perhaps also mediated through shifts in oxygen extraction curves, thrombocyte adhesiveness, rheology, and metabolism within the cell.

For how long should therapy last? This depends on the objectives. Symptomatic patients should naturally be treated for as long as therapy is accompanied by improvement. Asymptomatic patients without clinical findings, suggesting need of beta-blockade, should, in my opinion, be treated for as long as their risk for subsequent events is considered elevated. This implies continuous risk evaluation of the patients. Withdrawal of beta-blockade in patients with ischemic heart disease should be performed gradually, and the patients should be informed of rebound phenomena and observed for three weeks after withdrawal (18). What beta blockers should be used and what ancillary properties may be advocated? Those beta blockers showing a beneficial effect after acute myocardial infarction have been either selective or nonselective, thus indicating a common denominator in the beta$_1$-blockade. However, the selective beta blockers are not totally selective, and a beta$_2$ effect is probably achieved in the doses given. The common denominator for the studies is that adequate beta-blockade is achieved. Whether intrinsic sympathy activity (ISA) is beneficial or not is not solved; however, those studies in which beta blockers with a high level of ISA have been used have not shown a reduction in mortality. Thus, ISA does not seem to be an ancillary property that is especially wanted in this setting. Whether nonselective beta blockers using the beta$_2$-blockade and, thus, having an effect on potassium exchange, implies a better protection against VF is also not documented. Thus, in my opinion, when protection is considered, the target for therapy drugs where this has been shown should be used. These are in alphabetical order: metoprolol, propranolol, sotalol, and timolol. The doses used should be those given in the studies; however, individual titration to achieve adequate beta-blockade should be advocated.

REFERENCES

1. Norris, R. N., Barnaby, P. F., Brown, M. A., et al. (1984): Prevention of ventricular fibrillation during acute myocardial infarction by intravenous propranolol. *Lancet*, 2:883–886.
2. Herlitz, J., Elmfeldt, D., Hjalmarsson, A., et al. (1983): Effects of metoprolol on indirect signs of the size and severity of acute myocardial infarction. *Am. J. Cardiol.*, 51:1282–1288.
3. Rydén, L., Arniego, R., Arnman, K., et al. (1983): A double-blind trial of metoprolol in acute myocardial infarction: Effects of ventricular tachyarrhythmias. *N. Engl. J. Med.*, 308:614–618.
4. Hjalmarsson, A., et. al. (1985): The MIAMI Trial Research Group. Metoprolol in acute myocardial infarction (MIAMI). A randomized placebo-controlled international trial. *Eur. Heart J.*, 6:199–226.
5. The International Collaborative Study Group (1984): Reduction of infarct size with early use of timolol in acute myocardial infarction. *N. Engl. J. Med.*, 310:9–15.
6. Oyang, P., Brinker, J. A., Mellitz, E. D., et al. (1984): Variables predictive of successful medical therapy in patients with unstable angina: Selection by a multivariate analysis from clinical, electrocardiographic, and angiographic evaluations. *Circulation*, 70:367–376.
7. Telford, A. M., and Wilson, C. (1981): Trial of heparin versus atenolol in prevention of myocardial infarction in intermediate coronary syndrome. *Lancet*, 8232:1225–1228.

8. Muller J. E., Turi, Z. G., Pearle, D. L., et al. (1984): Nifedipine and conventional therapy for unstable angina pectoris: A randomized, double-blind comparison. *Circulation,* 69:728–739.
9. Tadani, U. (1984): Assessment of "optimal" beta-blockade in treating patients with angina pectoris. *Acta Med. Scand. (Suppl),* 694:178–187.
10. Kenny, J., Keath, P., Holmes, J., and Jewitt, D. E. (1985): Beneficial effects of diltiazem and propranolol, alone and in combination, in patients with stable angina pectoris. *Br. Heart J.,* 53:43–46.
11. Upford, J. V., Achras, F., and Jackson, G. (1985): Oral labetalol in management of stable angina pectoris in normotensive patients. *Br. Heart J.,* 53:53–57.
12. Bae, E., Arstila, M., Herkinen, R., et al. (1985): The comparison of the efficacy and tolerability of metoprolol, nifedipine and the combination in effort angina pectoris. Presented at the Davos conference on angina pectoris on myocardial infarction.
13. Tollins, M., Kjessler, E., and Pierpont, G. L. (1984): Maximal "drug therapy" is not necessary optimal in chronic angina pectoris. *J. Am. Coll. Cardiol.,* 3:1051–1057.
14. May, G. S., Eberling, K. A., Furberg, C. D., et al. (1982): Secondary prevention after myocardial infarction: A review of long-term trials. *Prog. Cardiovasc. Dis.,* 24:331–351.
15. Olsson, G., Rehnqvist, N., Sjögren, A., Erhardt, L., and Lundman, T. (1985): Long-term treatment with metoprolol after acute myocardial infarction. Effect on three-year mortality and morbidity. *J. Am. Coll. Cardiol.,* 6:1428–1437.
16. Olsson, G., and Rehnqvist, N. (1984): Ventricular arrhythmias during the first year after acute myocardial infarction: Influence of long-term treatment with metoprolol. *Circulation,* 69:1129–1134.
17. Lidell, C., Rehnqvist, N., Sjögren, A., Yli-Uotila, R. J., and Rønnevik, P. K. (1985): A comparative efficacy of oral sotalol and procainamide in patients with chronic ventricular arrhythmias. *Am. Heart J.,* 109:970.
18. Olsson, G., Hjemdahl, P., and Rehnqvist, N. (1984): Rebound phenomena following gradual withdrawal of chronic metoprolol treatment in patients with ischemic heart disease. *Am. Heart J.,* 108:454–462.

Hammersmith Cardiology Workshop Series, Vol. 3,
edited by A. Maseri, B. E. Sobel, and S. Chierchia.
Raven Press, New York © 1987.

Calcium Antagonists and Their Combination with Nitrates and Beta-Blocking Agents in the Treatment of Ischemic Heart Disease

Paul R. Lichtlen

Division of Cardiology, Hannover Medical School, LD-3000 Hannover, Federal Republic of Germany

Today, calcium antagonists are accepted as the third pillar in the medical treatment of ischemic heart disease, especially angina pectoris (1–8). Their mode of action, the way they reduce or inhibit ischemia, is well-known today (1,2,9–11). However, some of their effects, e.g., cardioprotection during ischemia or acute myocardial infarction, were mainly demonstrated in animal experiments (12,13) and still lack final proof in man. Calcium antagonists are drugs which, due to their inhibitory effect on the transmembraneous calcium influx across the potential operated calcium channel of vascular smooth muscle cells, primarily lead to relaxation of vascular smooth muscle tone and, by this, to arterial dilatation (2,14,15). This action is observed not only in arteries of all peripheral vascular beds (e.g., cerebral, visceral bed), but even more so in coronary arteries.

All clinically used Ca antagonists (verapamil, nifedipine, diltiazem) were shown to dilate both coronary arterioles as well as large epicardial coronary arteries and, by this, to increase regional myocardial blood flow in the poststenotic ischemic area (2,9,11,16). This occurs in the presence of a considerable decrease of myocardial oxygen consumption following the reduction in afterload (1). This behavior of regional myocardial blood flow is completely different from the one observed with nitrates (17) or beta-blocking agents (11), where regional myocardial blood flow in the ischemic region shows an autoregulatory decrease following the drop in myocardial oxygen consumption. Obviously, Ca antagonists, by dilating coronary arterioles, to a certain extent block autoregulation. However, this blockade is incomplete and, under the clinically used doses, leads only to an approximately 20% increase of resting flow (9,11,18). This is in contrast to dipyridamole where, even under small doses, resting flow was observed to increase to the maximum of coronary reserve so that during increased oxygen demand, induced by exercise or rapid atrial pacing, coronary flow showed no further increase (3). Under all three Ca antagonists clinically used, regional myocardial blood flow was found to increase further when oxygen demand was raised by exercise or rapid atrial pacing (9,11). This might explain why a steal phenomenon—defined as new appearance of angina pectoris due to a decrease of coronary flow in the poststenotic region in presence of an increase of coronary flow in the normal area—was never observed by us with Ca antagonists, in contrast to dipyridamole.

In addition to arteriolar dilatation, Ca antagonists were also found to dilate considerably eccentric coronary obstructions (15,19–21). This type of obstruction was found to retain a considerable amount of normal wall segments with intact smooth muscle cells (22) still able to dilate or constrict, i.e., to increase the degree of obstruction up to occlusion (coronary spasm) in a short interval (23). Hence, the anti-ischemic action of Ca antagonists can be attributed both to small as well as large coronary artery dilatation in the poststenotic area; this increase in oxygen delivery is supported by the decrease in wall tension, i.e., oxygen demand.

Besides the influence on smooth muscle tone, Ca antagonists, in animal experiments, proved to have a profound cardioprotective effect (12,13), and in man, to reduce myocardial contraction when administered directly into the coronary system (1,24). In animals, when given before induction of myocardial infarction, they are able to limit the infarct size (25), and when administered shortly after coronary artery ligation, they are able to prevent myocardial damage induced by Ca overload of ischemic myocardium (12,26); especially, mitochondrial function, ATP-production, and, by this, left ventricular contractility are preserved (12). In man, this clinically important effect of Ca antagonists is, however, difficult to measure and pertaining studies, so far, remain equivocal (27). This, however, does not exclude a considerable biological effect in man; improvement in techniques as well as the shortening of the often long interval between beginning of an infarct and subsequent treatment might eventually be conclusive with regard to infarct size limitation.

Ca ANTAGONISTS AND NITRATES

The combination of Ca antagonists with nitrates and beta blockers has been studied extensively during the past years. The combination with nitrates, at first glance, seems an unnecessary one as the primary effect of both drugs is smooth muscle relaxation. However, as shown on Table 1, nitrates mainly relax venous tone and reduce preload already in very low doses, whereas Ca antagonists primarily relax arterial smooth muscle tone. In addition, they act by different mechanisms; Ca antagonists reduce smooth muscle tone by inhibition of the transsarcolemmal Ca influx through the potential-operated channel (28,29). Nitrates, in contrast, act within the cell (30); they are transformed to nitrosoxide, which reacts with certain thiols to form nitrosothiol, which is the final activator of guanylate cyclase, necessary to transform GTP to cyclic GMP. The way the latter leads to smooth muscle relaxation is still debated (30). Table 1 summarizes the expected changes observed under the combined administration of Ca antagonists and nitrates; most of these effects were verified in man; some are still speculative and not substantiated by reliable studies. No studies on coronary blood flow so far are available in

TABLE 1. *Comparison of the hemodynamic effects of nitrates and Ca entry blockers alone and in combination*

	NITRATES	Ca-BLOCKERS	COMBINATION
PRELOAD	↓	—	↓
AFTERLOAD/ RESISTANCE	(↓) =	↓↓	↓↓
BLOOD PRESSURE	↓	↓↓	↓↓↓
HEART RATE	↑ =	↑ = ↓	↑↑ = ?
CARDIAC OUTPUT	↓	↑↑	↑ - ?
DEGREE OF OBSTRUCTION	↓	↓↓	↓↓↓
CORONARY FLOW	↓	↑	(↑) ?
MVO_2	↓	↓	↓↓
O_2-DEL/MVO_2	↑	↑	↑↑
ANGINA - REST	↑	↑↑	↑↑↑
- EXERCISE	↑	↑	↑↑ ?

Most of these data are based on the literature or our own experience; for some of them, special studies and clinical experience are still lacking.

man and, therefore, no comment on the behavior of coronary arteriolar tone is possible. This, however, is important, as nitrates in clinical doses are not increasing coronary blood flow and do not relax coronary resistance vessels, in contrast to Ca antagonists. In general, their combination, however, has a synergistic effect with regard to both afterload and blood pressure. Heart rate will increase depending on the Ca antagonists used. Dihydropyridines, especially nifedipine, show a marked reflex increase in heart rate after a drop in blood pressure in contrast to verapamil and diltiazem; it can therefore be expected that under these two drugs, both reducing sinus- and AV-nodal conduction, heart rate will remain unchanged or even decrease mildly.

Cardiac output decreases under nitrates due to the drop in preload, that is, venous return, and increases with Ca antagonists due to the peripheral arteriolar dilatation. It is probable that this effect of Ca antagonists will prevail and cardiac output will stay unchanged or even increase. Although the behavior of regional myocardial blood flow under the combination is still unknown, it is very probable that the relation between oxygen delivery and oxygen consumption is improved in excess and, that in general, the effect on ischemia will be a favorable one. This results from the fact that due to the decrease both in pre- and afterload myocardial oxygen consumption is reduced, whereas oxygen delivery most probably is mildly increased due to persisting arteriolar relaxation and the considerable dilatation of the large epicardial coronary arteries and eccentric obstructions. In addition, eccentric obstructions show a significant dilatation, often by more than 50% (2,15,19) and, in doing so, the combination often brings eccentric obstructions out of the critical range, i.e., renders them clinically asymptomatic. This coronary dilatory effect is much greater under the combination than when Ca antagonists or nitrates are administered alone (15). The combination will be favorable especially in Prinzmetal's variant form of angina pectoris, where today the combination represents the choice of treatment. In stable angina pectoris, the combined adminis- tration will allow the reduction of nitrate dose and, by this, decrease the tendency toward nitrate tolerance (30). In summary, the combined treatment with "coronary dilators" such as Ca antagonists and nitrates is especially recommended if vasospas- tic angina, ischemia due to a transient increase in vasomotor tone superimposed on high-grade eccentric obstructions, is present. However, a number of consider- ations also speak for a more liberal use in stable angina pectoris.

Ca ANTAGONISTS AND BETA BLOCKERS

The combination of beta blockers with Ca antagonists is far more used but also far more controversial. In contrast to a number of clinical studies demonstrating an improvement of angina pectoris, especially of stable angina (4,6,8,31,32), in combining beta blockers with nifedipine or verapamil (33–39), only a few studies on hemodynamics (33) or on the behavior of coronary blood flow exist (10). Therefore, the exact mechanism of the further improvement of angina pectoris under this combination is still at variance (35,40). From our own studies analyzing the effect of nifedipine on regional myocardial blood flow during rapid atrial pacing up to ischemia and angina pectoris (9,11), it appears that propranolol, in clinical doses, counteracts the vasorelaxing effect of the Ca antagonist (10,16). The increased coronary blood flow either decreased when the beta blocker was added or the beta blocker prevented the flow increase when the Ca antagonist was added. This observation is of considerable clinical importance and needs further explanation: in vascular smooth muscle cells, including the coronary arteries, calcium influx across the cell membrane is regulated by at least two channels, the potential- operated and the receptor-operated channel (Fig. 1), the latter depending on beta- and alphasympathetic stimulation. Beta stimulation, unlike in heart muscle where

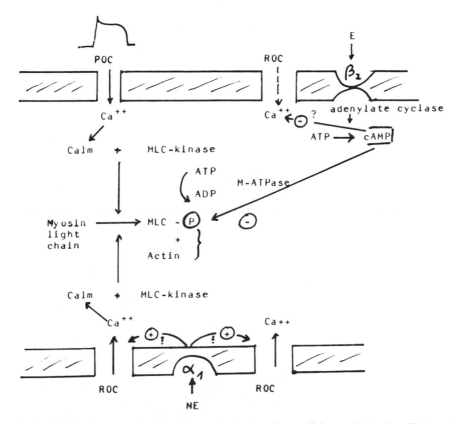

FIG. 1. Effects of various Ca channels on smooth muscle contraction and relaxation. Biochemical reaction leading to contraction and relaxation. POC, potential-operated channel; ROC, receptor-operated channel; Calm, calmoduline; E, epinephrine; NE, norepinephrine.

it leads to contraction, in vascular smooth muscle leads to relaxation, that is, to vasodilatation; today, it is believed that this effect is also mediated by cyclic AMP which, in smooth muscle cells, inhibits phosphorylation of the myosin light chain and by this leads to vasodilatation.

In contrast, postsynaptic alpha-1 and alpha-2 stimulation through norepinephrine opens, in some—up to now—unknown way, the receptor-operated channel and increases the Ca influx and, by this, the level of cytosolic calcium, which then, after binding to calmodulin through activation of the myosin light chain-kinase, leads to phosphorylation of the myosin light chain and to vasoconstriction. On the other hand, circulating norepinephrine and especially epinephrine lead to vasodilatation by stimulating beta-2 receptors, an effect which is completely inhibited by administration of beta-blocking agents (41). Calcium entering through the potential-operated channel, probably also depending on neurogenic stimuli (42), plays an additional important role with regard to phasic contraction of vascular smooth muscles; otherwise, Ca antagonists, acting mainly on the potential-operated channel,

DRUG	POC VC	ROC-β_2 VD	ROC-α_1 VC	VASOMOTION VC	VD
NO DRUG	+	+ +	+	↑	↑
Ca-ANT-AGONIST	∅	+ + (+)	+ (+)	↑	⇑
Ca-ANT-AGONIST + β-BLOCKER	∅	∅	+	↑	−

POC = POTENTIAL-OPERATED CHANNEL, ROC = RECEPTOR OPERATED
CHANNEL, VC = VASOCONSTRICTION, VD = VASODILATION

FIG. 2. Behavior of vasomotion of coronary arteries, depending on the various Ca channels.

would not have such a powerful inhibitory effect on smooth muscle contraction resulting in profound coronary arterial vasodilatation. This vasodilatory effect is either the result of unopposed overwhelming beta-2 tone, not suppressed by increased alpha-1 sympathetic tone, or it results from the lack of phasic and tonic Ca-mediated smooth muscle contraction and represents the basal smooth muscle tone. At any rate, if an increase in alpha-1 sympathetic tone occurs, it is balanced by beta stimulation which obviously is stronger than the alpha-1 effect and indirectly supports the action of the calcium-entry blocker (Fig. 2).

However, if in addition to calcium-entry-blockade also beta-blockade is applied, vasodilatation cannot be maintained any longer; in the absence of the beta-receptor-mediated inhibitory effect on phosphorylation of the myosin light chain after beta-blockade, smooth muscle contraction is the only reaction left, and this depends solely on alpha-receptor stimulation. Hence, the blocked calcium influx after administration of a Ca antagonist is then easily compensated by increased alpha-1 sympathetic tone, leading to calcium influx through the still functioning receptor-operated alpha-channel. This makes it very likely that already mild alpha-1 or alpha-2 stimulation through norepinephrine or other alpha-mediated stimuli (histamin, serotonin) lead to severe coronary constriction (spasm) and a decrease of coronary blood flow, in spite of the presence of Ca antagonists, as it was observed in our own flow measurements (10).

What this means for the treatment of angina pectoris has not yet become quite clear. Most of the studies combining beta blockers and Ca antagonists, so far, in

TABLE 2. *Comparison of the hemodynamic effects of Ca antagonists alone and in combination with beta blocking agents*

	CaA	BBL	CaA + BBL
MYOCARDIAL O$_2$-SUPPLY			
CORONARY FLOW	↑	↓	↓
CORONARY TONE - ARTERIOLES	↓	↑	↑
EPICARDIAL ARTERIES	↓	?	?
ECC. OBSTRUCTIONS	↓	?	?
MYOCARDIAL O$_2$-CONSUMPTION			
HEART RATE	↑ = ↓	↓	↓
CONTRACTILITY	↑ (↓)	↓	↓
WALL TENSION	↓	↓	↓↓
AFTERLOAD, BLOOD PRESSURE	↓	↓	↓↓
PRELOAD	= ↓	↑	↑=
CARDIAC OUTPUT	↑	↓	= (↑)
AV NODAL CONDUCTION	= ↓	↓	↓↓

Most of these effects were analyzed clinically.

spite of a reduction of coronary blood flow, by and large demonstrate a considerable improvement in exercise performance both with regard to time up to ST-depression as well as to total workload (37,39); this was demonstrated by a number of studies analyzing the percent increase in exercise performance during combination of calcium channel blockers [verapamil (37,38), nifedipine (8), and diltiazem (43)] with a beta blocker. These studies clearly demonstrated the highest improvement when the combination was compared with placebo and a somewhat smaller increase when compared with the beta blocker or the Ca antagonist alone. Nevertheless, although clinically this combination seems to work satisfactorily, a word of caution is appropriate (Table 2): obviously under the combination, blood pressure is further decreased due to the reduction in cardiac output, and this could become critical in patients with a low perfusion pressure and high proximal coronary resistance, e.g., in the presence of a critical left main coronary obstruction.

Furthermore, vasoconstriction under the combination prevails, maybe even more so than with the beta blocker alone; coronary vasomotor tone is increased, coronary flow is decreased, and the diameter of the critical eccentric obstruction is probably further reduced. This, however, is speculation, as so far no data are available on the effect of the combined administration of beta blockers and Ca antagonists on vasomotor tone of large epicardial arteries and, especially, on eccentric obstructions. Nevertheless, anecdotal observations from our and other laboratories in a number of cases, especially in patients with variant angina pectoris, but also in some patients with angina at rest and during exercise, indicate a marked increase in the number of anginal attacks at rest and even signs of coronary spasm when beta blockers were added to Ca antagonists (10,16). Finally, contractility is decreased, especially when combining verapamil with a beta blocker, and this could lead to latent or overt heart failure. On the other hand, myocardial oxygen consumption is further and substantially reduced, which is beneficial, of course, for the ischemic patient.

SUMMARY

The combination of Ca antagonists with nitrates seems to have very few "negative" effects: The decrease in perfusion pressure has to be observed very closely, especially in patients at the limit of their coronary reserve. The combination with beta blockers seems, however, more controversial, as vasoconstriction might prevail and even lead to coronary spasm and, in addition, blood pressure might also drop considerably. In addition, those Ca antagonists influencing AV-nodal conduction should be used with great care, as conduction defects might occur or be enhanced.

There is no doubt that Ca antagonists added new dimensions to the treatment of both stable and unstable angina pectoris, especially when increased coronary vasomotor tone prevails. The combination of Ca antagonists with either beta blockers or nitrates is possible and, in many patients, beneficial; however, one has to proceed with care and, therefore, fixed combinations should not be used.

REFERENCES

1. Simon, R. (1984): Calcium-antagonists: Effect of systemic and coronary hemodynamics. Z. Kardiol. (Suppl. 2), 73:79–88.
2. Lichtlen, P. R., Engel, J. H., and Rafflenbeul, W. (1984): Calcium-entry-blockers, especially nifedipine in angina of effort: Possible mechanisms and clinical implications. In: Calcium-Antagonists and Cardiovascular Disease, edited by L. H. Opie, pp. 221–236. Raven Press, New York.
3. Lichtlen, P. R. (1975): Coronary and left ventricular dynamics under nifedipine in comparison to nitrates, beta-blocking agents, and dipyridamole. In: Second International Adalat Symposium: New Therapy of Ischemic Heart Disease, edited by W. Lochner, W. Braasch, and G. Koneberg, pp. 212–224. Springer, Berlin, Heidelberg, New York.
4. Julian, D. G. (1985): Comparisons and combinations in antianginal therapy. Eur. Heart J. (Suppl. A), 6:37–45.
5. De Ponti, C., Mauri, F., Ciliberto, G. R., and Carù, B. (1979): Comparative effects of nifedipine, verapamil, isosorbide dinitrate, and propranolol in exercise-induced angina pectoris. Eur. J. Cardiol., 10:47–58.
6. Livesley, B., Catley, P. F., Campbell, R. C., and Oram, S. (1973): Double-blind evaluation of verapamil, propranolol, and isosorbide dinitrate against a placebo in the treatment of angina pectoris. Br. Med. J., 1:375–378.
7. Bala Subramanian, V., Bowles, M. J., Khurmi, N. S., and Raftery, E. B. (1982): Comparative evaluation of 4 slow channel-blockers with propranolol in stable angina pectoris. Circulation (Suppl. II), 66:18.

8. Ekelund, L. G., and Oroe, L. (1979): Antianginal efficiency of nifedipine with and without a beta blocker, studied with exercise-test. A double-blind, randomized subacute study. *Clin. Cardiol.*, 2:203–211.

9. Daniel, W. G., Engel, H. J., and Lichtlen, P. R. (1984): Effects of Ca antagonists on regional myocardial blood flow. In: *Ca Antagonism. International Symposium on Calcium-Antagonism*, edited by U. Althaus, D. Burckhardt, and E. Vogt, pp. 152–162. Universimed Verlag, Frankfurt.

10. Daniel, W. G., Reil, G. H., Schober, O., Creutzig, H., and Lichtlen, P. R. (1986): Effects of combined nifedipine and beta-blocker treatment on regional myocardial blood flow in coronary patients. In: *Sixth International Adalat Symposium*, edited by P. R. Lichtlen, pp. 414–421. Excerpta Medica, Amsterdam.

11. Engel, J. H., and Lichtlen, P. R. (1981): Beneficial enhancement of coronary blood flow by nifedipine; comparison with nitroglycerin and beta-blocking agents. *Am. J. Med.*, 71:658–667.

12. Nayler, W. G. (1983): The role of calcium in myocardial ischemia and cell death. In: *Calcium-Channel-Blocking Agents in the Treatment of Cardiovascular Disorders*, edited by P. H. Stone and E. M. Antman, pp. 81–105. Futura Publishing Company, Mount Kisco, New York.

13. Clark, R. E., Christlieb, I. Y., Henry, P. D., Fischer, A. E., Nora, Y. D., Williamson, Y. R., and Sobel, B. E. (1979): Nifedipine, a myocardial protective agent. *Am. J. Cardiol.*, 44:825–831.

14. Simon, R., Amende, I., and Lichtlen, P. R. (1982): Differential effects of nifedipine and nitroglycerin on hemodynamics in single coronary arteries in man. *Circulation*, *(Suppl. II)*, 66:119.

15. Lichtlen, P. R., Rafflenbeul, W., (1985): Effects of calcium-antagonists on fixed and dynamic obstructions in patients with severe coronary artery disease. In: *Cardiovascular Effects of Dihydropyridine-Type Calcium-Antagonists and Agonists*, edited by A. Flechenstein, C. Van Breemen, R. Groβ, and F. Hoffmeister, pp. 381–407. Springer, Berlin, Heidelberg, New York.

16. Lichtlen, P. R., Daniel, W. G., and Engel, H. J. (1985): Effects of the calcium-entry-blocking agents nifedipine, verapamil and diltiazem on regional myocardial blood flow in patients with severe coronary artery disease (*in press*).

17. Lichtlen, P. R., Halter, J., and Gatticker, K. (1974): The effect of isosorbide dinitrate on coronary flow, coronary resistance and left ventricular dynamics under exercise in patients with coronary artery disease. *Basic Res. Cardiol.*, 69:402–420.

18. Bourassa, M. G., Coal, P., Theroux, P., Tubaut, J. F., Genain, C., and Waters, D. D. (1980): Hemodynamics and coronary flow following diltiazem administration in anesthetized dogs and in humans. *Chest*, 78:224.

19. Rafflenbeul, W., and Lichtlen, P. R. (1982): The concept of dynamic coronary artery stenoses. *Z. Kardiol.*, 71:439–442.

20. Conti, C. R., Hill, J. A., Feldmann, R. L., Conti, J. B., and Peppine, C. J. (1984): Comparison of nifedipine and nitrates: Clinical and angiographic studies. In: *Calcium-Antagonists and Cardiovascular Disease*, edited by L. H. Opie, pp. 269–275. Raven Press, New York.

21. Rafflenbeul, W. (1983): Dilatation of coronary artery stenoses with diltiazem i.v. In: *New Calcium-Antagonists, Recent Developments and Prospects*, edited by A. Fleckenstein, K. Hashimoto, M. Herrmann, H. Schwarz, and L. Seidel, p. 181. Gustav Fischer, Stuttgart.

22. Freudenberg, H., and Lichtlen, P. (1981): The normal wall segment in coronary stenoses: a postmortal study. *Z. Kardiol.*, 70:863.

23. Maseri, A., Severi, S., L'Abbate, A., and Pesola, A. (1977): Variant angina: One aspect of a continuous spectrum of vasospastic angina. *Circulation*, 55/56:III–33.

24. Amende, I., Simon, R., Hood, W. P., Hetzer, R., and Lichtlen, P. R. (1983): Intracoronary nifedipine in human beings: magnitude and time course of changes in left ventricular contraction/relaxation and coronary sinus blood flow. *J.A.C.C.*, 2:1141–1144.

25. Reimer, K. A., and Jennings, R. B. (1985): Effects of calcium-channel-blockers on myocardial preservation during experimental acute myocardial infarction. *Am. J. Cardiol.*, 55:107B–115B.

26. Nayler, W. G. (1981): The role of calcium in the ischemic myocardium. *Am. J. Pathol.*, 102:262–270.

27. Clark, R. E., Christlieb, I. Y., and Clark, B. K. (1986): Use of nifedipine in cardioplegic solution for high-risk patients. In: *Sixth International Adalat Symposium*, edited by P. R. Lichtlen, pp. 406–411. Excerpta Medica, Amsterdam.

28. Fleckenstein, A., Janke, J., Döring, H. J., and Leder, O. (1975): Key role of calcium in the production of non-coronarogenic myocardial necroses. In: *Pathophysiology and Morphology of Myocardial Cell Alterations, Vol. 6*, edited by A. Fleckenstein and G. Roner, pp. 21–32. University Park Press, Baltimore, London, Tokyo.

29. Fleckenstein, A. (1984): Calcium-antagonism: history and prospect for a multifaceted pharmacodynamic principle. In: *Calcium-Antagonist and Cardiovascular Disease,* edited by L. H. Opie, pp. 9–28. Raven Press, New York.
30. Kukovitz, W. R., and Holzmann, F. (1983): Mechanism of nitrate-induced vasodilation and tolerance. *Z. Kardiol. (Suppl. III),* 72:14–19.
31. Bassan, M., Weiler-Ravell, D., and Sharev, O. (1982): The additive antianginal action of oral nifedipine in patients receiving propranolol. Magnitude and duration of effect. *Circulation,* 66:710–716.
32. Krikler, D. M., Harris, L., and Rowland, E. (1982): Calcium-channel-blockers and beta-blockers: Advantages and disadvantages of combination therapy in chronic stable angina pectoris. *Am. Heart J.,* 104:702–708.
33. Findlay, I. N., and Dargie, J. H. (1983): The effects of nifedipine, atenolol, and that combination on left ventricular function. *Postgrad. Med. J. (Suppl. II),* 59:70–73.
34. De Ponti, C., De Biase, A. M., Pirelli, S., et al. (1981): Effects of nifedipine, acebutolol, and their association on exercise tolerance in patients with effort angina. *Cardiology (Suppl. II),* 68:195–199.
35. Dietz, A., Walter, J., Ebner, F., Schramm, A., and Wiese, K. H. (1979): Treatment of coronary heart disease with a combination of nifedipine and beta-blocker. *Herzkreislauf,* 11:243–248.
36. Winniford, M. D., Huxley, R. L., and Hillis, L. D. (1983): Randomized, double-blind comparison of propranolol alone and propranolol-verapamil combination in patients with severe angina of effort. *J.A.C.C.,* 1:492–498.
37. Leon, M. B., Rosing, D. R., Bonow, R. O., Lipson, L. C., and Epstein, S. E. (1981): Clinical efficacy of verapamil alone and combined with propranolol in treating patients with stable angina pectoris. *Am. J. Cardiol.,* 48:131–139.
38. Subramanian, B., Bowles, M. J., Davis, A. B., and Raftery, E. B. (1982): Combined therapy with verapamil and propranolol in chronic stable angina. *Am. J. Cardiol.,* 49:125–132.
39. Leon, M. B., Rosing, D. R., Bonow, R. O., and Epstein, S. E. (1985): Combination therapy with calcium channel blockers and beta-blockers for chronic stable angina pectoris. *Am. J. Cardiol.,* 55:69B–80B.
40. Epstein, S. E., Cannon, R. O., Watson, R. M., Leon, M. B., Bonow, R. O., and Rosing, D. R. (1985): Dynamic coronary obstruction as cause of angina pectoris. Implications regarding therapy. *Am. J. Cardiol.,* 55:61B–66B.
41. Robertson, R. M., Wood, A. J. J., Vaughn, W. K., and Robertson, D. (1982): Exacerbation of vasotonic angina pectoris by propranolol. *Circulation,* 65:281–285.
42. Hensch, G., and Deussen, A. (1983): The effects of cardiac sympathetic nerve stimulation on perfusion of stenotic coronary arteries. *Circ. Res.,* 53:8–15.
43. Hung, J., Lamb, I. H., Connally, S. J., Intzy, K. R., Gori, M. L., and Schroeder, J. S. (1983): The effect of diltiazem and propranolol alone and in combination on exercise performance and left ventricular function in patients with stable effort angina: a double-blind randomized placebo-controlled study. *Circulation,* 68:560–567.

Hammersmith Cardiology Workshop Series, Vol. 3,
edited by A. Maseri, B. E. Sobel, and S. Chierchia.
Raven Press, New York © 1987.

Précis of the Discussion: Section XV

MEDICAL TREATMENT OF ISCHEMIC HEART DISEASE

Lawson McDonald

Richard Conti, in discussing the choice of a beta blocker, said that he usually starts with propranolol and, if necessary, he goes on to something else. Remarking on Transiderm-Nitro (nitroglycerin), he thought it was an expensive placebo. He added that he did not delay long in giving beta blockers and calcium antagonists to patients who had not responded optimally to nitrates. Asked about intravenous isosorbide dinitrate in refractory pump failure, Dr. Conti thought that it seemed to be less well tolerated than intravenous nitroglycerin. Lawson McDonald asked Richard Conti about the place of mononitrates; Dr. Conti said that he had no experience with them. Paul Lichtlen thought that they had only a theoretical advantage, and he was not sure that these expensive drugs were needed. Dr. Lawson McDonald commented that some people had very early serious side effects to initial doses of beta blockers and felt extremely unwell; he asked if anyone knew the mechanism. No one did.

Dr. McDonald asked about beta blockers after cardiac infarction: Should they be given intravenously, acutely, and chronically for longer than 36 months? Nina Rehnqvist said that she would give intravenous beta blockers if the patient was seen after a short delay (6 to 8 hr), and in the long term would judge particularly on evidence of ischemia. If their risk of dying was judged as low, beta blockers would be withdrawn. Desmond Julian agreed that premature ventricular contractions did have prognostic significance, but not necessarily of therapeutic significance. Richard Conti asked Nina Rehnqvist about the dose of Transiderm-Nitro. It was an individual dose titration, and between 5 and 20 mg of nitroglycerin was given. Dr. Conti thought this important, and that a patch of 5 mg might not do anything.

Paul Lichtlen was asked how the severity of stenosis was quantified and if the poststenotic flow was measured. He replied that the obstructions were measured with the Vernier caliper, and that coronary blood flow was measured from the Xenon technique. Richard Conti shared Dr. Lichtlen's concern about the use of beta blockers in patients with heart failure, but mentioned the communications from Gothenburg regarding the use of beta blockers in acute myocardial infarction with heart failure. Dr. Lichtlen had found heart failure a problem, and mentioned that in the Gothenburg study they were used in a low dose and in patients with cardiomyopathy. In replying to a question on the existence or otherwise of the calcium antagonist withdrawal syndrome, Paul Lichtlen said that he had never seen a true case of it.

Lawson McDonald raised the question of bypass grafting improving prognosis in ischemic heart disease. Richard Conti thought that it did so in some subsets, as did Nina Rehnqvist, David Kelly, and Paul Lichtlen. Dr. Lichtlen commented that the European study showed that this was so not only for triple-vessel disease, but also for double-vessel disease as long as the left anterior descending artery was involved. Dr. Conti reiterated what Attilio Maseri had said, namely, that all double-vessel disease is not the same, nor was triple-vessel disease. He stressed the importance of finding out whether or not there was concomitant evidence of ischemia. Spencer King thought that with a very high-grade lesion of the anterior descending artery, angioplasty or grafting would show an improvement in five-year survival. Burton Sobel said that surgery should not be used as a single modality, but with regard to other treatment that was given after surgery.

Lawson McDonald then asked the contributors a hypothetical question regarding two 40-year-old twin men, one with an exercise test that was borderline positive in all respects, and the other in which it was unequivocally positive. They were asymptomatic. Richard Conti, after repeating the exercise test on drugs, advised proceeding to angiography in someone who continued to show a positive stress test. If it remained borderline, however, he would talk things over with the patient. Others agreed with this approach. Paul Lichtlen said that he would investigate both, as there were very few studies on identical twins with coronary artery disease! Spencer King said that he personally would like to be investigated if he had even a little ischemia. Desmond Julian thought that the question was very difficult, and said that he would like to have full information about the individual, and that to make a decision solely on the exercise test was wrong. Floyd Loop, however, advised going ahead to an outpatient arteriogram.

Asked about the routine use of long-term beta blockers after myocardial infarction, with no contraindications, Floyd Loop said that he would initiate beta blockade for a substantial myocardial infarction, but would not ordinarily use it intravenously except for the relief of pain. Burton Sobel believed that the use of beta blockade was the most underutilized major medical advance after myocardial infarction. Desmond Julian agreed that it was underutilized, but thought that there were low-risk subsets which constituted 40% to 50% of the postinfarct population who were free of symptoms with exercise, free of hypertension, and in whom the infarct was relatively small. He would avoid treating them and thought the incidence of subtle side effects with treatment was quite high. Paul Lichtlen said that there was a low-risk group not needing beta blockade, and a high-risk group needing an arteriogram after cardiac infarction. David Kelly thought that every patient should have a beta blocker after myocardial infarction until they had been investigated in some way or other. Nina Rehnqvist did not think that the low-risk percentage was as high as 50%. Richard Conti stressed that the question referred to the routine use of beta blockers; physicians should not recommend the routine use of anything. He took the position of David Kelly and Desmond Julian.

Asked whether there was any cutoff in male and female patients, David Kelly's opinion was that coronary artery disease should be treated more conservatively with age, but that age, particularly with surgery that did carry an increased risk, should not be a final contraindication. Burton Sobel agreed and pointed out that it was physiological age, and not chronological, which was important. Floyd Loop agreed.

Lawson McDonald asked to what extent potential cerebrovascular disease should be investigated in these patients. Floyd Loop had found that it was not the stenotic flow-limiting lesions that were the problem, but the friability of the aorta during cross-clamping. Lawson McDonald asked if he would examine for carotid stenosis, for example. Dr. Loop would do so in a symptomatic patient, and some with loud bruits were investigated noninvasively. But many of these, even if they have carotid lesions, have operation without anything being done for the carotid.

The discussion turned to management in pump failure, and what criteria should be used to establish the optimal dose of a beta blocker. Paul Lichtlen emphasized that the heart rate should decrease by about 10%; hemodynamic measurements might be useful but could be misleading. Richard Conti agreed with Dr. Lichtlen; in pump failure, he found blood pressure, filling pressure, and cardiac output on a beat-to-beat basis to be of value. In a difficult patient, he started with intravenous nitroglycerin. Desmond Julian noted the delay inherent with Holter monitoring and the expense; he did not think it worthwhile. He thought exercise testing vital, and that there was a lot to be said for the ejection fraction.

The contributors were asked to discuss the place of intravenous blockers in acute myocardial infarction. Burton Sobel thought their place was limited; those with substantial tachycardia, which was not due to incipient ventricular failure or a pericardial effusion, might benefit. Desmond Julian noted that very large studies had failed to show a significant benefit, but that they had shown beta blockade to be safe. In selected patients they were good for controlling arrhythmias, pain, and tachycardia in the absence of failure.

Henry Neufeld asked whether two calcium blockers together might be helpful. Paul Lichtlen preferred to increase one drug rather than to add another. Nina Rehnqvist thought it unwise to combine two calcium blockers. She added that calcium antagonists had not been shown to improve prognosis. Richard Conti was not happy about the use of two calcium-blocking drugs together. Paul Lichtlen added that sometimes very high doses were needed: up to 480 mg of nifedipine daily. Attilio Maseri stressed that sometimes patients got better anyway with the passage of time, and that it was not necessarily the last therapeutic measure that had caused improvement.

The question of warfarin as prophylaxis was raised. Lawson McDonald replied that this was an enormous question. No member of the panel was prepared to answer it quickly.

Editorial comment: A. Maseri

A rational treatment should be based on the understanding of the prevailing causes of episodes of myocardial ischemia in the individual patient and of their relationship to prognosis. However, since this information often is not clearly available, the improvement of signs and symptoms of ischemia during daily life and during stress test is the most important yardstick by which to judge the effects of treatment. It may be difficult to distinguish the beneficial effects of any treatment, from placebo effects and from spontaneous remission, unless appropriate controlled studies are performed: placebo effect is important, and short or long periods of remission are frequent, both in chronic stable and in unstable angina. However, for patients the goal of treatment is the improvement or remission of signs and symptoms of ischemia independent of the mechanisms through which it does occur. Thus, when an apparently rational treatment is not effective, it should be modified empirically until improvement is obtained. The guidelines for a rational first line of treatment directed to relieving ischemia should be indicated by the prevailing pathogenetic mechanisms of angina in the individual patient.

It may be reasonable to consider the treatment of signs and symptoms of ischemia as separate from that only directed to improve prognosis, on the assumption that the achievement of a satisfactory relief of ischemia during spontaneous daily life and during maximal stress test is likely to improve prognosis (no matter how it is achieved). Thus, the dilemma of treating patients only for improving prognosis remains confined to those with few or no signs and symptoms of ischemia.

Hammersmith Cardiology Workshop Series, Vol. 3,
edited by A. Maseri, B. E. Sobel, and S. Chierchia.
Raven Press, New York © 1987.

Determinants of Survival in Ischemic Heart Disease on Medical Treatment

Desmond G. Julian

*Department of Cardiology, University of Newcastle upon Tyne, Freeman Hospital,
Newcastle upon Tyne, NE7 7DN, England*

Prognostication has become a subject of major concern to the practicing cardiologist. This is not only because the patient and his associates need to be informed as fully as possible about what to expect in the future, but also because the choice of therapy—whether it be drugs or surgery—depends critically upon the prognostic subset into which the individual falls.

It is for this reason that so much attention has been devoted to this topic in recent years, but we still have an inadequate body of knowledge upon which to base our decisions. Time and again the designs of therapeutic trials have been based upon assumptions that have subsequently been proved false. Nowhere was this more obvious than in the Coronary Artery Surgery Study (CASS), in which the mortality in those with three-vessel coronary disease was much less than had been expected (1). Braunwald attributes the low mortality in CASS to what he believes to be improving natural history of coronary disease (2). He wrote (2), ". . . it is particularly interesting to consider the steadily improving survival rate among medically treated patients with angiographically confirmed three-vessel obstructive coronary artery disease . . . The annual mortality rate for such patients was 11.4% in the late 60s . . . 4.8% in the early and mid-1970s, 3.5% in the European Coronary Surgery Study and only 2.1% in the recently reported CASS Study.''

While this is an attractive concept, there are excellent reasons for questioning this explanation. Before reviewing what we know about prognosis, it is worthwhile to refer to a thoughtful article by Goldman, Mudge, and Cook (3) on the problems of comparing the natural history of ischemic heart disease at different points in time and in different populations. They point to three types of errors that may confuse the issue.

The first is lead-time (starting-time) bias. The error here arises because patients who are diagnosed earlier in their course obviously live longer from the time of diagnosis than those diagnosed later. A good example of this relates to the prognostic significance of coronary arteriographic findings. In the 1960s, this investigation was usually undertaken only on patients who had had disabling symptoms over a long period. Now, particularly in the United States, it is performed as soon as possible after the diagnosis is suspected. This will inevitably affect the predictive value of the findings.

The second error is referral (transition) bias. The reasons for referral to a cardiologist change from time to time. Thus, when a new test or therapy becomes available only the sickest are sent. If the test or therapy appears efficacious, patients who have an inherently better prognosis are referred. Thus, when coronary care units were first opened, a disproportionately large number of patients with shock or heart failure were admitted; subsequently, much milder cases were referred, with an inevitable apparent reduction in mortality.

The prevalence-incidence (length) bias is the third type of error. Incidence studies include all patients who are observed to develop the condition being studied, and an accurate knowledge of their survival is obtained whether this be short or long. Prevalence studies concern the number of individuals with the specific condition in the community at a particular time. Prevalence, then, depends on both incidence and the distribution of survival times. Such studies are likely to include a greater proportion of cases with longer survival times. The natural history will then appear to be better than it actually is.

CHANGING DIAGNOSTIC METHODS

In addition to the three forms of bias enumerated by Goldman, Mudge, and Cook, I would like to add another: that resulting from changing diagnostic methods. In the case of myocardial infarction, methods of diagnosis have been changing progressively but almost imperceptibly over the years. This is particularly obvious in the case of enzyme studies. They have been in use for about 25 years, but during that time the number of tests used and their sensitivity and specificity have been changing continuously. Even if we use what is an apparently standardized definition, e.g., a rise to twice the upper normal level, this will be achieved more often if more frequent samples are taken, as the peak enzyme level is more likely to be recorded. Milder cases with a lower total enzyme release will thus be included as "definite" infarction, thereby lowering "mortality" by introducing a lower risk group of cases. This factor has undoubtedly contributed to the apparent fall in mortality in coronary care units.

MAJOR DETERMINANTS OF PROGNOSIS
IN ISCHEMIC HEART DISEASE

There can be no question that the major determinants of prognosis include the severity of fixed coronary arterial narrowings and the amount of myocardium that is potentially ischemic or actually infarcted. Most of the noninvasive indicators of prognosis that have been identified are related in one way or another to the extent of coronary stenoses or left ventricular function. Nonetheless, it is apparent that there are other important variables that have no direct relationship, such as age, diabetes, hypertension, and smoking habit. Furthermore, prognosis is critically dependent upon clinical context. Thus, patients with similar coronary anatomy may have completely different prognoses depending on whether they are suffering from stable angina, unstable angina, myocardial infarction—or sudden death!

NONINVASIVE INDICATORS OF PROGNOSIS

Although the information provided by coronary arteriography is unique, to obtain it is expensive and uncomfortable. Furthermore, it cannot be frequently repeated and it may be misleading. Thus, far too much has been inferred from the finding of "three-vessel disease" and, as a consequence, many patients have been mindlessly consigned to surgery. We, therefore, need other simple and cheap indicators of prognosis. I would like to focus on some of the most simple.

Symptoms

Although symptoms may be very misleading, these should not be ignored in regard to prognosis. Thus, in stable ischemic heart disease, Cohn et al. (4) have shown that when patients are matched for coronary anatomy and left ventricular function, those with significant symptoms fare worse than those without. In unstable angina, though the severity and duration of symptoms may not be a useful guide, the failure of symptoms to respond to treatment is ominous (5).

In myocardial infarction surprisingly little attention has been devoted to analyzing the severity and duration of pain and its consequences. One's clinical impression, however, is that the failure of severe pain to respond to analgesics is associated with extension of infarction and with shock.

Blood Pressure

In stable angina, hypertension is an important complicating factor, mortality being at least twice as high in those with raised pressure as in those without (6) (Table 1). In the context of myocardial infarction, both low systolic pressure (<100 mm Hg) and high pressure (>180 mm Hg) have been associated with increased mortality, particularly the former (7).

Normal ECG

Cardiologists feel that one of the important messages that they can convey to general practitioners is the uselessness of the resting ECG in the diagnosis in

TABLE 1. *Mortality in men with stable angina*[a]

	No.	Cardiac death
ECG abnormal		
BP+	30	29.8%
BP normal	68	11.8%
ECG normal		
BP+	43	6.2%
BP normal	134	1.6%

[a] Death, <30/12 of baseline (HIP study). (From ref. 6.)

angina. Although this is largely valid, the ECG is an invaluable clue to prognosis. It is intriguing to note that the gradient in prognosis between the patient with a normal ECG and normal blood pressure (6) and the patient with both features abnormal is at least as great as that between one vessel and left main disease demonstrated by coronary arteriography.

In unstable angina, a strictly normal ECG during the attacks of pain casts doubt on the diagnosis, but the nature of ECG changes when they occur is important. Thus, changes in the anteroseptal leads and profound ST depression, particularly if they do not return quickly to normal, are adverse prognostic features. In myocardial infarction, a normal ECG on presentation is an encouraging finding as it is likely that the extent of damage will be relatively slight and the risks of complications low (7).

Stress ECG

There is now an enormous literature on the prognostic value of the stress ECG both in angina and in myocardial infarction. Some of the evidence is conflicting; this probably relates to the differing selection of patients recruited and to the different protocols used. Nonetheless, it is clear in anginal patients that exercise-induced signs of ischemia relate importantly to prognosis.

A study by Bonow et al. (8) showed that exercise-induced ECG changes and a fall in ejection fraction separated patients with three-vessel disease into two groups with very differing prognoses. In the European Coronary Surgery Study (9) the beneficial effects of surgery appeared to be confined to those who had a positive exercise test.

The prognostic value of the exercise test in those who have survived myocardial infarction is still the subject of much study and dispute. Certainly, the appearance of ST changes at a low work load predicts angina in the forthcoming months, but how good a predictor of mortality it is, is less clear. Some like Theroux et al. (10) have found a strong correlation, whereas others have failed to find such a relationship, noting rather that the inability to complete a limited test, or a poor hemodynamic response to it, is indicative of a high complication rate.

CONCLUSION

The ability to define meaningful prognostic subsets has become an important component of cardiological practice. Although coronary arteriography supplies unique information, this investigation is often not necessary if the significance of noninvasive observations is appreciated.

REFERENCES

1. CASS Principal Investigators and Their Associates. Coronary Artery Surgery Study (CASS) (1983): A randomized trial of coronary artery bypass surgery. Survival data. *Circulation,* 68:951–960.
2. Braunwald, E. (1983): Effects of coronary artery bypass grafting on survival: implications of the Coronary Artery Surgery Study. *N. Engl. J. Med.,* 309:1181–1184.
3. Goldman, L., Mudge, G. H., Jr., and Cook, F. E. (1983): The changing "natural history" of symptomatic coronary artery disease: basis versus bias. *Am. J. Cardiol.,* 51:449–454.
4. Cohn, P. F., Harris, P., Barry, W. H., Rosati, R. A., Rosenbaum, P., and Waternaux, C. (1981): Prognostic importance of anginal symptoms in angiographically defined coronary artery disease. *Am. J. Cardiol.,* 47:233–237.
5. Gazes, P. C., Mobley, E. M., Faris, H. M., Duncan, R. C., and Humphries, G. B. (1973): Pre-infarctional (unstable) angina—a prospective study—ten year follow-up. *Circulation,* 48:331–337.
6. Weinblatt, E., Frank, C. W., Shapiro, S., and Sager, R. V. (1968): Prognostic factors in angina pectoris—a prospective study. *J. Chronic. Dis.,* 21:231–245.
7. Brush, J. E., Brand, D. A., Acampora, D., Chalmer, B., and Wackers, F. J. (1985): Use of the initial electrocardiogram to predict in-hospital complications of acute myocardial infarction. *N. Engl. J. Med.,* 312:1137–1141.
8. Bonow, R. O., Kent, K. M., Rosing, D. R., et al. (1984): Exercise induced ischemia in mildly symptomatic patients with coronary artery disease and preserved left ventricular function. *N. Engl. J. Med.,* 311:1339–1345.
9. European Coronary Surgery Study Group. (1982): Long-term results of prospective randomized study of coronary artery bypass surgery in stable angina pectoris. *Lancet,* ii:1173–1180.
10. Theroux, P., Waters, D. D., Halpen, C., Debaisieux, J. C., and Mizgala, H. F. (1979): Prognostic value of exercise testing soon after myocardial infarction. *N. Engl. J. Med.,* 301:341–345.

Hammersmith Cardiology Workshop Series, Vol. 3,
edited by A. Maseri, B. E. Sobel, and S. Chierchia.
Raven Press, New York © 1987.

When Can Coronary Surgery Help Survival?

Celia M. Oakley

Division of Cardiovascular Diseases, Royal Postgraduate Medical School,
Hammersmith Hospital, London W12 OHS, England

Coronary bypass surgery relieves angina by improving the blood supply to heart muscle territories which had been ischemic. Medical treatment reduces angina by increasing the efficiency of the heart but is much less effective than surgery in relieving symptoms and, in general, it does little to improve the defective blood supply.

That surgery relieves angina by correcting ischemia has been shown by comparing the effects of exercise testing on ST segment depression and thallium distribution before and after surgery as well as studies of segmental left ventricular function on exercise shown on nuclear blood pool images pre- and postoperatively. After surgery, evidence of ischemia can frequently no longer be elicited by any test. Medical treatment for ischemia rarely removes all evidence of it, and this is why it is also less effective than surgery in relieving angina.

It has not been possible for ethical reasons to conduct trials in which medical treatment of angina has been compared with no treatment. Patients recovering from myocardial infarction are often symptom-free but have been recognized to have coronary heart disease by the fact of the infarct, and the beta adrenergic blocking group of drugs has been shown in randomized trials to improve the prognosis in the first year following the episode. These drugs are effective in preventing ischemia-provoked arrhythmias (ventricular fibrillation [VF]) in experimental animals, and it is likely that their beneficial effect in the year after infarction is due to prevention of ischemia-provoked VF. Many patients would do well without any treatment, and it is likely that the subgroup of patients whose prognosis is improved by beta-blocking drugs after infarction are the same patients whose prognosis might have been even more improved by coronary bypass surgery or by angioplasty after infarction. This group of patients of seemingly good, but actually uncertain, prognosis may be recognized by exercise testing and coronary angiography.

Painless ischemia is common in coronary heart disease and is well demonstrated by exercise testing and ambulant ECG monitoring when ST segment depression may not be accompanied by pain. There is no evidence that painless ischemia confers a better prognosis than painful ischemia, and it has been shown in several studies that myocardial infarction, when painless, carries the same mortality and incidence of complications as typical infarction. Moreover, patients who have survived painless infarction have an increased incidence of painless ischemia. People with a "defective early warning system," as this has been called, are unlikely to be detected simply because they have no symptoms or atypical symptoms, but they presumably comprise the 25% of patients whose sudden deaths from VF appear to have been the first symptoms of coronary disease. No fewer than 50% of patients having their first infarct have suffered the infarct as the first symptom of their disease or following only a day or two of new and escalating angina. There is no evidence that the pathology of their infarcts differs from that of patients who have had previous stable angina, and it seems likely that previous ischemia caused by atheromatous narrowing preceded the infarct but never passed a high pain threshold.

SURGERY VERSUS MEDICAL TREATMENT

The effects of surgery on the survival of patients whose symptoms do not, of themselves, demand surgical relief are particularly difficult to evaluate. A method that is popular in the United States is to compare the survival curve of operated groups with the expected survival of a "normal" age and sex matched population, but to my knowledge no one has stratified the survival curve according to whether symptoms were present or absent before operation. A more difficult but probably better way to look at survival is by means of multicenter, randomized prospective clinical trials in which the effects of medical treatment only are compared with the effects of medical treatment plus surgery in various defined subsets of patients with coronary artery disease. The three big trials that have been carried out, the Veterans Administration (VA) study, the European study (ECSS), and the American study (CASS), differed in many ways, and the conflict between the results of the two most recent and best studies (ECSS and CASS) has caused much argument.

The ECSS showed an improvement in prognosis of the surgical patients as a whole compared with the medical group whereas CASS did not. The ECSS showed an advantage to surgically treated patients with three-vessel coronary artery disease over the five to eight years of follow-up as well as to patients with two-vessel disease, as long as it involved the proximal third of the anterior descending branch of the left coronary artery. CASS showed no statistically significant advantage in any subset. The VA trial had shown improvement in survival in patients with left main stem disease such that these patients were omitted from the CASS. The ECSS allowed inclusion of left main stem disease, but no patients with very severe left main stem stenosis were, in fact, included. All of those who were randomized had between 50% and 75% narrowing and did not start to die for the first two or three years (presumably the time it took for the stenosis to become critical), so that differences between medical and surgical treatment for left main stem disease were not statistically significant even though an escalating death rate was seen in the medically treated patients beginning only after the first two or three years.

The wide disparity between the results of the ECSS and CASS must be explained. The total number of patients randomized was about the same, and the patients as described were comparable; the surgical mortality was slightly higher in the ECSS and, therefore, militated against the success of surgical treatment in the ECSS, but the eventual mortality in the surgically treated patients was low and similar in both the ECSS and the CASS. The difference between the trials lies in the much higher mortality of the medically treated patients in the ECSS. In the CASS, the medical mortality was so very low that there was no way that surgical treatment could show an advantage. This lower mortality of the medical patients in the CASS compared with the ECSS cannot be explained by better medical treatment in CASS because, in fact, only 43% of the CASS patients were on beta blockers compared with 75% of the ECSS patients. The higher medical mortality of the ECSS patients indicated that they had more advanced disease and were a high-risk group. The medical mortality on the CASS registry was much higher than in the randomized patients and, indeed, similar to that in ECSS—83% over five years. The randomized patients in CASS, therefore, represented milder disease and a better prognosis group. The explanation for this is that patients with possible angina have coronary angiography very much earlier than do patients in Europe and than patients did at the time of the VA study in the United States. The European patients had, therefore, already "used up" much of their prognosis by the time they come to be randomized.

This change in referral practice as well as the beneficial effects of medical treatment would together account for the improvement in the medical prognosis seen since the 1960s, when the annual mortality of "three-vessel coronary artery disease" was between 11.4% and 15%. In the 1970s, the VA trial showed an annual mortality of three-vessel disease of only 4.8%. By the time of the ECSS, the mortality was 3.5% and in the CASS it had become only 2.1%. When coronary angiography began at the Cleveland Clinic only patients with long-standing crippling angina were referred. By the time of the CASS, the major centers in the United States investigated anyone with suspected coronary disease. None of the trials included exercise testing with blood pressure measurement in the protocols, and it is now acknowledged that observations on the extent of ischemia plus the coronary angiographic appearance together provide the best indicator of severity and of prognosis.

The prognosis of coronary artery disease is individually unpredictable from sudden death tomorrow to clinical stability over decades. Most of the victims of sudden death are found at post-mortem to have the kind of coronary disease that we now recognize angiographically as carrying a bad prognosis. That is, they have proximal and severe three-vessel disease, left main stem disease, or proximal stenosis of the anterior descending branch of the left coronary artery. Symptoms may have been absent, unchanging, or worsening. The results of any large randomized trial in a disease of infinite variations in symptoms, prognosis, and anatomic forms and with varying rates of progression represent a grotesque oversimplification. Inability to stratify patients both because of ignorance and because of the ensuing reduction of the numbers in any group means the inclusion of patients with widely dissimilar prognoses within the same descriptive categories and an inevitable clouding of the issues. The templates of those who need surgery for their survival may be obscured in these clumsy groupings by admixture with patients destined to do well anyway. The prognosis of left main stem disease is acknowledged to be benefited by surgical treatment, but this group might have emerged simply because it is easily described.

Relying on symptoms offers an easy and economical way of deciding which patients should be offered surgery, and the results of the CASS have been welcomed. It is unlikely that another massive trial will ever be organized and it would, in any case, take another decade before it reported and hence, like all the others, be criticized because it represented the prescribing practices and surgical techniques of an earlier era.

Patients with known or suspected coronary disease should be investigated by exercise testing and coronary angiography even when their symptoms are mild or absent, so that threatening disease shown by widespread, provokable ischemia and proximal disease in main coronary arteries can be recognized so that it can be treated either by transluminal angioplasty or by coronary bypass. Comparison of angioplasty with coronary bypass has not yet been made.

Hammersmith Cardiology Workshop Series, Vol. 3,
edited by A. Maseri, B. E. Sobel, and S. Chierchia.
Raven Press, New York © 1987.

Précis of the Discussion: Section XVI

DETERMINANTS OF PROGNOSIS IN ISCHEMIC HEART DISEASE

Attilio Maseri

David Kelly observed that an obvious reason for the relevant prognostic significance of an abnormal resting electrocardiogram is probably due to previous infarction and, therefore, it may be that the history of previous infarction is really the major prognostic indicator.

Along the same lines, Richard Conti expressed the opinion that the five times increase in mortality rate observed in hypertensive patients when they also had an abnormal electrocardiogram was probably related to the development of an infarction. Desmond Julian agreed but added that, unfortunately, "we have no evidence that controlling hypertension does any good to prevent infarction."

Attilio Maseri said, "You showed many examples where one variable is taken as a single prognostic discriminator. However, I believe that this is not necessarily a useful clinical exercise when patients are included in whom prognosis can be already assessed *a priori* on the basis of other obvious characteristics. For example, when you are considering the ECG, the history of previous infarction is probably the major prognostic indicator, as suggested by David Kelly and Richard Conti; accordingly, the predictive value of ejection fraction is certainly not independent from the history of multiple infarctions, of cardiac failure, or of the presence of an enlarged heart on the chest X-ray. Therefore, taking the example of ejection fraction, it would be more useful to establish its predictive value in patients in whom no other clues are available. In other words, it would be desirable to know the additional and independent information provided by the variables considered not already available from history, chest X-ray, and Q waves on the resting ECG. This is often attempted from a retrospective statistical analysis on pooled data, but it could be achieved more clearly and convincingly by including in prognostic studies homogeneous subsets of patients stratified, considering easily available parameters."

Desmond Julian responded, "I agree that some of these variables are very dependent on each other, for example, exercise test and symptoms are pretty closely related. On the other hand, age, blood pressure, and smoking habits, for example, are not. I think the trouble is that when statisticians start analyzing multiple risk factors they produce formidable and impossible formulae, plus the fact that translating from someone else's prognostic experience to your own is usually not terribly successful. I do not think one should try to be too precise but one should not ignore symptoms and one should not ignore exercise tests. All I am trying to say is that these add a considerable amount to coronary arteriogram and sometimes may mean it is unnecessary. If you have a postinfarction patient who is free of symptoms, has good left ventricular function, and a good exercise test, I personally do not think there is any indication for coronary arteriography.''

Raphael Balcon said, ''We have sat here for four days talking a lot and we have come to the conclusion that we don't know what variables predict survival and we don't know how they interact with each other, and now we are talking about stopping getting half of the data, which is the coronary arteriogram. Why don't you want to do a coronary arteriogram? I don't care whether you operate on the patient or not; I don't care what you do, but why don't you want to do a coronary arteriogram and have all the data? Then you can make some decisions.''

Paul Lichtlen: ''This is the concept that I have tried to get across to the politicians in Germany, although the waiting lists are already too long.''

Raphael Balcon: ''Most laboratories are doing five cases a day—let them all do 10 or 12 cases a day and you solve the first half of the problem.''

Celia Oakley: ''The productivity of our laboratory is lamentable and it is impossible to push it up.''

Desmond Julian: ''Raphael Balcon's views on this subject are well known and I have a certain sympathy with what he says, but I think one has to face the facts of life and the facts are that if you are going to do everybody who presents with angina this becomes a considerable expense. Moreover, it is not an entirely comfortable procedure and it isn't entirely free of risk. You have to justify it, although it would be lovely to have all the information possible.''

Referring to Celia Oakley's review, Richard Conti said, ''I agree that patients with significant left main coronary artery stenosis will benefit from surgery as well as patients benefit from pneumococcal pneumonia from penicillin, but it is interesting that you skipped over physiological assessment in those patients too, because if you go back to the VA trial (which, by the way, was with 96 patients), 50% mortality in three or four years meant 50% survival in three or four years in that group, too, and there must be some way to discriminate those; some had more disease than others, I suspect. The other point is that if the results had come out the other way, either there was no difference or that medicine was better than surgery, who would have believed that 96 patients would make a trial?''

Celia Oakley responded, ''In the European study left main stem disease could be randomized; our requirement was 50% narrowing or more, not 75%, and in analyzing the left main stem patients who were put into the trial, we found that nobody with very severe left main stem stenosis had been included. All the left main stems that had gone in had sort of 50% to 75% stenosis, which fulfilled the terms of the trial but didn't immediately threaten the lives of the patients. That is probably why the European trial with the rather small number of left main stem patients failed to show benefit from surgical treatment of left main stem stenosis, statistically. Thus, I take that point: patients have to have physiological assessment as well as the angiographic one certainly.''

Concerning the interpretation of the CASS study, Spencer King thought it important to consider that the number of patients included in the trial per center was, on the average, one per month. Thus, it seems reasonable to assume that the CASS trial was made up of a lot of patients who would normally be treated medically. Furthermore, a sizable group of patients with three-vessel disease was crossed over to surgery, which may have prolonged their survival.

About the practical management of post MI patients, Henry Neufeld asked specifically about the contributors' views regarding a 45-year-old patient who has had an uncomplicated myocardial infarction.

John Goodwin stated, ''I don't think I would do an exercise test straightaway, but I would certainly do one within perhaps three months. I would be interested in how much effort he does without symptoms and how far he gets into the effort test with a given amount of ST segment depression. If he did well with the exercise test without any symptoms, and ST segment depression, I would not investigate him any further. However, in someone who has had angina following the infarct, then I would do an effort test much earlier. I think it would also depend on what one's position is: If one is simply in the position of treating patients, say, in a community hospital, then I think one would not do effort testing nearly quite so frequently; but if you are working in a major center, then probably you would have a policy of exercise testing everybody within perhaps two weeks, but I am not sure that that is a policy that one should recommend for routine community hospital use.''

Henry Neufeld asked, ''Would you put him on beta blockers?''

John Goodwin answered, ''I would like to try and identify the people who are really going to benefit from beta blockers. It is very tempting to put everyone who has no contraindications on beta blockers, but if you do that you will be treating a lot of people unnecessarily I think. If you can identify the really important subsets that would be the right thing to do. The flesh being weak and being feeble, I am afraid I often do put people on beta blockers because the general evidence seems to suggest they help, but I am sure I shouldn't.''

Celia Oakley said, ''My patient with an uncomplicated infarct would already be on a beta blocker and he would have an exercise test before he leaves the hospital. If the exercise test is negative with a good hemodynamic response, I will take him off the beta blocker and repeat the exercise test after a week or so. If it is still negative I will leave him off the beta blockers and I won't do coronary angiography, but I will repeat the exercise test annually or six-monthly because we are dealing with a potentially progressive disease.''

John Goodwin asked, ''You shouldn't do an exercise test on a beta blocker, should you?''

Celia Oakley answered that the beta blocker doesn't mask the evidence of ischemia. Thus, if the exercise is positive it definitely represents an indication to coronary angiography.

Desmond Julian said, "First of all, I am very much in favor of early exercise testing because I think it is part of the rehabilitation of the patient, and I think it is a very important thing for both doctor and patient to know how much the patient can achieve before he goes home. I think an early exercise test, in my mind, if the patient is fit for it, is highly desirable; he may not be fit for it, of course, but that is a different matter. I am not happy about the results of exercise tests on beta blockers in terms of assessing the hemodynamic response, which I put a lot of weight on. It is very difficult to know what you can infer from the blood pressure response or the heart rate response in someone who is on a beta blocker. I think you get much better information if the patient is not on a beta blocker. The alternative system of withdrawing the drug and reassessing things, to my mind, is admirable but presents terrible logistical problems. We find it very difficult to get patients back to hospital a week later to do exercise tests off beta blockers."

Celia Oakley agreed but did not feel like "depriving patients of a drug which may be helpful just in order to be able to demonstrate that they do have ischemia."

Attilio Maseri agreed: "There is an advantage to exercising the patient before he leaves the hospital because it may be difficult to get him back later. It is safe as long as the exercise test is carefully supervised and interpreted. Until the patient is in the hospital and is in the subintensive care he is not necessarily on a beta blocker unless there be a reason for it. If he is on a beta blocker he should be exercised on the beta blocker. The patient should be continued on the beta blocker anyway because of the reason he was on it (hypertension, tachycardia not caused by failure). A negative submaximal test is a very good indication for short-term prognosis. However, about a month later the patient should have a maximal test off treatment in order to assess long-term prognosis." This comment was followed by several short questions and answers.

John Goodwin: "Can I clarify one point? You talk about early exercise testing, that is irrespective of whether they have angina or not, including the small, uncomplicated infarcts?"

Attilio Maseri: "Every single one, particularly the nontransmural infarctions. Yes."

John Goodwin: "And would you recommend that for every physician in any community hospital as routine?"

Attilio Maseri: "As long as they are capable of doing a carefully supervised exercise test by monitoring the blood pressure and the ST segment and stopping as soon as there is the first sign of ischemia because that is what you want. You don't want to see whether the patient develops 4 mm ST segment depression without pain."

Henry Neufeld then gave another example for discussion. The cardiologist has referred a patient who has a mean nomenclature three-vessel disease. He is asymptomatic and his angiogram shows 70% in three vessels.

Floyd Loop: "I would ask for the results of the exercise test."

Henry Neufeld: "It was mildly positive."

Floyd Loop: "According to the CASS randomized trial, a patient with normal ventricular function and three-vessel disease did not fare any better with surgical treatment than medical treatment. I don't believe that because 38% of their patients with three-vessel disease crossed from medical to surgical therapy, so my answer to you is that most probably, unless there were an unusual set of circumstances, that patient would be a candidate for surgery, in my opinion."

Contributors were asked the following question: How far should we push a patient to undergo surgery, for example, a 65-year-old man who has severe three-vessel disease demonstrated at angiography, an exercise test with 3 mm ST segment depression at 100 watts, and who was accepted for surgery? At the last moment he refuses operation and now, after three months on medical treatment, is absolutely symptom free and refuses further operation. How far should the patient be pushed to undergo operation?

Ken Taylor responded, "I think surgeons tend to never force anyone who is unwilling to have an operation, however clear the indications might appear."

Paul Lichtlen asked, "About 30% of all myocardial infarctions are over the age of 70 in most hospitals. Are all these getting beta blockers and all having exercise tests, or do you have another strategy in this large group of patients?"

Celia Oakley said that she thought it illogical not to treat a 70-year-old patient the same as everyone else, considering, however, that older patients require smaller doses of everything, including beta blockers.

Henry Neufeld posed the problem of a 70-year-old man who had a complicated infarct and an ejection fraction of 30%.

Ken Taylor responded, "I think in the absence of angina there is evidence from CASS that in patients with ejection fractions of, say, 35% or below who are not presenting with angina as a principal symptom, surgery does not improve prognosis or symptomatology over medical therapy. I think both are equally bad."

Floyd Loop: "I think this patient obviously needs medical support more than surgical therapy. But I have one general point about the elderly because this has become a big problem in the United States. Already the mean age of our isolated coronary bypass population has reached 62, so it has advanced some 12 years in the last 15 years; about 15% of our patients in the Midwest are above the age of 70, and that is climbing also. If a woman reaches the age of 70 it is likely that she has an average survival of 15 more years, and for a man it is about 11 years. Therefore, the elderly, in terms of a decision for and against surgery, are becoming an increasing problem."

Henry Neufeld: "So we cardiologists have here a problem because for those patients, in the first 2 months after acute infarction, the death rate would be about 50% of the mortality during the first year; an annual death rate in this population would be about 15%, so it would be 7.5% in the first 2 months."

Paul Lichtlen: "We would certainly study them with regard to their arrhythmia profile."

Desmond Julian: "I would like to know any form of treatment that actually affects prognosis in these patients, and I don't know any, so I can't see why I should investigate him."

Raphael Balcon: "Unfortunately, we have no evidence that doing any therapeutic maneuver in this group does any good because all studies performed so far specifically excluded this group. They were specifically excluded from surgery and, in my view, they are the group . . . likely to gain most from surgery."

Editorial comment: A. Maseri

As for most diseases, including coronary disease, management is aimed at relieving symptoms and at improving prognosis. The uncertainty about prognosis occupies a particularly prominent position in the minds of coronary patients and of their physicians so that the desire to avoid the possible occurrence of infarction and death, often more than symptoms, conditions emotionally diagnostic and therapeutic approaches. Indeed, with the exception of very severe forms of angina, symptoms in coronary patients may be mild; for most of them, anginal pain is not always unbearable, lasts a few minutes, may not occur every day, and may be even absent altogether for weeks or months. Yet infarction and sudden death, although often heralded by recent onset or sudden worsening of symptoms, not infrequently are the first manifestations of coronary disease or occur unpredictably in periods totally or relatively free from symptoms. Hence, the understandable urge to identify and prevent the risk of these baffling events.

However, while the success of treatment aimed at the relief of symptoms can be promptly judged from the degree of symptomatic relief, improvement of prognosis is much more difficult to assess because it would require some reasonable knowledge of the natural history of the varied disease forms and, hence, of the probability of risk in individual patients.

The available information on prognosis is rather inaccurate because patients are classified according to rather gross single parameters, either clinical or angiographic, in order to obtain groups sufficiently large for statistical analysis.

The relationship between anatomy, symptoms, and residual coronary flow reserve is not given sufficient consideration. On the one hand, it is usually assumed that patients with similar symptoms have a similar prognosis independent of the cause of ischemia or of their coronary anatomy. On the other, patients with similar coronary anatomy are thought to have a similar prognosis independently of the causes of ischemia, of the severity of symptoms, and of the severity of reduction of their coronary flow reserve. Prognostic studies that include patients at very low and at very high risk, together with patients at intermediate risk, suffer from the hidden assumption that the risk of the in-between patients is a continuous variable, linearly related with the parameters that separate very high and very low risk patients.

The assessment of prognosis should be based on all easily available clues rather than on a single parameter, even if obtained with the latest technique or indicated by sophisticated statistical analysis. Important clues often available from routine examinations appear to provide additive and independent information on prognosis: the severity of impairment of ventricular function (indicated by a history of previous infarction(s), Q waves on the ECG, heart size and lung fields on standard chest X-ray); the severity of coronary obstructions, not only in terms of anatomy, but also in terms of demonstrable impairment of coronary flow reserve (indicated by low threshold for exertional angina and positive stress test at low work load); the tendency to develop episodes of impairment of coronary flow (indicated by recent onset or worsening of angina, prolonged and frequent spontaneous episodes); and the tendency to develop potentially fatal arrhythmias (indicated by history of syncope, and episodes of severe ventricular arrhythmias).

Patients with mild or no signs and symptoms of ischemia have both mild impairment of coronary flow reserve (hence, noncritical lesions or good collaterals) and a mild tendency to develop transient impairment of coronary flow. Their prognosis might be good even in the presence of angiographically demonstrable coronary obstructions. The demonstration of an improvement of survival in this group following therapeutic intervention would require an extremely large number of patients and long follow-ups.

SUBJECT INDEX

Subject Index

University of London

Royal Postgraduate Medical School

European and American Cardiology at the Hammersmith
Discussions 1987
(Preliminary Programme)*

1–5 June 1987

BASIC MECHANISMS OF CARDIOVASCULAR DISEASES
IMPLICATIONS FOR THERAPY AND PREVENTION

Organised by the Division of Cardiology
Royal Postgraduate Medical School, London; and
Division of Cardiology, Vanderbilt University
Nashville, Tennessee

Course Directors
Attilio Maseri, M.D., F.R.C.P.
John Oates, M.D.

Codirectors
Sergio Chierchia
Graham Davies
Gottlieb Friesinger
Rose Marie Robertson
Kenneth Taylor

---

* Further information and application form available from: School Office, R.P.M.S. Hammersmith Hospital, Ducane Road, London W12 OHS, England.

Monday, 1 June

The Varied Causes of Acute Myocardial Ischaemia in Patients

*   Active and quiescent phases in IHD: Role of fixed and dynamic stenoses
    A. Maseri
*   Role of lipid plaques and thrombosis in the development of fixed coronary
    obstruction   M. Davies
*   Development, control, and protective role of coronary collaterals
    W. Schaper
*   The various stages of coronary atherosclerotic disease: A research and a clinical
    approach   V. Fuster
*   Mechanisms of variable coronary flow reserve in chronic stable angina
    S. Chierchia
*   Natural history of ischaemic syndromes   G. Friesinger

Panel: Old and new strategies to improve prognosis

Control of Coronary Vasomotion

*   Cellular control of contraction, relaxation, and impulse transmission in coronary
    smooth muscle   T. Bolton
*   Role of the endothelium in the control of coronary smooth muscle tone
    R. Busse
*   Neural control of coronary vasomotor tone   G. Burnstock
*   Growth factors: Atherogenic and vasoconstrictor effects   W. Colucci
*   Effects of intracoronary injection of peptides and other neurotransmitters in
    patients   G. Davies

Panel: Neural versus humoral control of coronary tone

Tuesday, 2 June

Mechanisms of Thrombosis and Constriction in Acute Coronary Occlusion

- Postmortem findings in acute coronary syndromes compared to controls
  M. Davies
- Blood-vessel wall interaction   V. Fuster
- Animal models of acute transient coronary occlusion   R. Robertson
- Coronary hyperreactivity to constrictor stimuli: The model of variant
  angina   A. Maseri
- Dynamic coronary occlusion in the early phases of infarction in man
  G. Davies
- Coronary thrombosis as an excessive repair process: Rate limiting steps
  K. Bauer

Panel: Systemic versus local factors in acute coronary occlusion

Consequences of Ischaemia: Necrosis and Arrhythmias

- Determinants of reversible cell damage   R. Roberts
- Reperfusion injury: Strategies for control   M. Forman
- Mechanisms of fatal arrhythmias during acute ischaemia in patients: Rationale
  for their prevention   S. Cobbe

Special Lecture

- Transition from stable coronary disease to sudden cardiac death   J. Oates

Panel: Perspectives for delaying cell death during ischaemia in man

Wednesday, 3 June

Mechanisms of Heart Failure

* Myocardial alterations and mechanisms of cardiac failure   P. Poole-Wilson
* Assessment of cardiac contractility in man   M. Kronenberg

Panel: Development of specific antifailure drugs

Staff Round

Special Lecture

* Thrombin-specific thrombolytic agents and suppression of the antifibrinolytic process   D. Collen

Prevention of Coronary Occlusion

* Platelet inhibition in coronary vascular disease   G. FitzGerald
* Remodelling of infarct-related coronary stenoses after acute infarction
  D. Hackett

Panel: Strategies for achieving prompt and persistent coronary recanalisation and for preventing reocclusion

Immunology in Cardiovascular Diseases

* Genetic conditioning of immune response   F. Bottazzo
* Inflammation and the failing heart: What don't we know?   B. McManus
* Value of myocardial biopsy for the diagnosis of myocarditis   E. Olsen

Panel: Treatment of myocarditis

Thursday, 4 June

Aspects of Blood Cell Responses During Cardiac Surgery

- Platelets, prostacyclin, and microembolism   K. Taylor
- Lung injury during cardiac surgery   D. Royston
- Brain injury during cardiac surgery   C. Blauth

Study of Receptors in Cardiovascular Diseases

- General principles for the study of cardiovascular receptors and their function   D. Robertson
- Study of cardiovascular receptors by positron emission tomography in man
  A. Syrota

Genetic Studies of Cardiovascular Diseases

Special Lecture

- The "classical," the "new gene," and basic ideas in genetics   P. Tolani
- Apolipoprotein gene structure: plasma cholesterol levels and atherosclerosis
  J. Scott
- Study of the genetic components of cardiovascular collagen diseases
  A. Child
- Study of the genetic components of idiopathic hypertrophic cardiomyopathy   W. McKenna
- Genetic versus environmental risk factors in IHD   K. Berg

Panel: IHD: One or multiple aetiologies?

Friday, 5 June

MINI-SYMPOSIUM

Coronary Spasm and Ca^{++} Antagonists

Special Lecture

- Calcium channels and calcium antagonists in the control of smooth muscle tone   H. Reuter

Panel: Variant angina revisited: One or more aetiologies?   M. Bertrand, S. Chierchia, A. L'Abbate, R. Robertson, G. Specchia, D. Waters

Clinical Forum: Case preparations

Demonstration of Routine and Research Techniques Developed or in Use at the Hammersmith Hospital for Cardiovascular Investigations

- Holter monitoring

- Exercise testing

- Provocative tests—methodology

- Angioplasty

- Quantitative angiography